Pharmacological and Therapeutic Aspects of Hypertension

Volume II

Authors

Austin E. Doyle
Professor of Medicine
University of Melbourne
Austin Hospital
Heidelberg, Victoria
Australia

Frederick A. O. Mendelsohn
Associate Professor of Medicine
University of Melbourne
Austin Hospital
Heidelberg, Victoria
Australia

Trefor O. Morgan
Professor of Medicine
University of Newcastle
Royal Newcastle Hospital
Newcastle N.S.W.
Australia

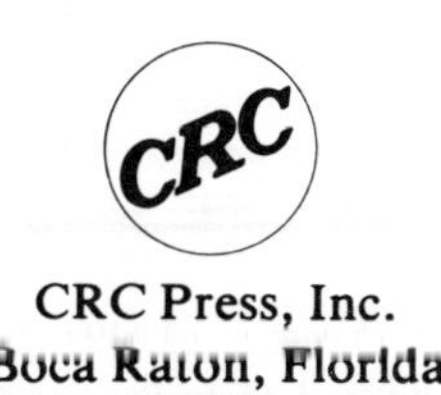

CRC Press, Inc.
Boca Raton, Florida

Library of Congress Cataloging in Publication Data

Doyle, Austin Eric.

    Pharmacological and therapeutic aspects of hypertension.

    Bibliography: p.
    Includes index.
    1. Hypertension—Chemotherapy. 2. Hypotensive
agents. I. Mendelshohn, Frederick A. O., joint author.
II. Morgan, Trefor O., joint author. III. Title.
LDNLM: 1. Hypertension—Drug therapy.
2. Hypertension—Physiology. 3. Antihypertensive
agents—Pharmacodynamics. WG340.3 D754p]
RC685.H8D69   616.1'32'061   78-27898
ISBN 0-8493-5385-8 (v. 1)
ISBN 0-8493-5386-6 (v. 2)

International Standard Book Number 0-8493-5385-8 (Volume I)
International Standard Book Number 0-8493-5386-6 (Volume II)

Library of Congress Card Number 78-27898
Printed in the United States

INTRODUCTION

There can be few better examples of the close relationship between pharmacology, therapeutics, and pathophysiology than hypertension. While it might logically be supposed that an understanding of pathophysiological mechanisms would lead to the development of pharmacological agents which are subsequently applied in the treatment of a disease, the development of an understanding of the pathogenetic mechanisms of arterial hypertension has followed almost the opposite course and has often been the result of, rather than the basis of, developments in therapeutics and pharmacology.

In this book, an attempt has been made to relate pathophysiological mechanisms to the pharmacology of drugs which have been observed to be therapeutically valuable. In many instances, the development of new drugs has led to new understanding of the complex processes which underlie the sustained elevation of arterial pressure. For example, the introduction of effective ganglion-blocking drugs almost 30 years ago was followed by the realization that many of the clinical manifestations of hypertension were the result of the raised pressure itself and that lowering blood pressure could reverse these. As a further example, the chance observation that clonidine, initially synthesized as a nasal vasoconstrictor, had marked antihypertensive properties was followed by a realization of the importance of norepinephrine as an important neurotransmitter within the cardiovascular regulatory centers in the brain, an observation which in turn led to the recognition that methyl dopa might also lower blood pressure via a central action.

More recently, the clinical observation that β-adrenoceptor-blocking drugs very effectively reduced blood pressure has stimulated intense activity in the production of new drugs with similar properties and has also provided an impetus to research designed to elucidate the mechanism of their antihypertensive actions.

In spite of the considerable advances in understanding of the nature of hypertension which have been made in the last few years, the treatment of hypertension remains largely empirical because in the individual patient, the precise mix of pathophysiological mechanisms is not often easily identified. Nevertheless, an understanding of the possible mechanisms, their interactions, and the ways in which these can be modified by drugs facilitates and improves treatment. It is hoped that this book will provide a bridge between an understanding of the disease process, the mechanism of action of drugs, and their practical application in treatment, both for those whose primary interest is the care of patients and for those working in the laboratory. Because the book is concerned primarily with this aim, it is by no means comprehensive, and areas of interest in the pathogenesis of hypertension such as the prostaglandins, encephalins, and kallikrein have been dealt with cursorily, if at all, since their current relationship, if any, to therapeutics is not yet clear. In areas which appear to be expanding rapidly, such as inhibitors of the renin-angiotensin system, an attempt has been made to anticipate possible developments. Even in these latter areas, however, it has been necessary to be selective and much detail has had to be omitted.

It needs to be emphasized that although an attempt has been made to provide a balanced view of the topic, the material presented and the interpretations of data represent attitudes which may not be universally held. We have attempted to put forth our own point of view in interpreting experimental work and ideas of pathophysiology, and the therapeutic section is largely based on our own experience. It is hoped that this work may be of assistance as a guide to the better management of patients with high blood pressure.

A. E. Doyle
Melbourne, August 1978

THE AUTHORS

Austin E. Doyle, M.D. is Professor and Chairman of the University of Melbourne, Department of Medicine, Austin Hospital, Heidelberg, Australia.
Dr. Doyle graduated in medicine in the University of London in 1946 and received his MD from the same University in 1950. He is a member of the International Society of Hypertension, Cardiac Society of Australia and New Zealand, Australasian Society of Nephrology, Australasian Society of Clinical and Experimental Pharmacology and Australian Physiological and Pharmacological Society. He is a Fellow of the Royal Australasian College of Physicians. His current research deals with autonomic mechanisms in hypertension and in the clinical application of anti-hypertensive drugs.
Frederick A. O. Mendelsohn graduated in medicine in the University of Melbourne in 1964. He received his MD in 1971 and his PhD in 1973 in the University of Melbourne. He is a member of the International Society of Hypertension, Australasian Society of Nephrology, Australian Society for Medical Research and Australian Physiological and Pharmacological Society. He is a Fellow of the Royal Australasian College of Physicians. His current research interests relate to the physiology of the renin angiotensin system and to steroid hypertension.
Trefor O. Morgan is Professor and Chairman of the University of Newcastle Department of Medicine at the Royal Newcastle Hospital, Newcastle, New South Wales, Australia.
Dr. Morgan graduated in medicine from the University of Sydney in 1960 and received his MD from the same University in 1972. He is a member of the International Society of Hypertension, Australasian Society of Nephrology, Australasian Society of Clinical and Experimental Pharmacology and Physiology. He is a Fellow of the Royal Australasian College of Physicians. His research interests include the role of sodium in clinical and experimental hypertension and kidney function at the single nephron level.

ACKNOWLEDGMENTS

It is a pleasure to acknowledge the help of various colleagues, who have read sections of the book and who gave much constructive criticism. The manuscripts were typed with skill and efficiency by Ms. Jan Strange and Ms. Ilsa Rand. I am particularly indebted to my colleagues Dr. Mendelsohn and Dr. Morgan for keeping to their deadlines for their own contributions.

This book could not have been undertaken without the period of study leave granted to me by the Council of the University of Melbourne, to whom I express my gratitude.

Finally, I express my thanks to Ms. Sybil Walters, who not only helped me with the resource material and corrected the final version, but who maintained her usual equanimity by coping with all that and her usual secretarial work.

TABLE OF CONTENTS

VOLUME II

Chapter 2
Vascular Smooth Muscle, Vascular Reactivity, and Drugs Which Affect Vascular Smooth Muscle

Chapter 3
Therapeutics of Hypertension

TABLE OF CONTENTS

Pharmacological and Therapeutic Aspects of Hypertension

Austin E. Doyle

Volume I

Sodium Intake and Hypertension
Trefor O. Morgan and Austin E. Doyle

The Renin-Angiotensin System
Frederick A. O. Mendelsohn

Volume II

The Autonomic Nervous System

Vascular Smooth Muscle, Vascular Reactivity, and Drugs which Affect Vascular
Smooth Muscle

Therapeutics of Hypertension

Principles of Management and the Use of Drugs

Clinical Applicatons of Agents which Block the Renin-Angiotensin System

Remediable Secondary Hypertension

Chapter 1

THE AUTONOMIC NERVOUS SYSTEM

I. PATHOPHYSIOLOGICAL MECHANISMS

A. Introduction

The autonomic nervous system plays an important role in the regulation of blood pressure under various conditions and has as one of its major functions the regulation of the circulation so as to preserve an adequate perfusion of vital organs, depending on their metabolic needs. In man the activity of the autonomic nervous system plays a particularly important role in maintaining the circulation in the upright posture, so as to prevent orthostatic falls in blood pressure. The integrated control of the circulation is achieved by mechanisms within the brain. The vasomotor centers in the brain stem receive information from the arterial baroreceptors situated in the carotid sinus and in the aortic arch, low-pressure pressor receptors in the atria and in the pulmonary circulation, and chemoreceptors which are activated by hypoxia. They are also influenced or modulated by higher integrating centers which are located in the hypothalamus, the limbic system, and the cerebral cortex. Circulatory regulation is effected through the autonomic innervation of the heart, arteries, and veins.

When discussing the role of the autonomic nervous system in hypertension, a distinction has to be made between any possible role which it may have as an initiating factor in the causation of high blood pressure and any role that the autonomic nervous system may have as a sustaining mechanism in hypertension which has been initiated by other processes. In considering either of these roles, disturbances leading to hypertension might be situated on the receptor side, within the integrative control mechanisms, or on the effector side. In considering the possible role of the nervous system in the pathogenesis of hypertension, a brief account of the function of this system in normal man and animals is needed, with some comment on the possible manner in which its function may change in hypertension. The problem of integrative neural cardiovascular control has been extensively reviewed by Korner.[1]

B. Autonomic Reflexes

1. Arterial Baroreceptor Reflexes

The major systemic arterial baroreceptors are situated in the carotid sinus and in the aortic arch where they are strategically placed to monitor arterial pressure to the brain.[2] They consist of sensory receptors which appear to be sensitive to the pressure and, consequently, stretch of the vessels. Elevations of pressure within the carotid sinus or the aortic arch lead to nerve impulses being generated in the afferent nerves. If a steady increase in pressure is generated experimentally, there is a large increase in the firing frequency in the baroreceptor afferent nerve fibers which subsides somewhat after about a minute or a minute and a half to a steady level. This level can then be maintained virtually unchanged for periods of up to an hour if the pressure within the carotid sinus or aortic arch continues to be elevated.[3] For any mean pressure, the firing rate is greater when the pressure is pulsatile than when it is constant.[2]

It appears that the main function of the arterial baroreceptors is to provide information concerning rises or falls in blood pressure which is transmitted via the baroreceptor nerves and the vagus nerve to the integrative control mechanisms situated within the brain stem. These baroreceptor mechanisms represent a major mechanism whereby blood pressure is monitored and presumably represent an important sensory component in the autonomic control of blood pressure.

When the pressure within the carotid sinus is increased, there is then increased vagal activity on the heart leading to slowing of the pulse. This is probably the major immediate response to increased intracarotid pressure.[4,5] On the other hand, decreases in carotid sinus pressure lead to activation of the cardiac sympathetic nerves[6] and increased constrictor effects on both resistance and capacitance vessels within the splanchnic circulation.[7,8] the muscle bed, and the skin,[8] together with an increase in the output of catecholamines from the adrenal medulla[9] and of antidiuretic hormone.[10]

2. Cardiac Mechano-Receptors

Stretch receptors which are present in the walls of the atria and the ventricles are stimulated either by distension or by falls in pressure within these areas.[11] The atrial receptors appear to be low-pressure receptors which predominantly give information concerning the state of filling of the atria and presumably, therefore, venous return to the heart. The receptors are situated within the atria and give bursts of activity which are synchronous with the a-wave of the atrial pressure pulse and with the v-wave.[11] There appears to be a relationship between the firing frequency and the height of these waves. Stimulation of the cardiac vagal afferent nerves, which include fibers of every type of nerve ending, all produce changes in the autonomic activity including that to the heart, kidneys, and vascular supply in the renal, muscular, and splanchnic beds. Distension of either the left atrium or the right atrium induces a reflex rise in heart rate.[12]

Left ventricular receptors seem less sensitive than those within the atrium and may be analogous to the baroreceptors situated in the great vessels. Stimulation of left ventricular baroreceptors evokes reflex bradycardia and a fall in blood pressure.[13]

3. Chemoreceptors

Chemoreceptors within the arterial system such as the carotid body, are sensitive to changes in the arterial oxygen[14] and carbon dioxide concentration and to pH,[15] and their firing rate is influenced by changes in these parameters and also by changes in blood flow and to chemoreceptors. The firing rate of arterial chemoreceptors can be greatly enhanced by arterial hypoxia or by rises in arterial P_{CO_2}. If the isolated chemoreceptors are stimulated with hypoxia plus hypercapnia, bradycardia due to increased vagal and diminished sympathetic activity occurs together with a rise in blood pressure, which is due to a rise in total peripheral resistance in all major vascular beds.[16] There is also an increased secretion of adrenal catecholamines.

4. Lung Inflation Receptors

Pulmonary stretch receptors, which are very sensitive to changes in transpulmonary pressure, are mainly located within the bronchi and bronchioles. Changes occur in autonomic nerve activity during the normal respiratory cycle as the result of phasic discharge from pulmonary stretch receptors. Stimulation of these receptors tends to antagonize the effects produced by stimulation of the arterial chemoreceptors and inhibits peripheral sympathetic constrictor tone in all peripheral vascular beds.[17]

C. Central Integrative Mechanisms

Afferent fibers from the heart and great vessels run in the ninth and tenth cranial nerves into the medulla where they pass through the middle and posterior portion of the tractus solitarius. They synapse primarily in the tractus and medial part of the nucleus of the tractus solitarius.[18,19] From this area, there are bilateral projections through complex multisynaptic pathways to the bulbar depressor region, activation of which produces vagal excitation and generalized sympathetic inhibition.

The nucleus of the tractus solitarius runs posterorostrally and lies just under the floor of the fourth ventricle. The mediocaudal part of the nucleus, which lies in the same frontal plane as the area postrema, contains catecholaminergic cell bodies and is also densely innervated by catecholaminergic nerve terminals.[20,21] At a more rostral level, there are no catecholamine-containing cell bodies, but there are many catecholaminergic nerve terminals. These regions have been shown to contain high concentrations of norepinephrine, epinephrine, and dopamine.[22,23] It seems that this center acts as an important cardiovascular inhibitor, for bilateral ablation of the nucleus of the tractus solitarius causes acute severe hypertension in rats[24,25] and chronic hypertension in cats.[26] Moreover bilateral transsection of the afferent fibers just before they enter the nucleus causes a similar type of hypertension in rats without destruction of the cells of the nucleus.[27,28] Electrical stimulation of the nucleus induces a fall in both blood pressure and heart rate in the rat, and injection of norepinephrine and epinephrine either bilaterally or unilaterally into the nucleus causes a fall in blood pressure and heart rate in anesthetized rats.[29] These effects are inhibited and can be reversed by the previous administration of phentolamine.[29] This suggests that noradrenergic receptor sites are located in the nucleus of the tractus solitarius and may modulate autonomic inhibitory control and reflex regulation of cardiovascular function. The most sensitive area of the nucleus either to electrical stimulation or to the application of α-agonists is the mediocaudal section which contains numerous catecholaminergic cell bodies.[29]

The medulla also contains noradrenergic reticular cell groups from which pathways arise which descend to innervate both the dorsal and ventral horns of the spinal cord and also the sympathetic lateral column.[30] These pathways appear to have a cardiovascular excitatory function. After the arterial baroreceptors have been denervated, the development of hypertension in the rabbit is accompanied by an increase in norepinephrine turnover and tyrosine hydroxylase activity in the spinal cord. This form of hypertension can be prevented by the intracisternal administration of 6-hydroxydopamine, which causes a selective degeneration of noradrenergic nerves which is most marked in the spinal cord.[31] These results suggest that these descending noradrenergic neurones are directly involved in the baroreceptor reflex arc. However, Haeusler and Lewis[32] found that intracisternally administered 6-hydroxydopamine did not inhibit the blood pressure response in the rat to bilateral sinus nerve stimulation. It is therefore not entirely certain whether the spinal noradrenergic neurones are an integral part of the baroreceptor reflex arc, or whether they are involved in a modulatory fashion.

There is also evidence for a large number of suprabulbar centers which are involved in cardiovascular regulation. These centers can be regarded as groups of interneurones between the afferent and efferent pathways of the medullary autonomic mechanisms. These supraoptic centers are situated in the hypothalamus, basal ganglia, limbic system, and the cerebral cortex.[1]

The interactions between the hypothalamic centers and the medullary vasodepressor area have been extensively studied. It seems that there are at least two areas within the hypothalamus which can induce cardiovascular changes and which can also strongly influence the baroreceptor reflex response. The hypothalamus is densely innervated with noradrenergic nerve terminals which arise predominantly from cell groups in the pontomedullary area.

In the posterior hypothalamus, electrical stimulation in the region of the defense center described by Hilton[33] leads to a pronounced rise in blood pressure and heart rate.[34] Stimulation of these areas also inhibits the bradycardia which results from activation of the baroreceptors.[33] It has been claimed that superfusion of this area in the cat with α-adrenoceptor antagonists inhibits the rise in blood pressure produced by stimulation of the posterior hypothalamus,[36] whereas superfusion with clonidine enhances the pressor response.[37] These results suggest that α-adrenoceptors in this area are involved in the pressor response to electrical stimulation.

The anterior hypothalamus appears to be involved in responses which are directly opposite to those in the posterior part of the area. Electrical stimulation of the anterior hypothalamus in cats causes a decrease in blood pressure[38,39] and markedly enhances the bradycardia which results from activation of the baroreceptors.[40] This hypotensive response is inhibited when this area is perfused with α-adrenoceptor antagonists,[39] which suggests that in the anterior hypothalamus the hypotensive effects are related to α-adrenoceptors. It seems likely that inputs from the cerebral cortex and limbic system as a result of such stimuli as pain or emotion may also operate through the hypothalamic centers to influence the baroreceptor responses, either to facilitate or inhibit them. These higher centers are also powerfully influenced by inputs from chemoreceptors and the lung inflation receptors, and Korner[1] has pointed out that both cortical and diencephalic autonomic mechanisms are continuously active, both during rest and normal reflex activity, so forming an effective addition to the centers in the pons and medulla. Korner suggests that the development of strong inhibitory systems in the cerebral hemispheres which are linked to the lung inflation input have a major effect in limiting excess autonomic activity and in this way allow the blood pressure control system to operate under normal circumstances as a relatively low power regulator. This ensures that as far as possible the blood flow needs of various organs are catered to by local autoregulatory mechanisms. During periods of stress, however, these higher centers are probably responsible for resetting the level to which blood pressure is regulated, so permitting increases or decreases in blood pressure as circumstances require. It is entirely possible that derangements in this system might be responsible for alterations in the set level to which blood pressure is regulated and so induce hypertension.

It appears that catecholaminergic mechanisms within the central nervous system play an important role in cardiovascular reflex responses, and it appears that in general α-noradrenergic stimulation induces depressor responses, although there are areas where the opposite is true. The relative roles played by norepinephrine, epinephrine, and dopamine in various areas of the brain have not been finally elucidated, but there appear to be areas where all three amines may play a significant role. These have particular relevance to the mode of action of antihypertensive drugs which act in the nervous system and which will be discussed in more detail in a later section.

D. Peripheral Mechanisms

The effector side of the autonomic nervous system consists of the vagal and sympathetic supply to the heart and the peripheral sympathetic nerves. The efferent limb of the vagal cardiac fibers arises in the dorsal nucleus of the vagus. Stimulation of these fibers leads to a slowing of the heart rate through an action primarily on the sinoatrial node. When the cardiac sympathetic supply is stimulated, it operates through β-adrenoceptors and leads to an increase both in heart rate and force of contraction of the heart muscle. In general, reflex responses affecting the heart operate through both mechanisms simultaneously with vagal stimulation and a corresponding reduction in adrenergic stimulation, or vice versa, occurring together.[4]

The efferent sympathetic fibers synapse within the autonomic ganglia from whence postganglionic fibers arise to supply arteries, arterioles, and veins. These postganglionic fibers are noradrenergic in nature, the neurotransmitter being norepinephrine. As the sympathetic nerve fibrils approach their terminals, they develop swellings or varicosities which have been shown by the use of fluorescent histochemical techniques

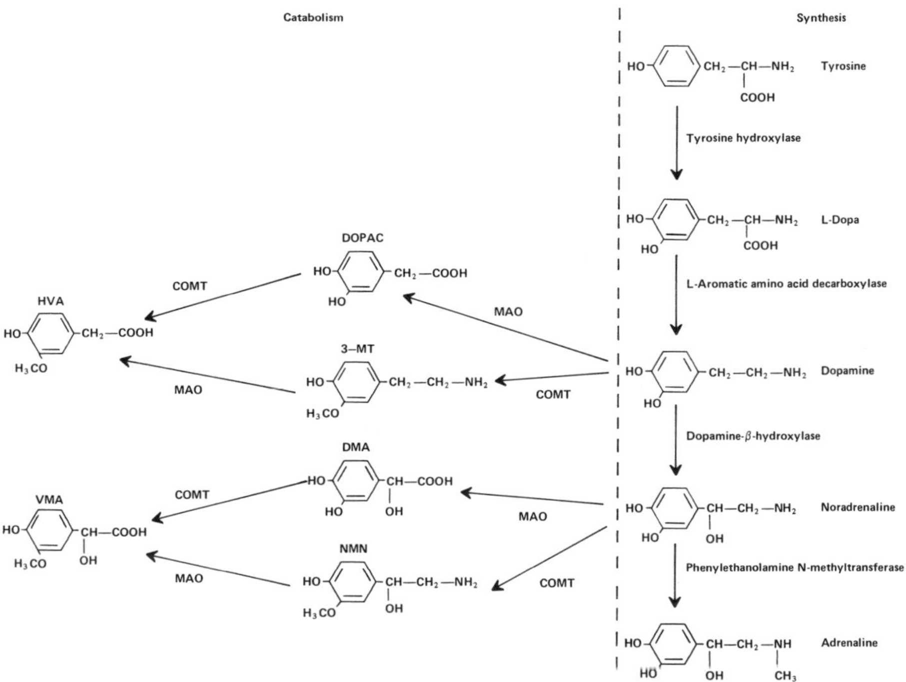

FIGURE 1.   Catecholamine biosynthetic pathway. The intermediates and the enzymes involved in the synthesis of norepinephrine and epinephrine, and some of the catabolites of dopamine and norepinephrine formed by the action of catechol-*O*-methyltransferase (COMT) and monoamine oxidase (MAO). Abbreviations: DOPAC — dihydroxyphenylacetic acid; 3-MT — 3-methoxytyramine; DMA — 3,4-dihydroxymandelic acid; NMN — normetanephrine; α-Methyl-3-MT — α-methyl-3-methoxytyramine; α-Methyl-NMN — α-methyl-normetanephrine; HVA — 4-Hydroxy-3-methoxyphenylacetic acid (homovanillic acid); VMA — 4-Hydroxy-3-methoxymandelic acid (vanillylmandelic acid).

to be rich in norepinephrine. The biosynthetic pathway for norepinephrine is shown in Figure 1.

The rate-limiting step in the biosynthetic pathway is the conversion of tyrosine to deoxyphenylalanine (DOPA) via the enzyme tyrosine hydroxylase.[41] Since catecholamines inhibit tyrosine hydroxylase, increased sympathetic nerve activity, by reducing catecholamine concentrations in the nerve cells, leads to increased tyrosine hydroxylase activity (Figure 2).

DOPA is converted to dopamine by the enzyme dopa decarboxylase which is present within the nerve cell cytoplasm. Dopamine is taken up into the granular storage vesicles which contain the enzyme dopamine-β-hydroxylase, which converts dopamine to norepinephrine. The newly synthesized norepinephrine is inactivated and stored within the vesicle by binding to a Mg-ATP complex.

Excitation of the nerve terminal is followed by a release of the contents of the granular vesicle, norepinephrine, dopamine-β-hydroxylase, and ATP into the synaptic cleft. This occurs as a result of exocytosis of the granule into the synaptic cleft. The exocytosis is enhanced by cyclic nucleotides, and the amount of released norepinephrine and dopamine-β-hydroxylase has been shown to be enhanced for any given degree of nerve stimulation either by inhibitors of phosphodiesterase or by analogues of cyclic AMP.[42,43] The process of norepinephrine release is accompanied by an influx of sodium and calcium into the cell cytoplasm and by an efflux of potassium. Although it has been claimed that prostaglandins of the E series may regulate release of neurotrans-

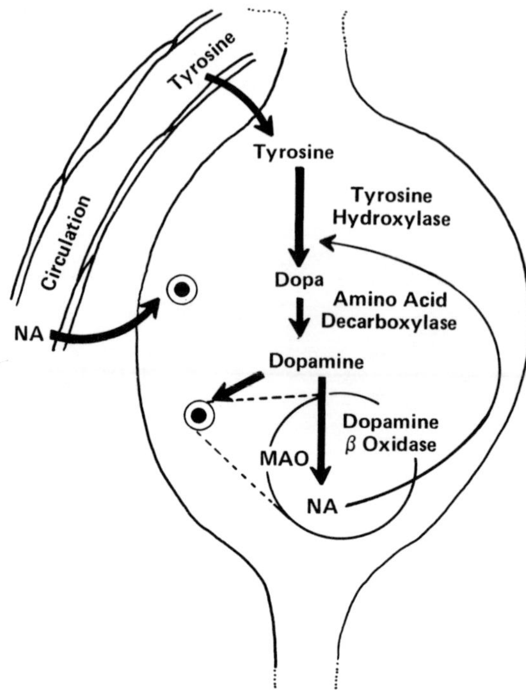

FIGURE 2.   Regulation of tyrosine hydroxylase activity by norepinephrine (NA) concentration within the nerve cell cytoplasm. (From Axelrod, J. and Weinshilboum, R., *N. Engl. J. Med.*, 287, 237, 1972. With permission.)

mitter, prostaglandin synthesis inhibition by indomethacin did not affect transmitter overflow in the cat spleen.[43]

Release of norepinephrine appears to be enhanced by the presence of angiotensin,[44] which has also been claimed to enhance catecholamine biosynthesis in sympathetic nerve endings.[45]

The magnitude of norepinephrine release is controlled in part by prejunctional receptors. The prejunctional α-adrenoceptor responds to released norepinephrine within the synaptic cleft to inhibit subsequent exocytotic release of transmitter in response to subsequent nerve impulses, thereby providing a negative feedback loop to modulate transmission[43,46] (Figure 3). It has been postulated that a similar prejunctional β-receptor is also concerned with modulating transmitter release, but as a positive feedback loop, so that released norepinephrine would enhance further norepinephrine release. l-Isoproterenol, but not d-isoproterenol, enhances the release of norepinephrine during nerve stimulation at low frequencies.[47] It has been suggested that these presynaptic β-receptors may be of the β_1 type, since they are blocked by the cardioselective β-adrenoceptor antagonist, metoprolol.[48]

It has been suggested that the negative feedback mechanism of the prejunctional α-receptor operates by a restriction of the calcium available for the excitation secretion coupling. It has been reported that inhibition of norepinephrine release obtained by exposure to exogenously administered norepinephrine is more pronounced when the calcium concentration in the medium is reduced.[49] The potentiation of the inhibition produced by α-receptor agonists by a reduction in the calcium concentration suggests that activation of these presynaptic α-receptors may reduce the availability of calcium, which is thought to be essential for the process of norepinephrine release.

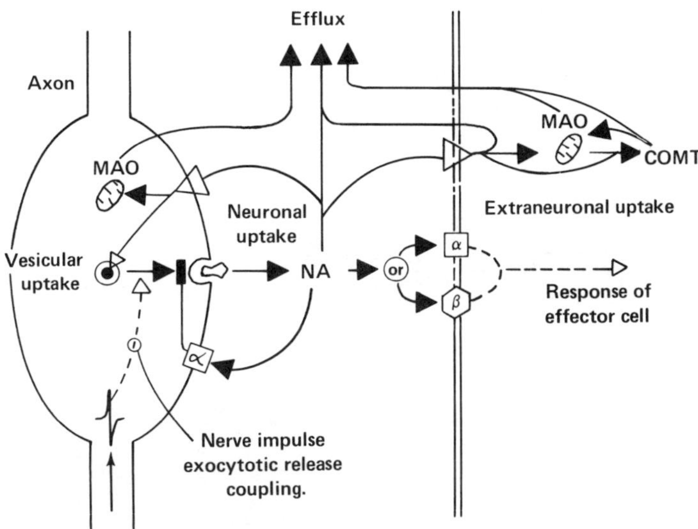

FIGURE 3. Diagrammatic representation of the of the actions and fate of norepinephrine released from noradrenergic nerve terminals.

Norepinephrine (NA) is released from noradrenergic vesicles in the neuron into the extracellular space by nerve-mediated exocytosis. The released norepinephrine acts postjunctionally on either α- or β-adrenoceptors to produce a response in the effector cell. Norepinephrine can also activate α-adrenoceptors on the nerve terminal itself to inhibit further exocytotic release of norepinephrine, thus forming a negative feedback loop to modulate transmitter release. The released norepinephrine diffuses away from the receptor sites and is also taken back up into the neuron for re-release. Excess norepinephrine in neuronal and extraneuronal sites is catabolized by the actions of monoamine oxidase (MAO) and catechol-O-methyltransferase (COMT) to inactivate metabolites which also diffuse away.

Exogenously applied α-adrenoceptor agonists further decrease exocytotic release of norepinephrine, whereas α-adrenoceptor antagonists increase this form of neurotransmitter release. (From Rand, M. J., McCulloch, M. W., and Story, D. F., *Central Actions of Drugs in Blood Pressure Regulation*, Davies, D. S. and Reid, J. L., Eds., Pitman Medical, Kent, U.K. 1975, 94. With permission.)

It appears that the facilitation of transmitter release which is produced by activation of the presynaptic β-receptors may be mediated through an increase in the levels of cyclic AMP in noradrenergic nerve endings. In support of this, it has been found that papaverine, which inhibits phosphodiesterase, enhances norepinephrine release during nerve stimulation, and the effect of papaverine on norepinephrine release is reduced by exposure to small amounts of propranolol.

The importance of the presynaptic receptors in either the pathophysiology of hypertension or in the mechanism of action of antihypertensive drugs has not yet been firmly established. It has been suggested, however, that α-receptor-blocking drugs which block both postjunctional and prejunctional receptors may be ineffective in the management of hypertension because blockade of the prejunctional receptors removes the inhibitory control of norepinephrine release and allows increasing amounts of norepinephrine to overcome the postjunctional receptor blockade. This had led to the suggestion that the major regulatory mechanism for norepinephrine release under physiological conditions is mediated via the presynaptic α-adrenoceptors.[49] It has also been suggested that the antihypertensive effect of β-adrenoceptor-blocking drugs is in part

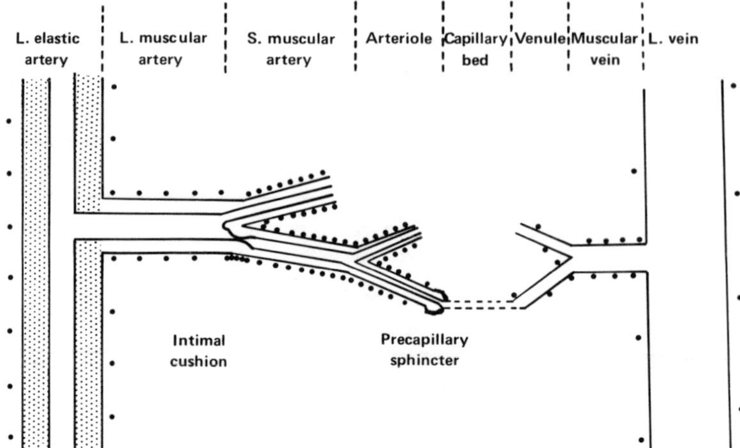

FIGURE 4.   Diagrammatic representation of innervation density in different regions of the vascular system. (From Burnstock, G., *Clin. Exp. Pharmacol. Physiol.*, Suppl. 2, 8, 1975. With permission.)

due to a decrease in norepinephrine release as a result of blocking of the presynaptic β-adrenoceptors which mediate the positive feedback mechanism, which enhances norepinephrine release.[48]

Norepinephrine released into the synaptic cleft acts on the postjunctional receptor to produce its physiological effects. Like the prejunctional receptors, the postjunctional receptors consist of two types, namely, the α-receptor and the β-receptor. In the peripheral vascular bed, the α-receptor is concerned predominantly with inducing constriction of smooth muscle while the β-receptor usually induces vasodilatation. It has been proposed that stimulation of the β-receptor involves the activation of adenylate cyclase with a consequent formation of cyclic AMP and a reduction in intracellular free calcium.[50,51] As discussed later, there are circumstances in some tissues where the concentrations of cyclic AMP appear to be independent of vascular smooth muscle dilatation or contraction. It has also been proposed that the stimulation of the α-receptor involves the activation of guanylate cyclase, with a consequent increase in the nucleotide cyclic GMP, which has been thought to have the effect of augmenting the release of activator calcium in vascular smooth muscle.[52] It is clear that the interaction between the neurotransmitter, norepinephrine, and its two receptors is complex. Plainly, the magnitude of the response of the vascular smooth muscle must depend on the concentration of norepinephrine within the synaptic cleft, the affinity between neurotransmitter and receptor, and the factors which lead to vascular smooth muscle contraction following receptor occupation.

Burnstock[53] has reviewed the patterns of innervation of vascular smooth muscle. There is considerable variation in the density of innervation of different parts of the vascular tree. Most large elastic arteries are sparsely innervated, and there is wide muscle-nerve ending separation of 1000 to 2000 nm. As muscular arteries decrease in size, the density of innervation increases, so that the small arteries and large arterioles are the most densely innervated. In these resistance vessels, the nerve endings are much more closely applied, with a cleft width of approximately 80 to 120 nm. Most precapillary arterioles are sparsely innervated (Figures 4 and 5).

There is also wide variation in the pattern of innervation in different vascular beds, the mesenteric and splanchnic bed being richly innervated,[54] while the coronary[53] or cerebral[55] vessels appear very sparsely innervated.

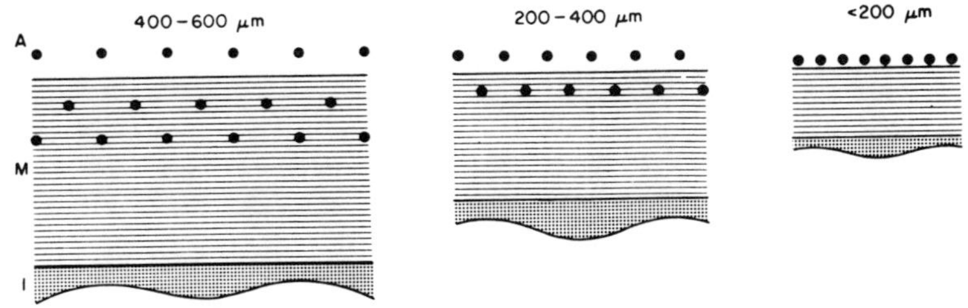

FIGURE 5.   Arrangement of nerves in arteries in different wall thickness. A, adventitia; •, nerve varicosities; M, media; I, intima. (From Burnstock, G., *Clin. Exp. Pharmacol. Physiol.*, Suppl. 2, 8, 1975. With permission.)

Most of the norepinephrine released into the synaptic cleft is retaken up into the nerve cell by an ion-dependent mechanism. It is likely that the reuptake process involves transport of both neurotransmitter and the potassium ion under the influence of the sodium pump. The reuptake of norepinephrine is inhibited by cocaine and by desipramine and dihydroergotamine. The reuptake process is stereospecific, but in addition to norepinephrine, epinephrine, dopamine, and amphetamine, metaraminol and other synthetic compounds can be taken up into the storage vesicles. Unbound norepinephrine within the cell body is metabolized by monoamine oxidase.

A small amount of the released norepinephrine diffuses from the biophase and finds its way into the circulation.

It is clear that the peripheral autonomic mechanisms which govern the interaction between sympathetic nerve excitation and the effector response are numerous and complex, and it is possible that quite minor derangements of this system could result in excessive autonomic effects which could lead to hypertension.

E. The Central Nervous System and Hypertension

There is no doubt that emotional and physical stimuli such as pain or exercise are capable of leading to rises in blood pressure in both normal man and animals. It has long been postulated that a possible cause for essential hypertension in man is that physiological stimuli induce either an excessive pressor response or an unusually sustained rise in blood pressure in susceptible individuals. There is considerable evidence that the blood pressure is more variable in people with hypertension, and this has been confirmed by a large number of studies using reflex stimuli such as controlled muscular exercise, the cold immersion of a limb, or difficult mental arithmetic done under pressure. Almost all these studies have revealed that hypertensive patients respond to such stimuli with larger rises in blood pressure than do normotensive people. The responses to such stimuli are probably analogous to the hypothalamic defense reaction. Brod and colleagues[56] have shown that the acute emotional stress induced in humans by difficult mental arithmetic induces the same hemodynamic pattern, with an increase in blood pressure and cardiac output, renal, splanchnic, and cutaneous vasoconstriction and muscular vasodilatation, as can be elicited in cats by electrical stimulation of the hypothalamus[57] or which occurs in cats during fighting.[58] Brod described a similar hemodynamic pattern in labile or borderline hypertension. Very similar findings were noted by Boyer, Doyle, and Fraser,[60] who studied the response of hypertensive and normotensive individuals to immersion of the foot in ice and water. In normal patients or in patients with labile hypertension, there was a rise in blood pressure accompanied by an increase in cardiac output and an increase in muscle blood flow. In patients with severe hypertension, however, the rise in blood pressure was usually accompanied by a fall in cardiac output and an increase in total peripheral resistance (Figures 6, 7, 8,

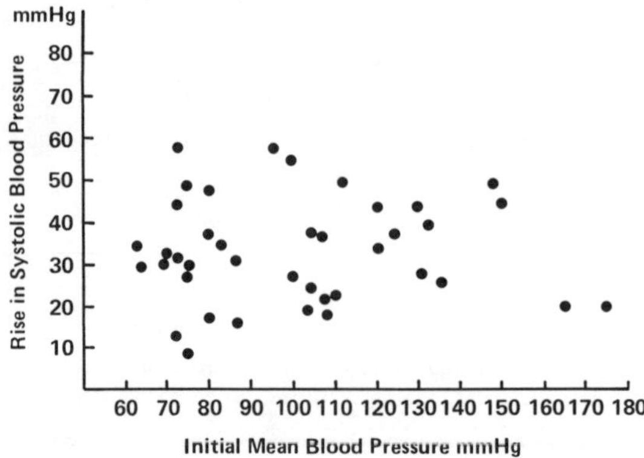

FIGURE 6.   Rise in systolic blood pressure during cold immersion compared with initial mean blood pressure of 41 subjects: 20 normal, 21 hypertensives. (From Boyer, J. T., Fraser, J. R. E., and Doyle, A. E., *Clin. Sci.,* 19, 539, 1960. With permission.)

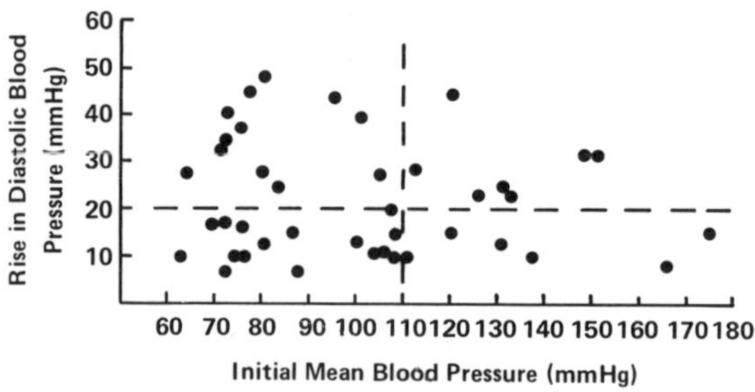

FIGURE 7.   Rise in diastolic blood pressure during cold immersion compared with initial mean blood pressure in 41 subjects: 20 normal, 21 hypertensive. Horizontal interrupted line indicates Hines' lower limit of hyperreaction (15). Vertical interrupted line provides alternative arbitrary classification according to blood pressure records during the tests. (From Boyer, J. T., Fraser, J. R. E., and Doyle, A. E., *Clin. Sci.,* 19, 539, 1960. With permission.)

and 9). It appears, therefore, that the hemodynamic response to emotional or painful stimuli may be qualitatively different in people with labile hypertension or in normal people than in those with severe hypertension. There have been numerous attempts to define a prehypertensive state by the use of blood pressure-raising reflexes. Hines and Brown[61] thought that an excessive response to cold immersion of the hand indicated a prehypertensive state, and that it strongly suggested the possibility of hypertension developing later in life. Although insufficiently adequate follow-up studies appear to have been done to confirm or deny this hypothesis, other workers using the cold pressor test could not demonstrate the clear separation between the two groups noted by Hines and Brown. Pickering and Kissin[62] found no difference in the responses of the hypertensive or normal subjects, and Alam and Smirk[63] and Russek and Zohman[64] found that while large pressor responses occurred frequently in hypertensive patients, some had responses within the normal range. These groups found that in normotensive subjects the proportion of individuals giving a large response increased with advancing

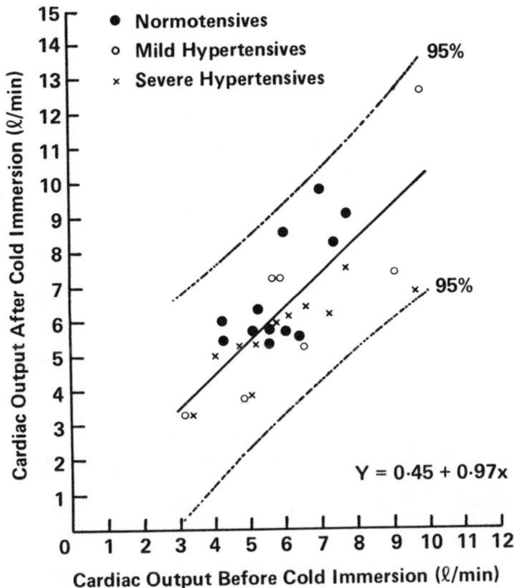

FIGURE 8.   Relationship between cardiac output estimations before and after cold immersion in 29 subjects. Interrupted lines indicate 95% confidence bands for prediction. (From Boyer, J. T., Fraser, J. R. E., and Doyle, A. E., *Clin. Sci.*, 19, 539, 1960. With permission.)

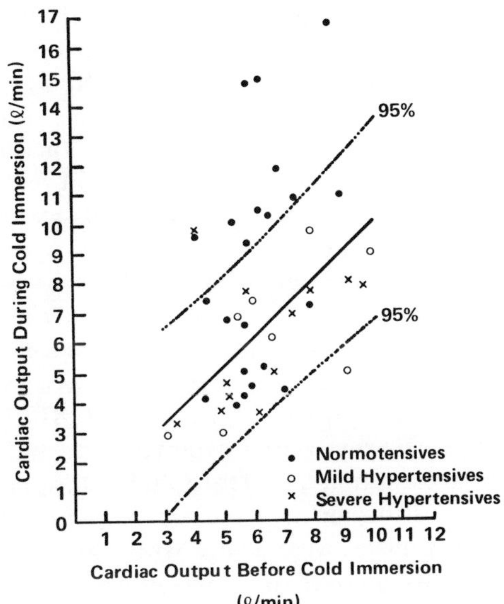

FIGURE 9.   Cardiac output of 41 subjects during cold immersion in relation to confidence bands established for the control values. (From Boyer, J. T., Fraser, J. R. E., and Doyle, A. E., *Clin. Sci.*, 19, 539, 1960. With permission.)

age and half the normal population above 50 years of age had responses which would be consistent with the hyperreactivity defined by Hines and colleagues. Exercise,[65] emotional stimuli,[66] or pain[63] usually produce rises in blood pressure, and these are often greater in hypertensive patients than in normotensive ones. Fowler and Guz,[67] using intra-arterial pressure recordings during standardized exercise, found that patients with mild or moderately severe hypertension had greater rises of blood pressure than normal people, but reported also that in very severe or in malignant hypertension, the rise in blood pressure was small or absent.

Both in hypertensive patients and in normal people, the blood pressure varies substantially during the day. Thus, during sleep[68] or on repeated measurement following sedation with barbiturates,[69] the blood pressure may fall considerably to a level which has been defined as the basal blood pressure.[69,70] Both in hypertensive patients and in normal people, the basal blood pressure is usually much lower than the level found on casual measurement. In a study of variation in arterial pressure throughout the day and night,[71] it was found that profound falls of arterial pressure occurred during sleep in both normal and hypertensive patients. The diurnal variation in pressure was apparently less in patients with secondary (mostly renal) hypertension than in primary (essential) hypertension. In patients with essential hypertension, the variation in blood pressure was less in the severely hypertensive patients than in the milder group. This observation may account for the observed difference between primary and secondary hypertension, since the latter included few patients with mild hypertension. The balance of evidence thus suggests that on the average the blood pressure varies more in hypertensive patients than in normotensive people. Some hypertensive patients, particularly those with severe disease, have rises or falls in blood pressure of no greater magnitude than the normal individual.

The undoubted relationship between genetic influences and blood pressure have been extensively studied by Smirk,[72] who has reported that the casual and basal blood pressures rise more in the first degree relatives of hypertensive patients in the decades following the 40th year. Smirk has also pointed out that casual blood pressures of identical twins tend to be very similar and reports discovering only one twin pair out of a total of 67 twin pairs in which one twin was hypertensive without the other being hypertensive. The fact that genetic factors seem to have a strong influence on blood pressure suggests that environmental factors leading to the defense reaction may have larger pressor effects in individuals genetically subject to hypertension than in those not predisposed in this way. There is certainly good evidence in the rat that selective breeding of animals with over average blood pressure leads to the development of a strain of spontaneously or genetically hypertensive rats.[73,74] It has to be emphasized that the link between genetic influences and the involvement of the central nervous system is tenuous in the extreme.

There is now clear experimental evidence in mice, squirrel monkeys, and baboons that persistent arterial hypertension can be induced by psychosocial factors or by operant conditioning. Henry and colleagues[75] studied the stimulating effects of a sustained disturbance of the social environment in socially deprived mice. When socially isolated males were placed with 16 normal females in population cages with intercommunicating boxes, the socially isolated animals became socially disturbed and fought vigorously with each other, and perhaps as a result of this developed a rise in blood pressure. In the groups that were exposed to this social interaction for up to 7 days, blood pressure returned to normal after approximately 4 days of post-exposure isolation. If the animals were made to undergo a period of 16 days of social interaction, the return to base line took 9 to 10 days. The blood pressure in these animals rose progressively up to a 21-day period, at which time social interaction was at a peak. Animals which were exposed to social pressures for 5 months and 9 months showed a persistent rise in blood pressure which fell only a little towards base line values even after the animals had been removed from the colonies and isolated again.

These experiments on socially disturbed mice are of particular importance in that they reveal that although brief exposure to a chronically disturbed situation led to a rise in blood pressure, early removal led to a prompt fall in blood pressure. Continued exposure led to persistent elevation of blood pressure, which then failed to fall even though the stimulus was removed. Of particular significance in these experiments is that in the animals whose blood pressure was elevated, heart weights were increased, and there was evidence of aortic arteriosclerosis and myocardial degeneration and fibrosis.

The relationship between environmental stimulation and genetic influences has been emphasized by the studies[76] which show that young spontaneously hypertensive rats raised from birth in a quiet, dark room in social isolation failed to develop an arterial blood pressure as high as that found in rats raised in normal circumstances. Herd and colleagues[77,78] have described the development of arterial hypertension in the squirrel monkey during operant conditioning experiments. The monkeys were trained to press a key which turned off a light associated with the delivery of a painful stimulus. As training progressed and each animal began to press the key rapidly, the number of painful stimuli delivered decreased, but the mean arterial blood pressure rose, and eventually in four of the six animals the mean arterial blood pressure was elevated before, during, and after each session, even when painful stimuli were not delivered. These behavioral experiments in animals provide strong evidence for the possibility that hypertension can be produced or aggravated by psychosocial or behavioral influences and provide some evidence for a direct link between these and genetic influences in the rat.

There have been numerous studies designed to determine whether there is evidence in favor of a primary psychological mechanism in the pathogenesis of essential hypertension in man. For obvious reasons, these experiments have been necessarily less direct. Higher blood pressures were observed in front-line troops for periods of about 3 months after combat,[79] and elevated arterial pressures were noted following the Texas City explosion.[80] There have been numerous attempts to characterize the personality type of hypertensive patients. Thus, Wolf and colleagues[81] identified a characteristic pattern of "readiness to take offensive action" which they believed derived from latent hostility. These authors thought that hypertensive patients preferred action to reflection, were tense and suspicious, but did not appear to be overtly aggressive. Hambling[82] and Van der Valk[83] also concluded that hypertensive patients were latently enraged persons. Harburg et al. have found a high correlation between raised blood pressure and environmental factors. They studied the incidence of hypertension of the inhabitants of high and low stress areas in Detroit.[84] Those individuals who lived in areas with a low socioeconomic status, high crime and violence rates, high density, and high rates of marital stress had the highest blood pressures, particularly among blacks. Harburg found that suppressed hostility was related to high blood pressure levels and to the percentage of men who were hypertensive and lived in black, high stress areas.

There are very real difficulties in interpreting personality studies in established hypertensive patients, since it is entirely possible that knowledge of hypertension may itself lead to personaltiy changes. There is, however, no doubt that both in patients with established hypertension and in those with normal blood pressures, everyday events have a substantial effect on the actual levels of blood pressure. Sokolow and colleagues[85] used continuously recorded blood pressures which they related to daily life events in patients with essential hypertension. Pulse rates and blood pressures tended to be high when the subjects were alert or anxious or were working against time and tended to be lowest when the patient was relaxed. Similar variability was noted by Bevan et al.,[86] who showed considerable variability of blood pressures in both hypertensive and normal people (Figure 10). Pain, anxiety, and coitus all caused marked elevations in blood pressure.

To summarize, it is clear that a wide variety of emotional stimuli leads to rises in blood pressure in most people. These elevations of blood pressure tend to be transient, but the possibility exists that repeated elevations of blood pressure as a result of emotional or physical stimuli operating through the central nervous system may lead in man to the gradual persistent elevation of blood pressure. The evidence that this occurs in animals is fairly strong, and it seems likely that some of these mechanisms may also prevail in man, although this is quite unproven.

F. The Role of the Autonomic Nervous System in Hypertension

There is clear evidence that in almost all forms of hypertension the autonomic nervous system remains responsible for the control of blood pressure and regulation of the distribution of blood flow. Thus, in human hypertension, normal circulatory reflexes are intact so that, for example, the assumption of the upright posture does not lead to orthostatic hypotension. Blood flow to specific organs is not generally different from that in normal people, and the blood pressure, although more variable in hypertensives, appears to be regulated although to an elevated level. These well-known facts carry the implication that the high blood pressure is regulated by the autonomic nervous system to its new raised level. This fact, however, should not be taken to imply that the autonomic nervous system is necessarily primarily responsible for the elevation of blood pressure, for it is becoming clear that in many types of hypertension the autonomic nervous system may play a secondary role in maintaining high blood pressure primarily raised by other factors.

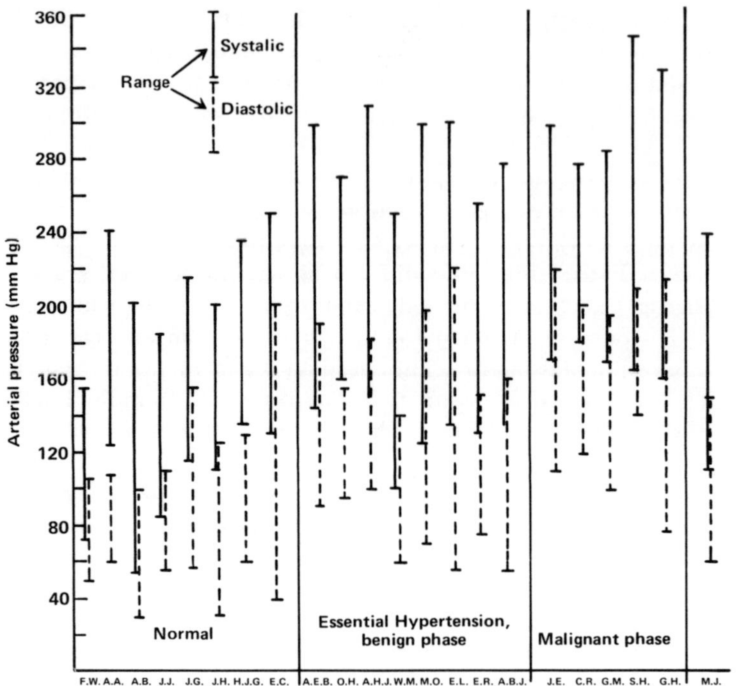

FIGURE 10. Extreme range of arterial pressure in individual subjects. (From Bevan, A. T., Honor, A. J., and Sott, F. H., *Clin. Sci.*, 36, 329, 1969. With permission.)

Changes in the activity of the autonomic nervous system, both at a central and peripheral level, have also been shown to occur in a wide variety of models with experimental hypertension. Although these experimental models have many characteristics in common with human hypertension, it cannot be assumed that any of them precisely mimic the somewhat heterogeneous situation in man. Moreover, although changes occurring as a result of induction of experimental hypertension may be significant in pathogenesis, the possibility always remains that the changes observed are secondary to the development of high blood pressure. Since the majority of these changes relate to disturbances in catecholaminergic mechanisms, many of them have direct relevance to antihypertensive drugs and so will be discussed in some detail here.

1. Central Autonomic Mechanisms in Experimental Hypertension

There is considerable evidence that norepinephrine is an important neurotransmitter in the brain and spinal cord.[87] The mapping of specific noradrenergic tracts within the central nervous system had been made possible by the development of histochemical fluorescent methods for the localization of catecholamines.[20] There are high concentrations of catecholamine-containing cells in the medulla and pons.[23] Many of the nerve fibers originating in these cell bodies terminate in the hypothalamus and the limbic system, while others descend to terminate in the reticular formation in the spinal cord. There are high concentrations of catecholamines in the nucleus of the tractus solitarius and the vasodepressor area of the medulla.[21] It now seems clear that not only is norepinephrine an important neurotransmitter in the central nervous system, but that dopaminergic nerves are common in the basal ganglia and limbic system, and there is some evidence also that epinephrine[23] and 5-hydroxytryptamine[29] may also act as central neurotransmitters.

A number of methods have been evolved to study the involvement of catecholaminergic neurones in the central nervous system. These include the administration of either catecholamines[88] or their receptor blockers[89] into the cerebrospinal fluid, electrical and iontophoretic stimulation with recording of evoked potentials, the measurement of metabolism, turnover of catecholamines and the activity of related enzymes,[90] and the use of chemicals that selectively impair the function of or destroy catecholaminergic nerves. This latter method has been extensively used. In particular, 6-hydroxydopamine has been used to produce selective ablation of central catecholaminergic nerves by causing selective degeneration of the nerve endings and depletion of their transmitter stores.[91,92] 6-Hydroxydopamine has the advantage that it does not readily cross the blood-brain barrier so that when given intrathecally or intracisternally, its effects are confined to the central nervous system. In normal animals, the central administration of 6-hydroxydopamine leads to a fall in blood pressure which lasts for a few hours and which has been attributed to stimulation of central α-receptor mechanisms by the 6-hydroxydopamine itself.[91] After a few hours, blood pressure gradually rises and it appears that 6-hydroxydopamine has no long-term effects on the arterial blood pressure of normotensive animals. This contrasts with its actions when given parenterally and combined with adrenalectomy in that a substantial fall in blood pressure occurs in normotensive animals.[93] It therefore appears that in normotensive animals at least, central adrenergic mechanisms play little part in the maintenance of blood pressure. As will become evident, this situation appears to alter in most varieties of experimental hypertension.

It has long been known that denervation of the carotid sinus and the aortic arch baroreceptors produces a neurogenic hypertension which is extremely labile and is usually accompanied by tachycardia.[94,95] Chalmers and Wurtman[90] have shown that the development of this type of hypertension in rabbits did not alter the endogenous catecholamine content of various regions of the brain, but did, however, lead to an increased turnover of tritiated norepinephrine both in the hypothalamus and in the thoracolumbar region of the spinal cord. Tyrosine hydroxylase activity was normal in the hypothalamus, but was increased to approximately twice the control levels in the spinal cord of the hypertensive animals. These authors suggested that these changes reflected increased activity of the bulbar and spinal neurones, and that one of the normal functions of the baroreceptors was to inhibit the physiological activity of the descending noradrenergic neurones which terminate in the sympathetic lateral horn of the spinal cord and that section of the baroreceptor nerves overcame this tonic inhibition. In subsequent experiments Chalmers and Reid[92] demonstrated that the destruction of the central catecholaminergic neurones with intracisternally administered 6-hydroxydopamine could prevent the development of neurogenic hypertension usually induced by sinoaortic section.

Doba and Reis[24] reported that bilateral electrolytic lesions of the nuclei of the solitary tract resulted in an immediate rise in blood pressure. The hypertension was associated with a marked increase in total systemic peripheral resistance and an increased central venous pressure. All rats died of pulmonary edema (Figure 11). The rise in blood pressure could be abolished by phentolamine, due probably to block of α-receptors, since removal of the adrenal glands did not affect the course of the hypertension. These authors postulated that this syndrome of acute neurogenic hypertension resulted from the release of preganglionic sympathetic neurones from inhibition by arterial baroreceptors. The hypertension depended on the integrity of structures lying above the midbrain and could be abolished by midcollicular decerebration. They suggested that the baroreceptors engaged in long loop cardiovascular reflexes with higher brain centers, most probably the hypothalamus. They suggested that this area[34] could be an

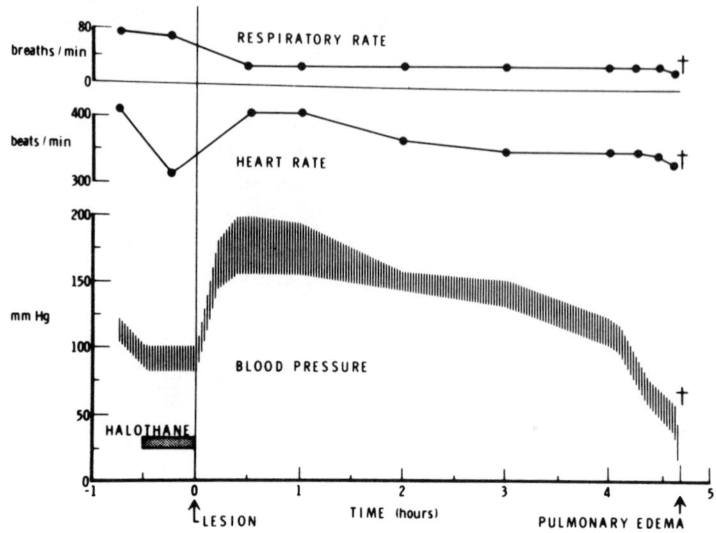

FIGURE 11. Time course of changes in systemic arterial blood pressure, heart rate, and respiratory rate in a representative unanesthetized rat after production of bilateral lesions in the NTS. Just prior to death the rat developed pulmonary edema. (From Doba, N. and Reis, D. J., *Circ. Res.*, 32, 584, 1973. With permission.)

important site of interaction between behaviorally determined cardiovascular events and baroreceptor reflexes. In subsequent studies, the same authors[25] demonstrated that the previous administration of intracisternally administered 6-hydroxydopamine prevented this hypertension. Moreover, local injection of 6-hydroxydopamine into the nucleus of the tractus solitarius of rats produced an increase in arterial blood pressure which lasted for about 14 days. It appears that both of these types of neurogenic hypertension depend on the removal of inhibitory pathways. In the one instance, the baroreceptor reflexes provide a tonic inhibition of the medullospinal sympathetic tracts, while in the other, ablation of the nucleus of the tractus solitarius appears to remove a chronic inhibitory control on blood pressure levels.

Additional evidence for the similarity between sinoaortic section and lesions of the nucleus of the solitary tract were produced by Nathan and Reis,[26] who observed the development of chronic labile hypertension in cats following lesions of the middle third of this area. They concluded that the hypertension was probably produced by disinhibition of sympathetic activity through central interruption of the baroreceptor reflexes. They further suggested that the higher pressures during the day might have been due to environmental stimuli absent at night (Figure 12).

Wing and Chalmers[96] have studied the role of central serotonergic neurones and circulatory control in rabbits, giving intracisternal injections of 5,6-dihydroxytryptamine (5,6-DHT) to cause degeneration of central serotonergic nerve terminals and depletion of serotonin stores. In normal rabbits, 5,6-DHT given intrathecally produced falls in mean arterial pressure which were maximal one week after injection, and central serotonin levels were reduced to less than half in the spinal cords of the rabbits treated with 5,6-DHT, compared with the levels in controls. The same authors found that pretreatment with 5,6-DHT prevented the increases in mean arterial blood pressure and heart rate which normally occur after sinoaortic denervation in rabbits. In rabbits with established neurogenic hypertension following baroreceptor denervation, treatment with intracisternal 5,6-DHT caused a rapid and persistent fall in mean arterial

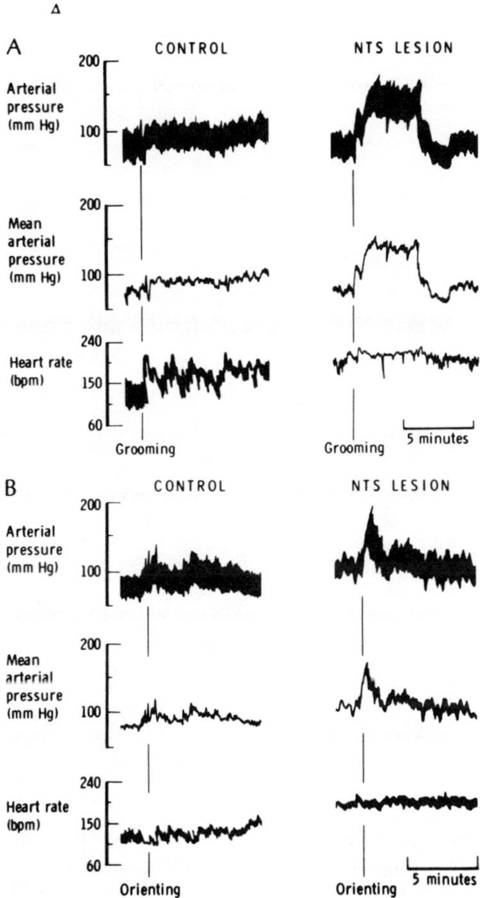

FIGURE 12. Effect of lesions of the nucleus tractus solitarius (NTS) on the changes in arterial pressure and heart rate associated with grooming (A) and orienting (B). The light vertical lines indicate the onset of the particular behavior. The responses were measured prior to the placement of NTS lesions (control) and after placement of the lesions (NTS lesion) in the same cat. (From Nathan, M. A. and Reis, D. J., *Circ. Res.*, 40, 72, 1977. With permission.)

blood pressure and heart rate, but did not interfere with the development or maintenance of the hypertension that followed bilateral wrapping of the kidneys with cellophane. The authors suggested that central serotonergic neurones participate in the baroreceptor reflex arc and that the integrity of these neurones appears to be necessary for the development of sustained neurogenic hypertension.

It is now evident that the baroreceptor reflexes are modified in both experimental and clinical forms of hypertension. Direct evidence for resetting of the carotid sinus baroreceptor reflexes was first obtained in renal hypertensive dogs by McCubbin, Greene, and Page (Figure 13),[97] and in rabbits with renal hypertension by Angell-James[98]. Records of nerve activity from the carotid sinus nerves indicated that both the threshold and the range of responses were shifted upwards in the hypertensive animals so that baroreceptor reflexes were acting to maintain rather than reduce the

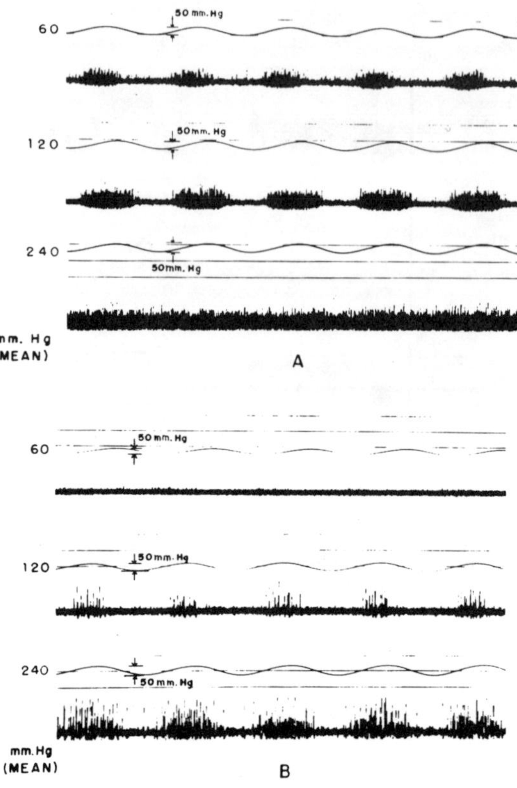

FIGURE 13.   Recordings of nerve activity from the afferent carotid sinus nerves at various levels of blood pressure in A (upper section) normotensive dogs and B (lower section) renal hypertensive dogs. (From Mc-Cubbin, J. W., Green, J. H., and Page, I. H., *Circ. Res.*, 4, 205, 1956. With permission.)

hypertensive levels. The resetting process occurs within a few hours or days of the rise in arterial pressure.

The resetting process occurs within a few hours or days of the rise in arterial pressure.

Angell-James described three types of fibers from which inpulses could be recorded from aortic arch receptors in the rabbit. Approximately two thirds of the fibers had a critical threshold pressure, below which there was no discharge. In the normal rabbit, this threshold pressure was approximately 50 mmHg. In about 20% of fibers, inter-mittent discharge was observed, while in the remainder, there was a plateau-type threshold in which the discharge frequency did not increase with pressure immediately, but only after a pressure rise of about 40 mmHg beyond the threshold. In renal hyper-tensive rabbits, the threshold pressure for the discharge of impulses rose from 52 mmHg in normal rabbits, whose blood pressures were about 87 mmHg, to 106 mmHg in renal hypertensive rabbits, whose blood pressures were approximately 174 mmHg (Figure 14).In the hypertensive rabbits, not only was the threshold elevated, but for any given increment in aortic arch pressure, there was a lower increment of impulse frequency (Figure 15). Angell-James also examined the pressure volume curves of aor-tae from rabbits with renal hypertension and from normal rabbits. The resting volume of the aortae of the hypertensive rabbits was slightly larger than that from normal rabbits, and increments of volume induced much greater rises in pressure in the hyper-

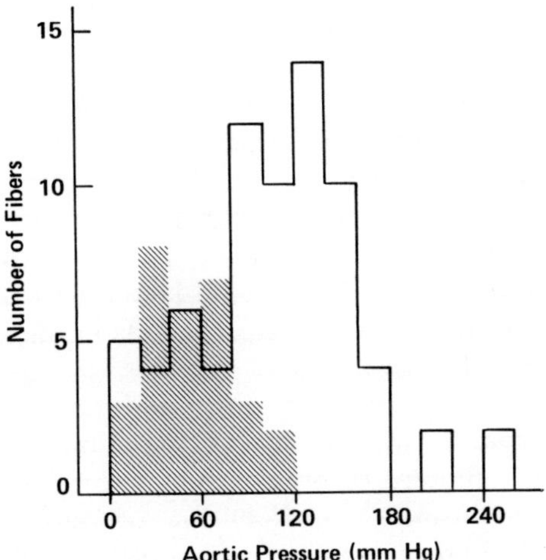

FIGURE 14.   Histogram of the number of fibers plotted against their threshold pressure: 29
fibers from 17 normal rabbits (cross-hatched
blocks) and 71 fibers from 8 rabbits with hypertension (open blocks) were tested. (From Angell-
James, J. E., *Circ. Res.*, 37, 149, 1973. With permission.)

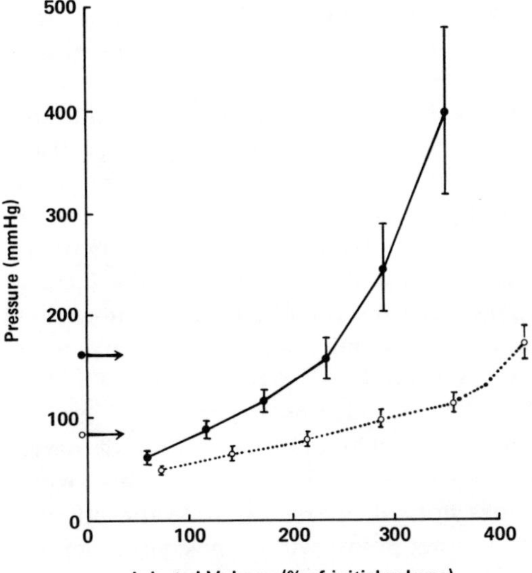

FIGURE 15.   Graph of the mean aortic pressure plotted against the injected volume (expressed as a percent
of the original volume measured at zero pressure). Eight
tests in four normal rabbits (open circles, broken line)
and eight tests in six rabbits with hypertension (solid
circles, solid line) were performed. The bars indicate the
standard error. The arrows indicate the means blood
pressures of the two groups. (From Angell-James, J. E.,
Circ. Res., 37, 149, 1973. With permission.)

tensive rabbits than in the normal ones, indicating that the vessels had become less distensible. Histological examination of the arteries demonstrated increased amounts of collagen and some fragmentation of the elastin. In a few sections there appeared to be areas in which the nerve fibers were fragmented. These changes in baroreceptor function did not develop immediately, but developed within a few days of the development of hypertension, suggesting that the baroreceptor dysfunction occurred as the result of hypertension rather than being a cause. It may be due in part to changes in water and electrolyte composition, which would increase the stiffness of the arteries, or it could in part be the result of pathological lesions in the arterial walls or damage of receptors due to necrosis or other injury.

Studies in man have been necessarily less direct and have depended on the measurement of the effects of baroreflex activity in reducing pulse rate. In man, sudden intravenous injections of small amounts of pressor substances which have no direct action on the heart, such as angiotensin or phenylephrine, produce brief increases in systolic pressure which lead via the baroreceptor reflex to corresponding slowing of the pulse. In normotensive patients, there is marked slowing of the pulse as the systolic pressure is raised. In hypertensive patients, there appears to be diminished baroreflex sensitivity. Bristow et al.[99] reported that although control heart rates were similar in the low and high pressure groups, in the hypertensives, further elevations of blood pressure, induced by either angiotensin or phenylephrine, produced little slowing of the heart (Figure 16). These changes not only occurred in hypertension, but tended to develop with increasing age of normotensive subjects, due presumably to a reduction in compliance of the arteries as a result of aging. The validity of these results in man have been strengthened by the observations of Korner,[100] who measured mean arterial pressure and heart period, which is a derivative of pulse rate, in normotensive and renal hypertensive rabbits, using an inflatable balloon within the aorta. The curves which he derived were very similar to those obtained in normal and hypertensive man by Bristow et al.,[99] and in subsequent experiments in normal and hypertensive patients, using the valsalva response (Figure 17), Korner[100] has also produced very similar curves. Further confirmation that the resetting of the receptors can be caused by hypertension was obtained by Kezdi,[101] who showed that if one carotid sinus was protected from the effect of raised pressure by anastomosing it to a jugular vein and tying the common carotid artery below the sinus so that the intrasinus pressure was maintained at about 40 mmHg, the subsequent development of renal hypertension induced by wrapping the kidney in cellophane was followed by evidence of resetting in the unprotected carotid sinus, but not in the protected one. The fact that the baroreceptors can be demonstrated to be reset during experimental hypertension of renal origin clearly provides one mechanism whereby the autonomic nervous system can regulate blood pressure to hypertensive levels. The fact that this mechanism has been demonstrated to be present does not, of course, exclude the possibility that other adaptive changes may be present at other points within the central nervous system.

In renal hypertension, activation of the renin-angiotensin system might operate through autonomic mechanisms to elevate the blood pressure. There are several ways in which this could operate. First, there is evidence that perfusion of the vertebral artery in dogs with angiotensin in small doses leads to elevation of the blood pressure and that this effect can be abolished by ablation of the area postrema. The infusion of angiotensin into the vertebral arteries reduces the degree of inhibition of vasomotor tone induced by stimulation of baroreceptor afferents from the carotid sinus.

A reduction of sensitivity of the baroreceptors as a result of hypertension might induce disinhibition of the central sympathetic pathways in much the same manner that sinoaortic nerve section or lesions of the nucleus of the solitary tract appear to do.

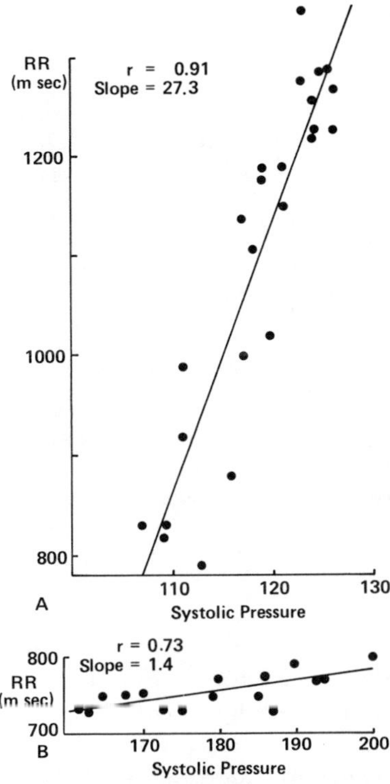

FIGURE 16. Relationship between individual systolic arterial pressures (mmHg) and subsequent pulse intervals (R-R, in milliseconds) when pressure was transiently increased by the sudden injection of angiotensin. (A) Results of one injection in a subject with a resting mean arterial pressure of 74 mmHg. (B) Results of one injection in a man with mean pressure of 119 mmHg. The difference in slopes of the regression lines is evident. Abbreviation: r = correlation coefficient. (From Bristow, J. P., Honor, A. J., Pickering, G. W., Sleight, P., and Smyth, H. S., *Circ. Res.*, 29, 48, 1969. With permission.)

The extent to which central catecholaminergic mechanisms participate in the development or maintenance of renal hypertension is by no means clear, and conflicting data have been obtained. There seems to be general agreement that destruction of central catecholaminergic nerves, using injections of 6-hydroxydopamine into the CSF, prevents the development of hypertension both in the rabbit[92] and in the rat with contralateral nephrectomy.[102] However, although Lewis et al.[103] reported that intracisternally administered 6-hydroxydopamine also caused the high blood pressure to return to near normal levels when given 18 weeks after renal wrapping had resulted in chronic renal hypertension in the rabbit, Dinch et al.[104] found no effect in rats when 6-hydroxydopamine was injected into the cerebral ventricles of chronic renal hypertensive animals. As has been previously mentioned, the administration of 5,6-dihydroxytryptamine appears to have little effect either on the development or the persistance of renal hypertension in the rabbit.

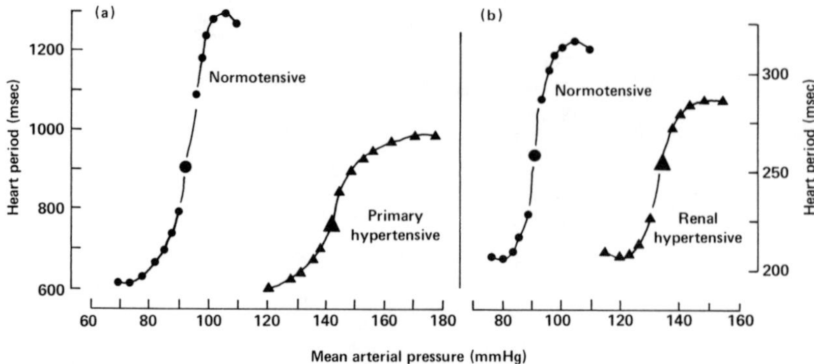

FIGURE 17.   Mean arterial pressure — heart period curves derived from 14 normotensive subjects and 4 hypertensive subjects in the age range 19 to 29 years. The curves on the right were derived from 28 sham-operated normotensive rabbits and 21 renal hypertensive rabbits studied 4 to 6 weeks after wrapping both kidneys in cellophane. (A) Man; (B) rabbit. (From Korner, P. I., *Clin. Exp. Pharmocol. Physiol.*, Suppl. 2, 171, 1975. With permission.)

Ayitey-Smith and Varma[105] showed that in totally immunosympathectomized rats, renal hypertension could be induced for a short time, but failed to be maintained. They suggested that the acute phase might be dependent on the renin-angiotensin system, but that the maintenance of chronic renal hypertension required the autonomic nervous system to be functioning. In the spontaneously hypertensive rat, the intraventricular administration of 6-hydroxydopamine to mature animals with established hypertension induced a transient fall in blood pressure which lasted for 4 to 5 days only.[104] On the other hand, the same treatment of 7-week-old spontaneously hypertensive rats reduced the blood pressure for a period of 5 weeks, while in control untreated animals, the blood pressure rose considerably during this period.[88]

The presence of epinephrine and phenylethanolamine *N*-methyltransferase has been found in the brain stem and in some hypothalamic nuclei. It has been reported that there is an elevation of the enzyme in certain areas of the brain stem in young spontaneously hypertensive rats. This raises the rather speculative possibility that epinephrine might be concerned in the brain stem in the development of spontaneous hypertension.[106]

It has been claimed that deoxycorticosterone and sodium hypertension in rats is associated with an increase in the activity of the peripheral sympathetic nerves and the adrenal medulla. The interaction between central adrenergic mechanisms and this form of hypertension is not entirely clear. Finch, Haeusler, and Thoenen[104] claimed that the intraventricular injection of 6-hydroxydopamine given 7 to 10 days before the administration of DOCA and sodium chloride completely prevented the development of hypertension. However, the administration of 6-hydroxydopamine had no effect on the blood pressure of rats whose blood pressures had already risen as a result of the administration of DOCA and sodium chloride, even though the norepinephrine content of the hypothalamus, the medulla, and the remaining parts of the brain were substantially reduced by the 6-hydroxydopamine, as was the tyrosine hydroxylase activity. These authors concluded that the intraventricular injection of 6-hydroxydopamine, while preventing the development of various forms of experimental hypertension, was ineffective in established hypertension. They suggested that central noradrenergic and/or dopaminergic structures might be involved in the initiation of hypertension, but seemed to be of no importance once hypertension had been established.

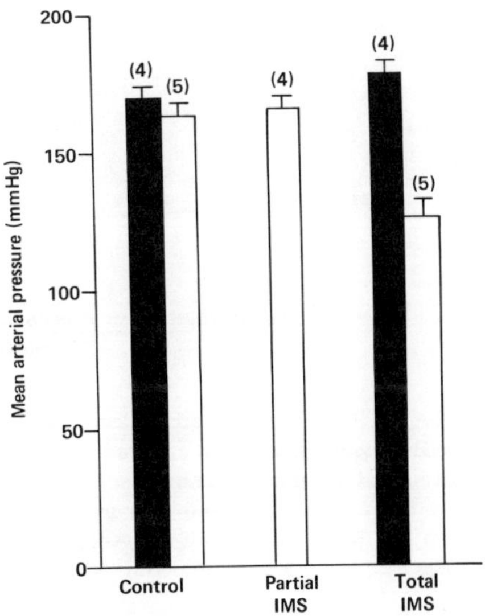

FIGURE 18.   Mean arterial pressure of normal (control), "partial" immunosympathectomized (partial IMS), and "total" immunosympathectomized (total IMS) rats after attempting to produce renal hypertension. Femoral arterial pressure was measured after recovery from ether anesthesia. Arterial pressure was determined at 30 (filled columns) and 50 days (open columns) after renal artery constriction. Vertical lines represent one half the S.E. Numbers in parentheses are the numbers of rats in the group. (From Ayitey-Smith, E. and Varma, D. R., *Br. J. Pharmacol.*, 40, 175, 1970. With permission.)

Rather similar findings have been reported by Reid et al.,[107] who also found that pretreatment with 6-hydroxydopamine given into the brain ventricular system prevented the rise in blood pressure in uninephrectomized rats given DOCA and salt (Figure 18). The rats which developed hypertension also had rises in plasma norepinephrine levels. Those in whom the rise in blood pressure was prevented by centrally administered 6-hydroxydopamine did not. Nakamura, Gerold, and Thoenen[108] found that DOCA sodium hypertensive rats had a decreased turnover of norepinephrine in the hypothalamus and brain stem, but increased turnover in the heart, suggesting that decreased activity of the noradrenergic mechanisms may reflect an attempt to decrease noradrenergic activity and compensate for the increased blood pressure. It appears that central autonomic mechanisms are essential for the early development, but not the maintenance, of this form of hypertension.

To summarize, there appears to be evidence that central autonomic mechanisms may be actively involved in the initiation of hypertension in a wide variety of experimental models. This appears to be so in the DOCA sodium hypertensive rat, the spontaneously hypertensive rat, and the renal hypertensive rabbit. There seems to be general agreement also that central adrenergic mechanisms play an important part in the development of neurogenic hypertension. It appears, however, that the mechanisms which maintain the raised level of blood pressure may be different from those which initiated the rise, and the majority of experiments suggests that gross inactivation of central

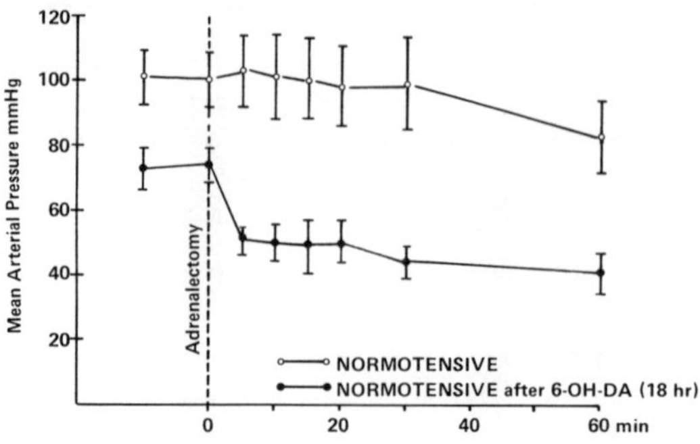

FIGURE 19.   Acute effects of adrenalectomy on the mean arterial pressure (mmHg) in anesthetized intact or sympathectomized normotensive animals. Each curve is the mean ± SE of six treated and four untreated animals. (From de Champlain, J. and van Ameringen, M. R., *Circ. Res.*, 31, 617, 1972. With permission.)

adrenergic neurones by the use of 6-hydroxydopamine has little effect on the subsequent maintenance of established hypertension. It is possible that in all forms of hypertension the development of the raised pressure is followed by a reduction in baroreceptor input, which is then associated with an impairment of the normal inhibitory function of the nucleus of the tractus solitarius and of the descendingbulbar spinal sympathetic fibers. Such a mechanism would link the various forms of experimental hypertension and in particular those of neurogenic hypertension and DOCA salt hypertension. The extent to which these experiments have relevance to the human situation is by no means certain. It is nevertheless possible that a similar mechanism might occur in man and that rises in blood pressure, no matter how initiated, may lead to the active participation of the central autonomic nervous system.

2. Peripheral Autonomic Mechanisms in Experimental Hypertension

6-Hydroxydopamine given peripherally to animals causes a generalized functional sympathectomy by producing degeneration of the peripheral sympathetic nerves. The role of the autonomic nervous system in the control of blood pressure has been studied using this technique.[93] It was found that the administration of 6-hydroxydopamine to normotensive rats and dogs produced a fall of blood pressure of about 30 mmHg, when compared to control untreated normotensive animals. Importantly, in such sympathectomized animals, subsequent removal of the adrenal medulla or the administration of α-receptor blocking drugs produced a rapid further fall of blood pressure (Figures 19 and 20). It has been suggested, therefore, that circulating catecholamines of adrenal origin maintain the blood pressure in sympathectomized animals. In support of this, Mueller et al.[109] have shown that following chemical sympathectomy with 6-hydroxydopamine, there is a sharp increase in the synthesis of catecholamines by the adrenal medulla. As a corollary, removal of the adrenal medulla leads to a sharp increase in norepinephrine turnover in peripheral sympathetic nerve fibers. It appears, therefore, that in normal animals the peripheral sympathetic nervous system and the adrenal medulla act together to maintain blood pressure levels. Whether this is done through arteriolar constriction raising peripheral resistance or by venoconstriction altering the capacitance vessels is not as yet clear. As has been stated in the preceding section, there is considerable evidence that central catecholaminergic mechanisms play a role in a variety of models of experimental hypertension. There is likewise evidence for the participation of the peripheral sympathetic nervous system, particularly in hy-

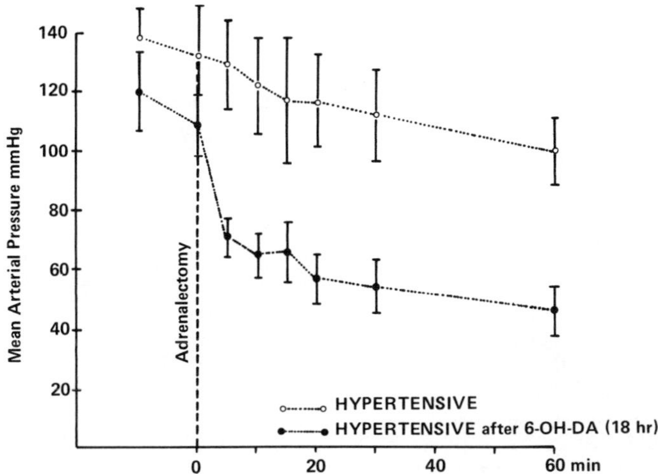

FIGURE 20. Acute effects of adrenalectomy on mean arterial pressure (mmHg) of anesthetized intact and sympathectomized hypertensive rats Each curve is the mean ± SE of six treated and four untreated animals. (From de Champlain, J. and van Ameringen, M. R., *Circ. Res.*, 31, 617, 1972. With permission.)

pertension following deoxycorticosterone sodium administration, but also in some other forms of experimental hypertension.

In deoxycorticosterone and sodium hypertension, the most important studies on the role of the peripheral autonomic nervous system have been performed by Axelrod and de Champlain and colleagues.[110-115] Rats treated by a weekly subcutaneous injection of DOCA (10 mg combined with 1% sodium chloride as drinking fluid) developed a significant increase in blood pressure during the second week of treatment which continued to rise for 4 to 6 weeks. In such animals, it has been shown that there is a marked reduction in the retention and storage of norepinephrine (Figures 21 and 22) in the peripheral sympathetic system, together with a marked increase in the turnover rate and the synthesis rate of norepinephrine. These changes occur in the heart and in the adrenal medulla, and more recent studies by de Champlain and colleagues[114] have demonstrated that there are increases in the circulating catecholamine levels in this model of hypertension. The same group has demonstrated that the intraneuronal distribution of norepinephrine is also disturbed, in that the fraction of soluble and free norepinephrine was greater in the heart of hypertensive rats at various times after the administration of tritiated norepinephrine, suggesting that greater amounts of physiologically reactive norepinephrine are accessible to receptor sites in this condition. It appears that the activation of the sympathetic nervous system occurs very early in the development of hypertension in this model. It has been found that a significant increase in cardiac norepinephrine turnover rate preceded the elevation of blood pressure, and plasma catecholamines were increased considerably a few days after the commencement of treatment with DOCA and sodium at a time when the blood pressure had not risen.

Chemical sympathectomy by 6-hydroxydopamine given peripherally resulted in a greater lowering of blood pressure in the DOCA salt hypertensive animals than in normal animals (Figure 23). Moreover, in animals sympathectomized at birth and treated weekly thereafter by injections of 6-hydroxydopamine, treatment with DOCA and sodium for 6 weeks did not cause an elevation of the blood pressure above normotensive levels, and Ayitey-Smith and Varma[105] have shown that this form of hyper-

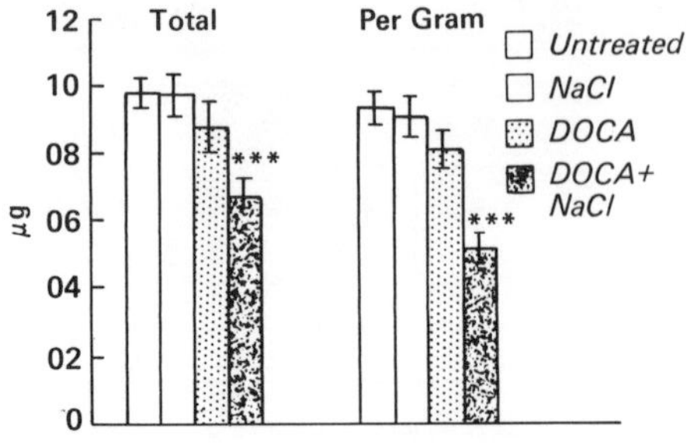

FIGURE 21. Endogenous norepinephrine levels in the hearts of rats treated with DOCA, saline, or both. Groups containing 10 to 18 animals were used and the results are expressed as the mean in mg ± SEM (vertical bars). (From de Champlain, J., Krakoff, L. R., and Axelrod, J., *Circ. Res.*, 20, 136, 1967. With permission.)

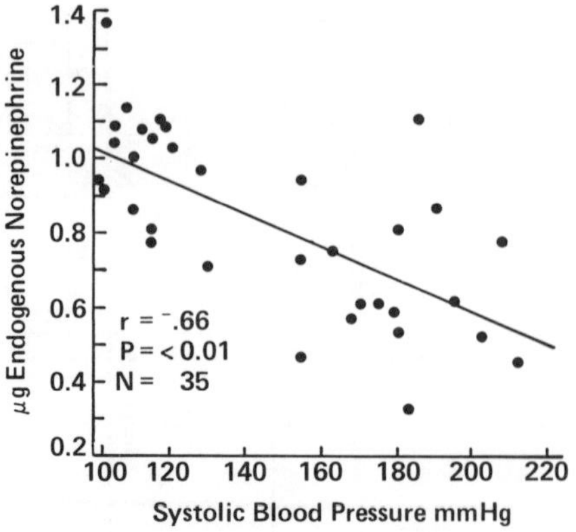

FIGURE 22. Correlation between systolic pressure and endogenous norepinephrine levels in the hearts from hypertensive and control animals. Each blood pressure is the mean of 2 separate determinations done 3 and 1 days before the killing. Norepinephrine is expressed as microgram per heart. (From de Champlain, J., Krakoff, L. R., and Axelrod, J., *Circ. Res.*, 20, 136, 1967. With permission.)

tension cannot be induced in totally immunosympathectomized animals. However, a number of authors have failed to confirm the latter findings. Thus, Finch and Leach[116] were unable to prevent the development of hypertension in DOCA and sodium-treated rats who had been pretreated with 6-hydroxydopamine, and Clarke and colleagues[117] likewise obtained negative results. It has been suggested that the reasons for these discrepancies were that the sympathetic nervous system might have regenerated,[118] since in the original observations of de Champlain and colleagues, 6-hydroxydopamine was administered at weekly intervals to maintain sympathectomy.

The mechanism whereby the peripheral autonomic nervous system is activated in this form of hypertension has been attributed by de Champlain, Krakoff, and Axelrod[115] to a relationship between sodium balance and the capacity of the nerve granules to bind and store norepinephrine. These authors demonstrated that sodium depletion enhanced the capacity for norepinephrine storage in the heart, whereas a high sodium diet or the use of DOCA decreased the storage capacity. They suggested that the state of sodium balance might be important in modulating the storage capacity of the nerve and regulating the availability of physiologically active norepinephrine. The same authors point out that since active transport and ionic shift are involved in the numerous functions of the nerve, it may be that the regulation of ionic balance is critical for the functioning of the storage and release of the nerve transmitter.

These disturbances in catecholamine binding and release may be related to the problem of vascular responsiveness to norepinephrine, which has been shown to be enhanced in this particular form of hypertension[119,120] as well as others (Figure 24). A reduced capacity to store catecholamines might lead to an increased concentration of catecholamines within the synaptic cleft as a result of diminished uptake. This situation would be enhanced if the turnover and release of catecholamines from nerve endings were increased. On the other hand, sodium depletion usually leads to a diminution in vascular responsiveness which might be related to augmented storage and diminished release of catecholamines on nerve stimulation. As has been discussed earlier, the re-

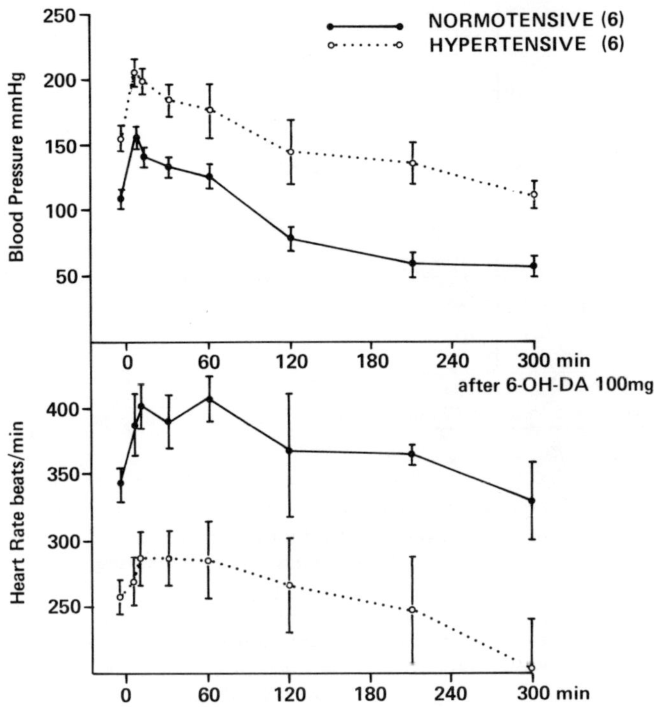

FIGURE 23. Cardiovascular responses in anesthetized normotensive and hypertensive (DOCA and sodium) rats during the first 5 hr after 1 i.v. injection of 6-OH-DA. (From de Champlain, J. and van Ameringen, M. R., *Circ. Res.*, 31, 617, 1972. With permission.)

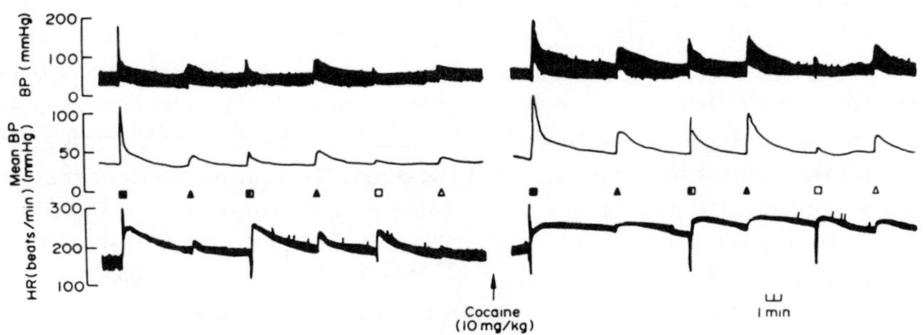

FIGURE 24. Records of pulsatile blood pressure (BP, upper channel), mean blood pressure (mean BP, center channel), and heart rate (HR, lower channel of a pithed, DOCA-salt-treated rat. Responses are shown to spinal stimulation and to norepinephrine before and after a dose of cocaine. Stimulation was with frequencies of 5 (■), 2 (▣) and 0.5 (□) Hz for 10 sec periods, and norepinephrine was injected in doses of 0.5 (▲), 0.2 ▲ and 0.1 (△) µg/kg. The time between panels was 10 min. (From Dusting, G. J., Harris, G. S., and Rand, M. J., *Clin. Sci. Mol. Med.*, 45, 571, 1973. With permission.)

lationship between body sodium content and hypertension is a complex one. However, these experiments indicate an additional possible mechanism for the development of hypertension in man. They may also be relevant to other forms of hypertension, since Guyton and colleagues[121] have proposed that a diminished capacity to excrete sodium is a fundamental property of most hypertensive situations (Chapter 1, Volume 1).

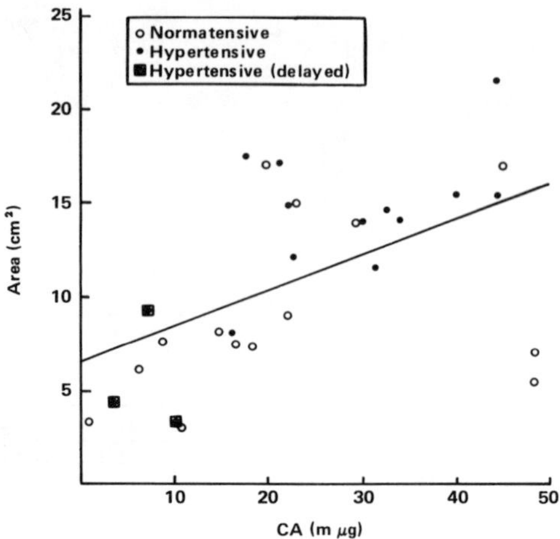

FIGURE 25.   Area of vasoconstrictor response obtained in skin of normotensive and hypertensive animals is plotted against total CA released during stimulation at 20 cycles/sec. Delayed hypertensive animals are those that did not develop an elevated blood pressure initially, but which were subsequently hypertensive. Regression equation is Y = 6.6 ± 0.19 X. (From Zimmerman, B. G., Rolewicz, T. F., Dunham, E. W., and Gisslen, J. L., *Am. J. Physiol.*, 27, 798, 1969. With permission.)

In experimental renal hypertension, an increased norepinephrine turnover in the heart has been reported.[122-124] Although the changes in norepinephrine turnover were similar to those found in DOCA hypertensive animals, endogenous norepinephrine levels were normal in most tissues, including the heart.[125,126] It has been reported that in rats and dogs with renal hypertension the stimulation of sympathetic fibers induces a greater vasoconstrictor response in various vascular beds, which is also associated with the release in larger quantities of norepinephrine at the nerve endings.[127,128] It is possible that this relates to the presence of the activated renin-angiotensin system, since even at low concentrations of angiotensin the vascular response to sympathetic stimulation has been reported to be potentiated,[129] and the quantity of transmitter released for a given number of nerve impulses was also found to be increased.[130] It has also been claimed that subpressor doses of angiotensin increase norepinephrine turnover in the heart.[131]

Chemical sympathectomy with 6-hydroxydopamine leads to a sustained fall in blood pressure in rats with one-kidney hypertension. The blood pressure does not fall to the same level as can be achieved by the removal of the remaining kidney in combination with 6-hydroxydopamine, suggesting that an additional factor might be present in renal hypertension[132] (Figure 25).

Ayitey-Smith and Varma[105] have studied the effects of immunosympathectomy on the development of one-kidney hypertension in the rat. They noted that in totally immunosympathectomized rats who had received two injections of antiserum to nerve growth factor, some rise in blood pressure was observed during the first 30 days after renal artery constriction, but that this hypertension could not be sustained beyond this period. These workers interpreted these findings to suggest that the initial phase of renal hypertension was independent of the sympathetic nervous system and might pri-

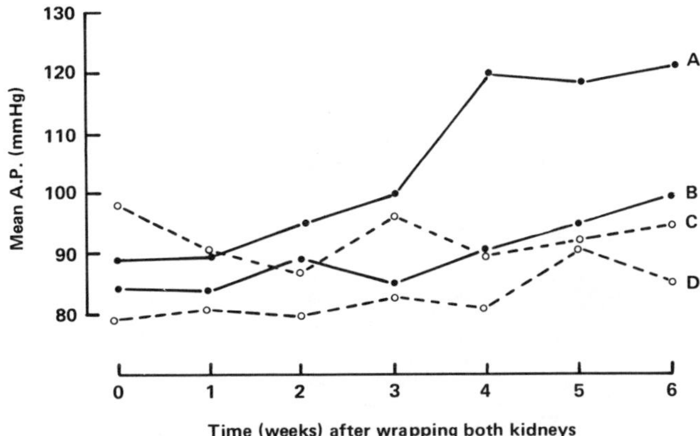

FIGURE 26.   The average mean arterial pressure (A.P.) of the four groups of animals (A-D). (From Lewis, P. J., Reid, J. L., Chalmers, J. P., and Dollery, C. T., *Clin. Sci.*, 45, 1155, 1973. With permission.)

marily involve the renin-angiotensin system, whereas the late phase of renal hypertension depended on sympathetic activity.

Recently, Dargie et al.[102] reported that an increase in circulatory plasma norepinephrine levels can be demonstrated to be present in rats made hypertensive by clipping one kidney and contralateral nephrectomy.

Although the situation in renal hypertension is complicated, there seems no doubt that the autonomic nervous sytem participates in the regulation of blood pressure in this experimental model. Whether this is due to a central or a peripheral interaction of angiotensin with the autonomic nervous system, whether it reflects alterations in sodium balance, or whether it is a secondary response to the development of hypertension acting via diminished baroreceptor is unclear. It is likely that all three factors play a part in activating the autonomic nervous system in this model.

In the spontaneously hypertensive rat, it appears that the autonomic nervous system is similarly activated. Thus, Smirk[133] found that immunosympathectomy prevented the development of hypertension in the New Zealand strain of genetic hypertensive animals, while in the Japanese strain of spontaneous hypertensive rats, direct recording of the electrical activity or section of the left splanchnic sympathetic nerves of spontaneously hypertensive rats showed that peripheral sympathetic tone was markedly increased compared with that of control animals.[134] An increased norepinephrine turnover rate has been demonstrated in the heart of young spontaneously hypertensive rats.[135] On the other hand, Louis and colleagues[136] found norepinephrine turnover and synthesis rates to be decreased in the hearts of spontaneously hypertensive rats, but these experiments were made difficult to interpret by the absence of appropriately inbred control animals. It appears that as in other forms of experimental hypertension, there is evidence for the participation of the autonomic nervous system in the development of hypertension (Figure 26).

3. Autonomic Mechanisms in Human Hypertension

Perhaps the strongest evidence for participation of autonomic mechanisms in patients with hypertension is the very effective control of blood pressure which can be obtained by drugs which interfere with the autonomic nervous system. There is evidence that in human hypertension elimintion of peripheral autonomic control of blood pressure by autonomic blockade induces very much larger falls of blood pressure in hypertensive patients than in normotensive. Doyle and Smirk[137] studied the effects of

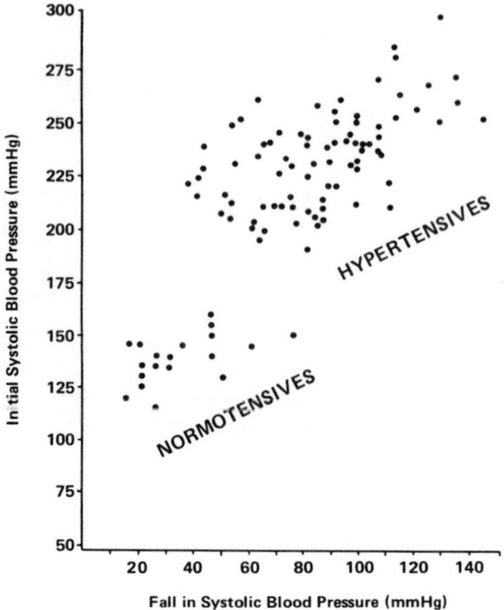

FIGURE 27. The relation between the initial level of the casual systolic blood pressure and the fall in systolic blood pressure (horizontal posture) following a "maximal" i.v. dose of hexamethonium. The results include normotensives and hypertensives. (From Doyle, A. E. and Smirk, F. H., *Circulation*, 12, 543, 1955. With permission.)

large intravenous doses of hexamethonium bromide in recumbent hypertensive and normotensive patients. The falls in blood pressure induced in hypertensive patients were on the average much larger than in normotensive (Figure 27). There was considerable variation in the extent to which the blood pressure fell between different individuals, suggesting that variation in autonomic activity might be an important component in the hypertensive process in some, but not all, hypertensive patients. The same authors noted that if the blood pressure was elevated by small doses of angiotensin infused intravenously, the effects of ganglion blockade given subsequently were substantially reduced. These observations suggested that the exaggerated falls in blood pressure induced by ganglion blockade did not merely reflect the elevated levels of blood pressure, but represented an exaggerated neurogenic component. Korner and colleagues,[138] using propranolol, atropine, phentolamine, and guanethidine, confirmed the results obtained by Doyle and Smirk[137] and further demonstrated that in hypertensive patients there was a substantial fall in total peripheral resistance (Figure 28). Both groups of workers drew attention to the fact that even after large falls of blood pressure had occurred with interruption of the peripheral autonomic nervous system, the remaining levels of blood pressure were considerably higher in hypertensive than in normotensive patients, suggesting that the whole of the rise in blood pressure could not be accounted for in most patients by autonomic factors alone. The interpretation of the excessive falls of blood pressure induced by interruption of the autonomic nervous system is difficult and is complicated by the fact that there appears to be an exaggerated response of peripheral mechanisms, including the arterioles to pressor stimuli in hypertension, so that the larger falls in blood pressure might merely reflect this increased vascular reactivity.

More direct evidence for the involvement of the autonomic nervous system in the

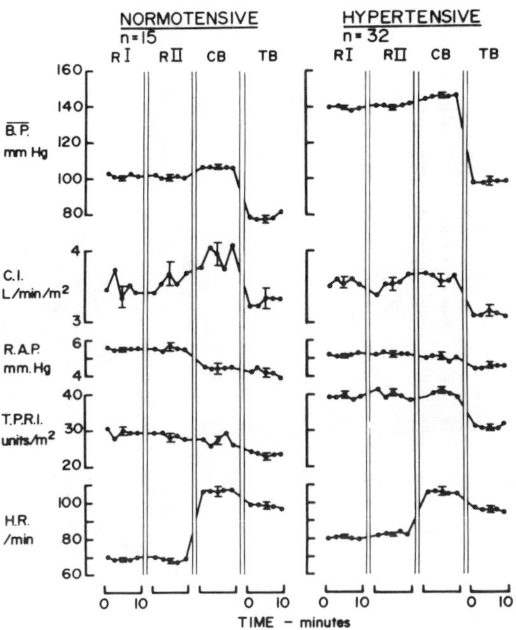

FIGURE 28. Mean values of the different circulatory variables obtained during first and second resting periods (RI and RII) and periods of 'complete' cardiac (CB) and 'total' autonomic (TB) block in 15 normotensive and 32 hypertensive subjects. $\overline{BP}$ and $\overline{RAP}$ = mean arterial and right arterial pressures; CI = cardiac index; TPRI = total peripheral resistance index; HR = heart rate. Each point is the mean of all observations of each group at that time interval. The symbol in the middle of each period is ± 1 SE, of the mean response at a single time interval, within subjects. For resting period I the standard error is calculated as SE(A) in Statistical Methods, while at other periods, it is calculated as SE(B). (From Korner, P. I., Shaw, J., Uther, J. B., West, M. J., McRitchie, R. J., and Richards, J. G., *Circulation*, 48, 107, 1973. With permission.)

maintenance of established hypertension in man has been derived from studies of catecholamines in hypertensive and normotensive patients. These studies have been facilitated by the development of sensitive radioenzymatic assays.[139] A number of authors have now reported elevations of plasma catecholamines or plasma norepinephrine in essential hypertension. Thus, Engelman et al.[140] reported increased levels of total catecholamines in peripheral circulating blood in hypertensive patients. About 75% of their patients with essential hypertension had higher than normal plasma catecholamine levels. De Quattro and Chan reported a smaller but still significant excess of plasma catecholamines over those in control subjects,[141] suggesting that about 25 to 30% of hypertensive patients had raised plasma catecholamines. de Champlain et al.[142] found an increase in plasma catecholamines in some hypertensive patients who tended to have higher blood pressures and a greater increase in heart rate in response to the erect posture (Figure 29). Using a modification of the radioenzymatic technique, Louis, Doyle, and Anavekar[143] found that although plasma epinephrine levels were normal in hypertensive patients, the plasma norepinephrine levels were significantly elevated, and the level of plasma norepinephrine in patients 3 days after admission to hospital correlated significantly with the height of the diastolic blood pressure (Figure

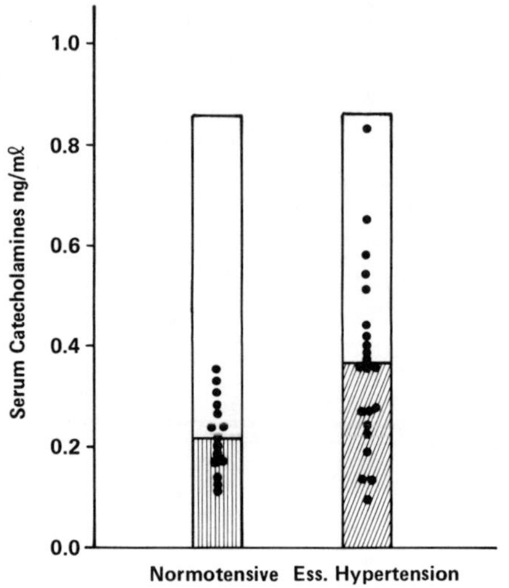

FIGURE 29.   Serum catecholamine levels in normotensive subjects and in patients with essential hypertension. The shaded area at the bottom of each rectangle represents the average level for all values in each group. (From de Champlain, J., Farley, L., Cousineau, D., and van Ameringen, M. R., *Circ. Res.*, 38, 109, 1976. With permission.)

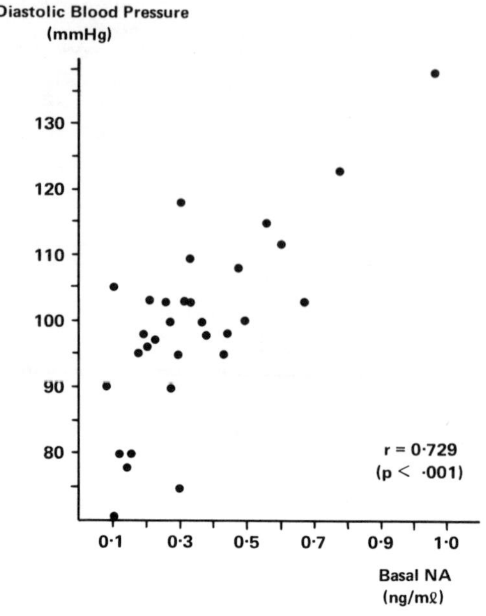

FIGURE 30.   Relation between resting diastolic blood pressure (BP) and basal plasma norepinephrine (NA) in patients with essential hypertension. (From Louis, W. J., Doyle A. E., and Anavekar, S. N., *N. Engl. J. Med.*, 288, 599, 1973. With permission.)

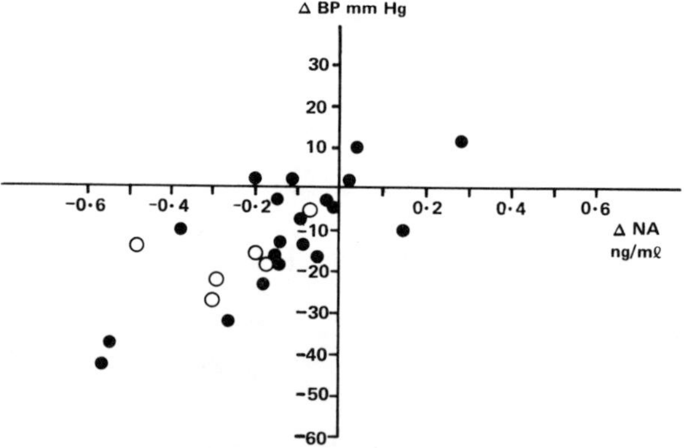

FIGURE 31.   The relationship between change in diastolic blood pressure and change in plasma norepinephrine (NA) levels (r = 0.704, p < 0.001) following the i.v. administration of pentolinium (•) or clonidine (O) in patients with essential hypertension. (From Louis, W. J., Doyle, A. E., Anavekar, S. N., and Johnston, C. I., *Hypertension, Current Problems*, Distler, A. and Wolff, H. P., Eds., Georg Thieme Verlag, Stuttgart, 1973, 269. With permission.)

30). Moreover, the subsequent administration of either pentolinium, a ganglion blocking drug, or clonidine, a centrally acting drug,[147] reduced both blood pressure and plasma catecholamines. Patients with the highest resting catecholamines had both the largest falls in blood pressure and the largest falls in plasma norepinephrine, suggesting

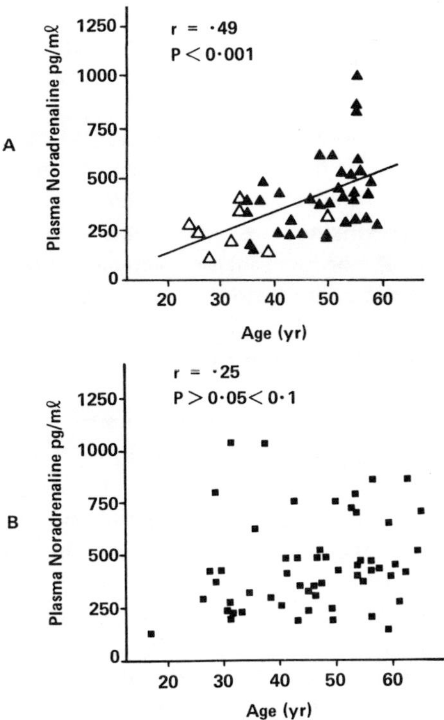

FIGURE 32. (A) P.N.A. and age: hormotensive, recumbent. (B) P.N.A. and age: hypertensive, recumbent. ▲ = civil servants; △ = other controls. Age vs. norepinephrine: civil servants, r = 0.42, p < 0.01; total controls, r = 0.49, p < 0.001. (From Sever, P. S., Birch, M., Osikowska, B., and Tunbridge, R. D. G., *Lancet,* 1, 1078, 1977. With permission.)

that the activity of the autonomic nervous system was contributing significantly to the level to which the blood pressure had risen (Figure 31).

The significance of the finding of elevated levels of norepinephrine in hypertensive patients has been disputed more recently.[144] It has been reported that plasma norepinephrine levels show a significant positive correlation with age,[144] and it has been suggested that the earlier results obtained might be due merely to the fact that the earlier authors studied older hypertensive and younger normotensive control patients. Similar findings have been reported by Ziegler et al. However, Sever et al.[144] found a significant correlation between basal norepinephrine levels with age in normotensive patients, but found that in hypertension the correlation was not present, because the younger hypertensive patients had elevated plasma norepinephrine levels (Figure 32).

Distler, Phillip, and Cordes[146] have studied the interactions between sympathetic responsiveness and blood pressure responses to norepinephrine in patients with essential hypertension. They found that in normotensive patients, there was an inverse relationship between circulating levels of norepinephrine and the sensitivity of the individual to intravenously administered norepinephrine. In hypertensive patients in whom plasma norepinephrine levels were higher, they found a similar inverse relationship, but the relationship was disturbed so that for any resting level of norepinephrine, the response to exogenously administered norepinephrine was increased. The higher the initial level of blood pressure, the greater was the shift in the relationship. Interestingly, although a similar inverse relationship could be demonstrated between plasma renin levels and the response to exogenously administered angiotensin, patients with renal hypertension and elevated levels of plasma renin did not show any evidence of altered sensitivity to angiotensin.

As has been stated previously, only a small fraction of norepinephrine released from autonomic nerve terminals finds its way into the circulation, most being either retaken up into adrenergic nerve terminals or inactivated by local enzymatic degradation. The finding of increased norepinephrine levels in the plasma of hypertensive patients might reflect an increased release of norepinephrine from adrenergic nerve terminals or might imply a diminished enzymatic degradation or decreased reuptake. Any of these mechanisms might lead to an exaggerated constrictor effect by virtue of an excessive amount of norepinephrine being available within the synaptic cleft. Geffen et al.,[148] using a radioimmunoassay, were able to measure an immunoreactive component of dopamine-β-hydroxylase in the plasma of hypertensive patients and showed that a significant relationship existed between the amounts of dopamine-β-hydroxylase measured by radioimmunoassay and the plasma levels of norepinephrine in patients with essential hypertension. This observation strongly suggests that the raised levels of plasma norepinephrine found in hypertensive patients are due to increased release of the neurotransmitter rather than to disturbances in reuptake or enzymatic degradation. A number of other workers using enzymatic methods for measuring dopamine-β-hydroxylase have been unable to confirm these findings,[149,150] perhaps because of the very considerable variation which exists among different individuals in the levels of the active enzyme in the circulation.[151] It seems very likely that the findings of Geffen et al. can be explained by the fact that an immunoreactive fragment of released dopamine-β-hydroxylase fortuitously gives an indication of release of this substance, whereas the enzymatic methods do not.

The findings of Distler et al.[146] also suggest that elevated norepinephrine levels are likely to be due to increased release rather than to increased enzymatic degradation or reduced uptake, for under either of these circumstances, exogenously administered norepinephrine should give larger pressor responses in those with the higher endogenous norepinephrine levels. The fact that lower responses were found would suggest that the exogenously administered norepinephrine was competing for receptor sites at the postjunctional receptor, with an increased local pool of norepinephrine due to increased release.

The finding of exaggerated falls in blood pressure following interference with peripheral autonomic mechanisms, coupled with the elevation of circulating levels of plasma norepinephrine in hypertensive patients, strongly suggests that in established hypertension in man, a very important component of the elevated blood pressure is maintained by autonomic mechanisms. It is interesting to note that most studies have demonstrated that plasma norepinephrine levels are higher in patients with fixed and stable hypertension than in patients with labile hypertension, suggesting that the participation of the autonomic nervous system may be as a sustaining mechanism. If this were the case, the situation would be very analogous to that found in DOCA salt in renal hypertension in rats and in the genetic or spontaneous hypertensive rat.

It seems that in hypertension, whether experimental or human, almost all methods or mechanisms of inducing hypertension involve the participation of the autonomic nervous system, either at central or at peripheral levels. In human hypertension, it is possible that in some instances the central nervous system acts as a prime initiator and that in other varieties, the autonomic nervous system assumes a sustaining role. In either event, it is clear that by the time hypertension has become established, autonomic mechanisms become important and in many patients may assume a dominant role in the maintenance of hypertension. Under these circumstances, it is perhaps not surprising that the most effective therapeutic agents for the treatment of hypertension have proved to be agents which interfere either with central or with peripheral autonomic activity.

II. ANTIHYPERTENSIVE DRUGS AFFECTING THE AUTONOMIC NERVOUS SYSTEM

A. Introduction

The great majority of effective antihypertensive drugs so far available have actions which interfere with the function of the autonomic nervous system, either at central or peripheral levels and in many instances, at both. The section that follows gives a brief account of the pharmacology and clinical pharmocology of individual drugs and their analogues. Although the section is divided broadly into centrally acting and peripherally acting drugs, in some instances, as for example with methyldopa and perhaps the β-adrenergic blocking agents, both mechanisms may be involved. The order in which these agents are dealt with does not reflect their value in therapeutics.

Elucidation of the action of the antihypertensive drugs has proved to be of considerable importance to the study and the understanding of the mechanisms involved both in experimental hypertension and in human hypertension. This is particularly true of the actions of clonidine, which have given a great impetus to the study of the central mechanisms of circulatory control. There are also many situations in which a supposed initial mode of action of a drug has had to be modified as a result of observations of the antihypertensive property of individual drugs in patients. For example, the mode of antihypertensive action of the β-adrenoceptor blocking drugs is still not by any means elucidated. As a further example, α-methyldopa, although initially introduced as a decarboxylase inhibitor, has since been found to have numerous effects both on the peripheral and the central autonomic nervous system, and prazosin, initially synthesized as a phosphodiesterase inhibitor, now appears to act predominantly as a peripheral α-adrenoceptor blocking agent. For these reasons, the classifications of the drugs which follow are to some extent arbitrary and may have to be modified subsequently as further information on the mode of action of these drugs becomes available.

B. Drugs Affecting the Central Autonomic System

1. Clonidine

Clonidine (Figure 33) is an imidazoline derivative originally synthesized as a nasal decongestant. It has potent α-agonistic activity, but lowers blood pressure at very low doses both in man and animals.[152] Given intravenously, clonidine induces a transient initial rise in blood pressure (Figure 34) followed by a prolonged fall in blood pressure.[153] It appears that the initial elevation in blood pressure after i.v. administration is due to a direct α-agonistic action, which induces peripheral vasoconstriction. The antihypertensive action of clonidine appears to be predominantly due to its effect on central adrenergic mechanisms.[154] Low doses of clonidine administered into the vertebral artery reduce blood pressure[155] (Figure 35) and prevent the hypertensive response to carotid occlusion. The antihypertensive action of clonidine persists in animals with midbrain section, but transsection of the brain or of the spinal cord caudal to the medulla abolishes its antihypertensive effects.[154]

It appears that the antihypertensive action of clonidine is due to a specific α-agonistic action on the inhibitory centers situated within the brain.[156]

Using superfusion studies on different medullary areas, Sinha and colleagues[159] were able to demonstrate reduction in blood pressure and bradycardia in the cat. Superfusion of the nucleus of the solitary tract with clonidine at a total dose of 3 μgm induced both a fall in blood pressure and bradycardia. The hypotensive and cardiac-slowing

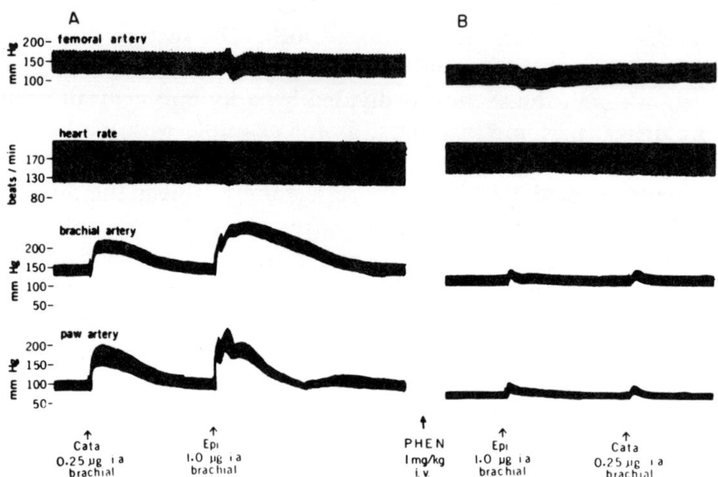

FIGURE 33.   Clonidine.

FIGURE 34.   Effect of Catapres (CATA) and epinephrine (EPI), injected into the brachial artery, on brachial and paw artery pressures in a perfused forepaw of a 10.0 kg dog before (A) and 10 min after (B) administration of phentolamine. Flow = 65 mℓ/min. (From Constantine, J. W. and McShane, W. K., *Eur. J. Pharmacol.*, 4, 109, 1968. With permission.)

effects began to appear 3 min after the commencement of clonidine superfusion and fell progressively for 90 min. Prior treatment with piperoxan in a total dose of 50 µgm antagonized this effect. Superfusion of the lateral pressor area of the reticular formation with clonidine at the same dose induced a fall in blood pressure, but only slight bradycardia. Again, the antihypertensive effect could be prevented by prior treatment with piperoxan. Superfusion of the dorsal nucleus of the vagus induced progressive bradycardia, but little, if any, hypotensive effect. The bradycardia appeared within 3 min of the commencement of the superfusion and continued for 90 min. Piperoxan superfusion also antagonized the slowing effect on the heart. These results seem to demonstrate that in the medullary region, clonidine acts on at least three sites and that the responses at each site are different. The fact that piperoxan, an α-receptor-blocking drug, antagonized all the effects of clonidine, strongly suggests that the α-agonistic action of clonidine is responsible for both the hypotensive and cardiac-slowing effects in these areas. These results confirm those of de Jong,[160] who has shown that microinjection of norepinephrine into the nucleus of the solitary tract induces hypotension and bradycardia which could be antagonized by phentolamine. The fact that clonidine appears capable of exerting its antihypertensive and bradycardiac action through the sympathoinhibitory centers in the medulla does not exclude the possibility that in intact animals or man, other sites of action within the brain may be involved. Particularly, there may be actions on the hypothalamic centers[161] and even the cerebral cortex. There is certainly evidence to suggest that the action of clonidine is widespread within the

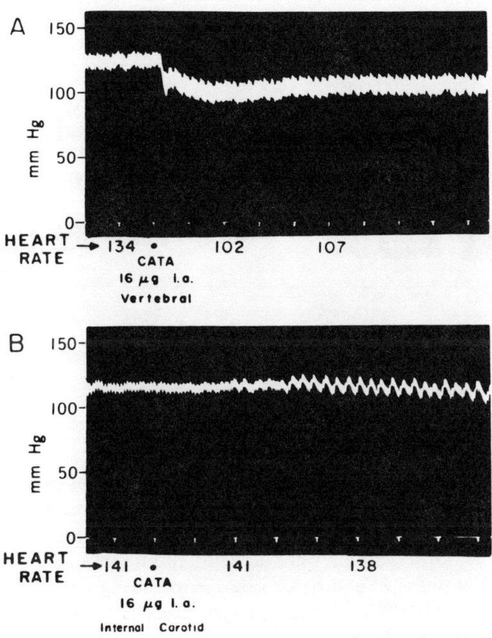

FIGURE 35. Effect of Catapres®, 16 µg, injected into the vertebral artery (A) or internal carotid artery (B), on the systemic blood pressure and heart rate of dogs, 9.9 and 9.6 kg body weight, respectively. Time marks = 1 min. (From Constantine, J. W. and McShane, W. K., *Eur. J. Pharmacol.*, 4, 109, 1968. With permission.)

brain. In the earliest animal experiments performed by Hoefke and Kobinger,[153] a sedatory effect was observed, and symptoms of sedation can be observed, not only in patients but also when the drug is given to dogs, cats, rabbits, rats, and mice. In young chicks in whom the blood-brain barrier is not fully developed, the systemic administration of clonidine induces sleep.[162] It is interesting that in these animals both norepinephrine and α-methylnorepinephrine also induces a sleep-like state,[163] presumably by passage into the brain. These effects can be inhibited by phentolamine[164] These observations suggest that clonidine has an action on the higher centers and that its effects are not confined to the medullary centers. Moreover, the inhibition of salivation, which has as its clinical manifestation the production of dry mouth, also appears to be centrally mediated. Rand, Rush, and Wilson[165] reported that parasympathetic salivary secretion stimulated by electrical impulses of the chorda tympani (Figure 36) and carbachol could not be blocked by clonidine and that conditioned salivation was inhibited by the prior administration of clonidine (Figure 37).

The antihypertensive effects of clonidine can be readily demonstrated in normal animals.[166] Clonidine also induces sharp falls in blood pressure in the conscious renal hypertensive cat and the spontaneously hypertensive rat.

Pharmacokinetic studies indicate that clonidine is well absorbed after oral administration. Peak blood levels occur in 3 to 5 hr. Approximately half of the dose of clonidine administered into man is excreted unchanged in the urine, and in patients with impaired renal function, the plasma half-life is correspondingly increased.

Clonidine appears to reduce arterial pressure by interfering with the autonomic nervous control of cardiac output and vascular resistance presumably by a central

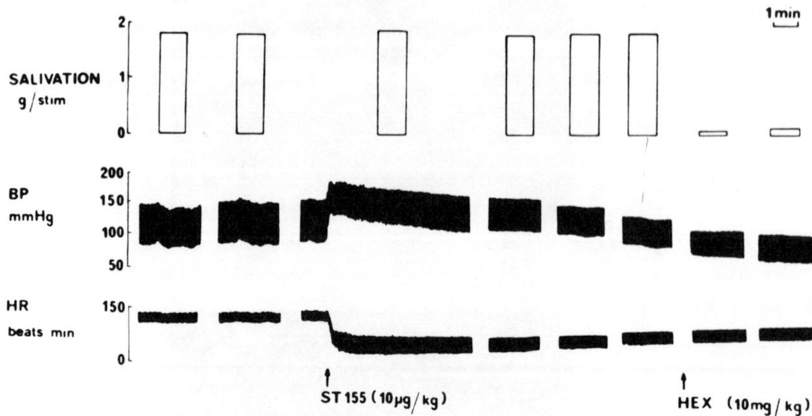

FIGURE 36.   Salivation induced by stimulating the chorda tympani in an anesthetized dog. The weight of saliva secreted from the duct of the left submaxillary gland in response to stimulation of the chorda with 1-msec pulses at 20/sec for 30 sec is indicated in the upper records. Observations were made at 10-min intervals, and corresponding sections of the blood pressure and heart rate records are given below. St 155 (10 µg/ kg) and hexamethonium (HEX 10 mg/kg) were injected intravenously at the points indicated. (From Rand, M. J., Rush, M., and Wilson, J., *Eur. J. Pharmacol.*, 5, 169, 1969. With permission.)

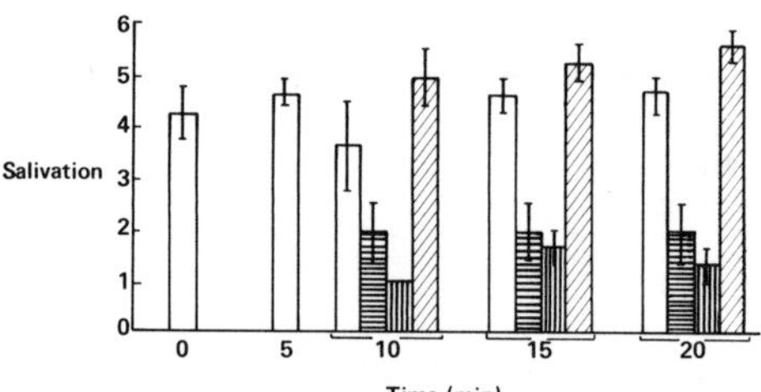

FIGURE 37.   Inhibition of conditioned salivation by St 155. The ordinate represents the degree of salivation on a rating scale. Observations were made at 5-min intervals. The mean degree of salivation in 4 experiments with each of 3 conditioned dogs is given by the heights of the columns at times 0 and 5 min. The vertical strokes represent the standard errors. Intravenous injections were given at 8 min. Thereafter, the columns represent mean degrees of salivation in each of three dogs; open columns, after saline; horizontal hatching, after 5 µg/kg of St 155; vertical hatching, after 10 µg/kg of St 155; diagonal hatching, after sufficient methohexitone to produce marked sedation (2 to 6 mg/kg). (From Rand, M. J., Rush, M., and Wilson, J., *Eur. J. Pharmacol.*, 5, 169, With permission.)

action.[166,167] There is usually a decrease in heart rate and sometimes a fall in cardiac output. There is often a fall in total peripheral resistance.[168] The fall in blood pressure is usually similar in the supine and erect postures, and the pressor responses to the Valsalva maneuver and to exercise are not abolished.[169] Given intravenously, clonidine

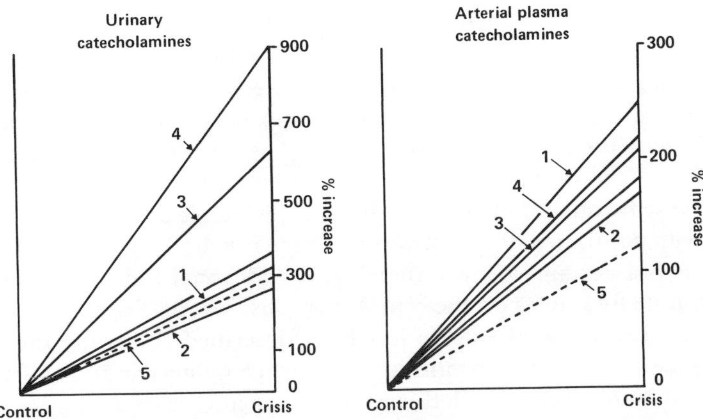

FIGURE 38. Percentage change in urinary and arterial plasma catecholamines from control (on clonidine) to crisis (rebound) period. Numbers on graph refer to individual patients. Broken line represents the reserpine-pretreated patient. Heavy line is mean of the five estimations. (From Hunyor, S. N., Hansson, L., Harrison, T. S., and Hoobler, S. W., *Br. Med. J., 2*, 209, 1973. With permission.)

induces a sharp fall in plasma catecholamines which correlates in extent with the magnitude of the fall in blood pressure.[147] Plasma renin activity and plasma renin concentration are not affected by the acute administration of clonidine,[170] but long-term administration may be associated with a fall in plasma renin activity.[171] There is usually little change in renal blood flow or glomerular filtration rate.[172]

Clonidine usually causes marked sedation and severe dryness of the mouth and eyes, both of which appear to be of central origin. An interesting and unusual phenomenon is the occurrence of sudden rebound hypertension which occurs in some patients following cessation of clonidine.[173] These patients develop headaches, insomnia, vomiting, tachycardia, tremor, and anxiety, which is accompanied by a marked rise in blood pressure and increased urinary catecholamine excretion (Figure 38). This syndrome responds to the administration either of phenoxybenzamine or phentolamine. Its mechanism of production is unknown. It is possible that it is analogous to the acute hypertensive response which develops following ablation of the nucleus of the solitary tract[24] in the rat, but there is as yet no firm evidence to support this possibility.

2. Reserpine

Reserpine is one of the alkaloids of *Rauwolfia serpentina*. Although it has been used therapeutically in Indian medicine for some centuries, it was not until 1952 that it was used in the Western world for the treatment of hypertension.[174-178] Reserpine acts at the adrenergic nerve terminal and affects both central and peripheral adrenergic nerves. It appears to act at the binding site at which norepinephrine is stored, perhaps at the granular membrane within the storage vesicles where intragranular norepinephrine is bound to ATP in a 4:1 M ratio.[179] This action appears to cause the release of bound norepinephrine. The released norepinephrine is thought to be metabolized by monoamine oxidase within the neurone, so that over a period of 24 to 48 hr after the administration of reserpine, there is a gradual decrease in the norepinephrine content of the nerve terminals. It appears that the action of reserpine on the storage granules may be irreversible and that following a single dose, full recovery may not occur for up to 14 days until newly synthesized storage granules are available.[180] Depletion of norepinephrine from the noradrenergic nerve terminals leads to a diminished response to tyramine and to other indirectly acting sympathomimetic agents and is associated with supersensitivity to the effects of exogenously administered noepinephrine.[181] In addition to causing depletion of norepinephrine, reserpine also leads to depletion of both epinephrine and 5-hydroxytryptamine in both nervous tissue and in platelets.[179]

Reserpine reduces the sympathetic responses to nerve stimulation. In large doses, it leads to flushing of the face, nasal congestion, salivation, and diarrhea. There is usually some bradycardia and a fall in blood pressure, which is of slow onset and increases progressively with continued administration. There is usually no postural fall in blood pressure.[175] It is not certain whether there is an additional central adrenergic action. There are undoubtedly effects on the central nervous system. Sedation is common and severe mental depression with suicide has been described following the use of large doses of reserpine.[182] Like the phenothiazines, reserpine may induce Parkinson's disease. This is presumably due to depletion of the basal ganglia of dopamine.

Reserpine appears to be rapidly absorbed in the gastrointestinal tract and is concentrated in adrenergic nerve tissue. There appears to be little, if any, relationship between plasma levels and antihypertensive effect. The antihypertensive effects appear, however, to be dose related.

A possible relationship between the long-term use of reserpine and an increased incidence of breast cancer has been found in three centers.[183-185] The findings suggest that the long-term treatment with reserpine increases the risk of breast cancer by between two and three times. The suggestion has been made that this may be due to increased prolactin release, but the association has not been found with methyldopa, which also stimulates prolactin release. The data linking the long-term use of reserpine with breast cancer are suggestive enough to have had the effect of inducing caution in the long-term use of reserpine, particularly in view of the fact that alternative and probably superior drugs are available.

3. α-Methyldopa

α-Methyldopa was originally introduced as an inhibitor of the enzyme DOPA decarboxylase and was initially used to reduce the synthesis of 5-hydroxytryptamine in patients with carcinoid tumors. Sjoerdsma et al.[186] showed that in such patients the administration of α-methyldopa led to increases in urinary 5-hydroxytryptophan. Subsequently, it was noted that the administration of α-methyldopa to hypertensive patients led to a reduction in blood pressure. This antihypertensive action was originally also attributed to inhibition of DOPA decarboxylase with a postulated consequent decrease in the stores of norepinephrine.[187,188] Subsequently, Carlsson and Lindqvist showed that α-methyldopa was itself converted to α-methyldopamine and subsequently to α-methylnorepinephrine, and Day and Rand[190] postulated that the hypotensive effect of α-methyldopa might be due to replacement of norepinephrine in peripheral nerves by the less potent α-methylnorepinephrine, which would act as a false transmitter. It now appears, however, that α-methylnorepinephrine is almost as potent an agonist as norepinephrine itself.[191] The most favored current hypothesis for the action of methyldopa is that it is converted within the central nervous system to α-methyldopamine and α-methylnorepinephrine and that the latter substances exert an inhibitory effect by virtue of their α-agonist actions on the inhibitory medullary centers in much the same way as do clonidine and norepinephrine itself. Heise and Kroneberg[192,193] and Heise[194] have developed a technique of perfusion of the cat cerebral ventricle. These authors were able to show that perfusion of the cat cerebral ventricles with norepinephrine and α-methylnorepinephrine produced almost identical dose-response curves for the reduction of blood pressure. The hypotensive effects of tyramine were similar. The hypotensive actions of norepinephrine and α-methylnorepinephrine were inhibited by the administration of phentolamine. Likewise, cocaine and reserpine diminished the hypotensive responses to tyramine. Heise[194] has described similar depressor effects which occur when dopamine was perfused through the cat cerebral ventricles and has also shown that the hypotensive activity of dopamine could be inhibited by haloperidol, although it was unaffected by phentolamine. Furthermore, the infusion of norepinephrine was unaffected by haloperidol, suggesting that there are both noradrenergic and dopaminergic inhibitory centers within the brain. It appeared that the optimal hypotensive activity for norepinephrine was most pronounced in the posterior part of the third and the anterior part of the fourth ventricle, whereas the dopamine response was most prominent if the distribution included the anterior part of the third ventricle. These effects did not seem to be due to local vasoconstriction, since ventricular perfusion experiments with angiotensin II resulted in a dose-dependent blood pressure rise. Rather similar results have been obtained by Finch et al., using α-methylnorepinephrine and norepinephrine[195] (Figures 39 and 40). It appears from these results that the central action of α-methyldopa may be mediated both by α-methyldopamine and α-methylnorepinephrine, both of which are present in high concentrations in the central nervous system after the administration of this drug. There may, in addition, be peripheral actions of α-methyldopa related to dopa decarboxylase inhibition and to the accumulation of α-methylnorepinephrine in peripheral autonomic nerve endings. It appears, however, that the central effects are most likely to be of importance, since peripheral decarboxylase blockade by the use of methyldopa hydrazine, which would interfere with the peripheral actions of methyldopa, does not diminish the hypotensive effect of methyldopa.[196] It is of interest that the hypotensive action of methyldopa does not appear to be enhanced by the use of methyldopa hydrazine, whereas that of l-dopa is.[197] The possibility that a peripheral action of α-methyldopa is significant in its antihypertensive effect therefore cannot be entirely excluded.

α-Methyldopa appears to be rapidly absorbed from the GI tract. Peak plasma levels of unaltered drug occur within 2 hr with a half-life of 3 to 4 hr and approximately half of the oral dose appears to be absorbed.[198] There appears to be considerable individual variation in absorption rate between different people. α-Methyldopa is predominantly excreted in the urine either unchanged or as α-methyldopamine. Patients with impaired renal function require lower doses.

Blood pressure usually begins to fall within 2 to 3 hr after an effective dose of α-methyldopa, and some persistent antihypertensive action is usually demonstrable for up to 12 to 24 hr.[198] There is usually an acute small fall in cardiac output, but the major changes are a reduction in peripheral resistance.[199] Long-term studies by Lund-Johansen[200] have revealed that the predominant change following α-methyldopa is a fall in total peripheral resistance with little alteration in cardiac output. There is often a small fall in plasma renin activity following effective antihypertensive treatment.

In small doses, methyldopa usually induces little orthostatic hypotension, and the falls in blood pressure occur equally with the patient lying and standing. Many patients only require small doses, but a few need considerably larger doses, and in these patients some orthostatic hypotension is usually present. There is no ready explanation for the differences in sensitivity to methyldopa. It may be that in some patients small doses, affecting mainly central mechanisms, are effective, while in a minority, doses large enough to interfere in some way with peripheral adrenergic mechanisms are needed. The mechanism of any peripheral actions are not yet clear. In particular, the relative affinities of α-methylnorepinephrine for the presynaptic and postsynaptic receptors have not been reported, but such changes in affinity might offer an explanation for a peripheral action of α-methyldopa.

Methyldopa is well tolerated by most patients, although complaints of drowsiness

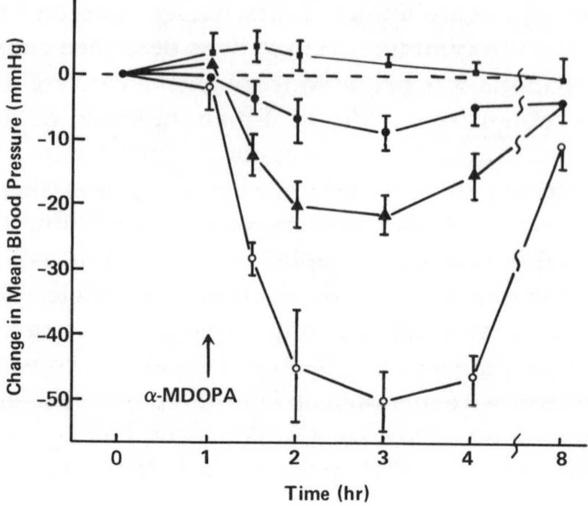

FIGURE 39.   Effect of intraventricular administration of α-methyldopa, 3 mg (O); tolazoline i.c.v., 200 μg (□); tolazoline, 200 μg given 60 min before α-methyldopa, 3 mg (●); tolazoline i.c.v., 75 μg given 60 min before α-methyldopa, 3 mg (▲) on the resting blood pressure of conscious renal hypertensive cats. Each point represents the mean; vertical bars indicate S.E. mean; n = 6 for all groups. (From Finch, L., Hersom, A., and Hicks, P., *Recent Advances in Hypertension,* Milliez, P. and Safar, M., Eds., Boehringer Ingelheim, Reims, 1975, 73. With permission.)

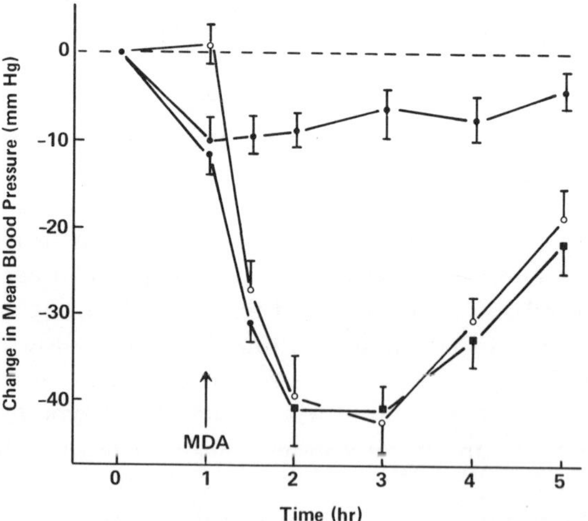

FIGURE 40.   Effect of intraventricular α-methyldopamine, 0.5 mg (O); flupenthixol, 1 mg/kg i.p. (●); flupenthixol, 1 mg/kg i.p. 60 min before intraventricular α-methyldopamine, 0.5 mg (□) on the resting blood pressures of conscious renal hypertensive cats. Each point represents the mean; vertical bars indicate S. E. mean; n = 6 for all groups. (From Finch, L., Hersom, A., and Hicks, P., *Recent Advances in Hypertension,* Milliez, P. and Safar, M., Eds., Boehringer Ingelheim, Reims, 1975, 73. With permission.)

are common. Fluid retention and weight gain may occur, leading to the syndrome of false tolerance, which can usually be overcome by the concomitant administration of a diuretic.

4. Diazepam

It has been reported that diazepam and other benzodiazepines inhibit pressor responses obtained by stimulation of the hypothalamus. The reduction of cardiovascular responses seems to be due to a centrally mediated reduction in evoked efferent sympathetic activity, with little or no effect on peripheral sympathetic structures.[201,202] It was further reported that medullary pressor responses were less inhibited than induced hypothalamic responses. Stimulation of the posterior hypothalamus causes hypertension and tachycardia in cats, and diazepam, which had only a slight effect on resting blood pressure and heart rate, caused progressive inhibition of responses to this stimulation.[203] In the same animals, diazepam produced little effect on the responses to bilateral carotid artery occlusion. No effects of diazepam could be found when the paramedial reticular formation was stimulated. It seems from these studies that diazepam has no action on medullary centers. The authors suggested that the benzodiazepines had no significant antihypertensive activity per se, but rather that they reduced evoked cardiovascular responses from supramedullary sites without significantly affecting tonic sympathetic outflow. They suggested that they might be effective in preventing stress-induced rises in blood pressure which may lead to sustained hypertension. In spite of these suggestions, diazepam has not been shown to inhibit the development of hypertension in the spontaneously hypertensive rat.

5. Recently Developed Drugs

There are a number of newer drugs, apparently with actions on the central nervous system. Although in some instances the pharmacological studies which have been reported have been fairly extensive, few have been extensively studied clinically as yet. They are included in this section in the anticipation that some of them may prove in the future to be clinically significant.

a. BS 100-141 (Sandoz Laboratories) (Figure 41)

This substance is N-amidino-2-(2,6-dichlorophenyl) acetamide hydrochloride. The drug has close structural and pharmacological similarities to clonidine, being an α-agonist which when injected intravenously produces short dose-dependent pressor responses, which can be blocked by pretreatment with phentolamine, but not by pretreatment with reserpine. Infusions of the drug into the vertebral artery and intracerebroventricular injection caused reduction of blood pressure, which could be prevented by phentolamine. The fall in blood pressure was accompanied by bradycardia and by reduction in peripheral sympathetic nerve activity.

There is some evidence that the site of action of this drug within the brain may be different from that of clonidine. Topical application of clonidine to the ventral surface of the medulla produces large falls of blood pressure, whereas the topical application of BS 100-141 (at the same site) was ineffective. It is also claimed that BS 100-141 produces less sedation in conscious animals than does clonidine.[204]

Clinical studies have been undertaken in a small number of patients. The drug seems to be as effective as clonidine in reducing blood pressure, and it is claimed that it induces much less sedation than clonidine. It appears to produce inhibition of salivation to about the same degree as clonidine.

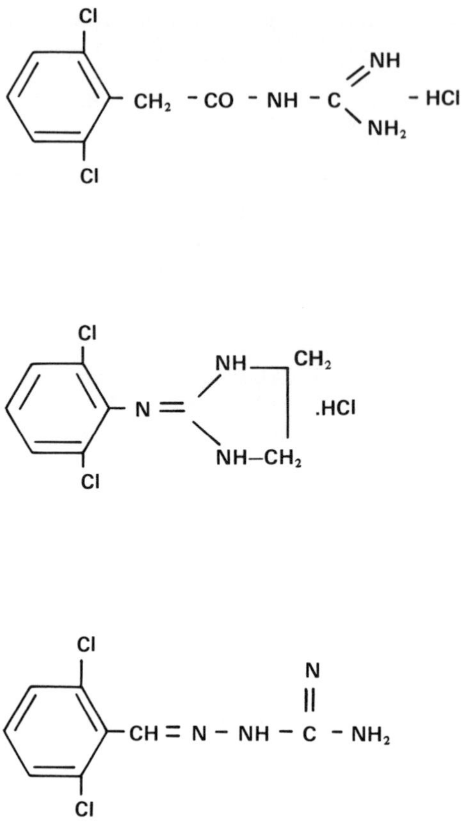

FIGURE 41.

b. Indoramin (Wyeth Laboratories)

Indoramin is (3-(2-(4-benzamidopiperid-1-yl)ethyl indole acetate. It has been shown to reduce blood pressure in both normotensive and hypertensive man[205-207] and animals. It is not entirely clear at present whether the predominant blood pressure-lowering activity is due to central or peripheral mechanisms. The compound possesses α-receptor blocking activity in isolated organ preparations and reduces the pressor response to epinephrine, but not norepinephrine, and intra-arterial administration leads to vasodilatation. However, it has been reported that the fall in blood pressure which follows systemic administration was associated with a fall in heart rate and efferent sympathetic nerve activity at higher doses, but not with lower doses. Indoramin had no effect on carotid sinus nerve activity.

Initial clinical trials have demonstrated that in a dose of 200 mg, indoramin induces a hypotensive effect on the response to exercise and also induces slowing of heart rate, both at rest and during exercise. It reduced the pressor effects of intravenously administered norepinephrine. Given chronically by oral administration for 4 weeks, there was an initial fall in both supine and erect diastolic pressure, which diminished with continued administration. The mode of action of this compound is not yet firmly established.

c. Guanbenz (Wyeth Laboratories)

Guanbenz is 2-6-dichlorobenzylidene amino guanidine acetate (Figure 41). It bears some structural similarity both to clonidine and to guanethidine and has been claimed to possess both a central action in reducing sympathetic outflow and a peripheral adrenergic blocking action. Experimental studies have shown that guanbenz at a dose of 1 µg/kg reduces both spontaneous peripheral sympathetic nerve activity and also that which follows stimulation of the posterior hypothalamus in the cat. However, at lower doses, it appeared to enhance both the peripheral sympathetic nerve activity and the pressor response to posterior hypothalamic stimulation.[208]

A clinical trial with guanbenz has been reported,[209] using a double-blind cross-over study against placebo. In doses of 16 mg daily, guanbenz produced only a small fall in diastolic pressure (6 to 9 mmHg). Eight patients noted marked sleepiness, and one, tremor. In two patients, the guanbenz was discontinued because of side effects. These preliminary results are not encouraging. It seems unlikely that this drug will prove useful clinically.

C. Drugs Affecting the Peripheral Autonomic System

1. Ganglion-Blocking Drugs

Transmission within the autonomic ganglia is effected by acetylcholine, and most of the drugs which block ganglionic transmission appear to do so by competitive inhibition of acetylcholine. The ability of tetraethyl ammonium to block the effect of ganglionic stimulation has been known for many years, but this drug had such a brief action and was so poorly absorbed in the GI tract that little clinical interest developed in the substance. In 1959, Paton and Zaimis described the pharmacological actions of the *bis*-trimethyl ammonium salts, and soon after this the C5,6 members of the series, pentamethonium and hexamethonium, were used in the treatment of severe hypertension. The ganglion-blocking drugs block transmission in both parasympathetic and sympathetic ganglia, and the degree of blockade is dose dependent. Importantly, the duration of ganglion blockade is also dose dependent, so that small doses induce partial and transient blockade, whereas large doses induce more profound interruption of ganglionic transmission, which persists for much longer. Alimentary absorption of the quaternary ammonium compounds is incomplete and variable, so that many of these agents needed to be given by injection, either intramuscularly or subcutaneously. In the majority of patients, the ratio of the oral and the i.v. LD_{50} of the quaternary ammonium ganglion-blocking drugs is about 20:1. The secondary amines, mecamylamine and pempidine, are much better absorbed, giving an oral to i.v. LD_{50} ratio of about 4:1.[211] The drugs are excreted predominantly by renal elimination. The excretion of mecamylamine is inhibited by the concurrent administration of benthodiazine diuretics or by acetazolamide and is enhanced by acidification of the urine.

Ganglion-blocking drugs produce impairment of sympathetic control of both arteries and veins, with a result that orthostatic hypotension is an intrinsic part of the action of the drugs. Cardiac output is usually somewhat reduced. The magnitude of the fall in blood pressure which occurs in the recumbent position is very variable from one patient to the next. In some patients, small doses of ganglion-blocking drugs induce substantial falls in blood pressure in both the recumbent and erect positions, whereas in other patients, even large doses fail to reduce the recumbent blood pressure to any important extent, and the main fall of blood pressure occurs on the assumption of the erect posture. It seems likely that these variations in response relate to the extent of the activity of the autonomic nervous system, for factors such as fever, hypovolemia, sodium depletion, hemorrhage, and the concurrent administration of diuretic agents all enhance the response to these drugs, whereas fluid retention reduces their effects. This latter fact is of significance in inducing tolerance to these drugs, since they usually induce a fall in renal blood flow and sodium excretion and often lead to marked fluid retention. Cerebral and coronary blood flow are usually not greatly affected unless the blood pressure falls excessively, when fainting or ischemic myocardial pain may develop. True pharmacological tolerance to the effects of ganglion-blocking drugs also occurs in that repeated administration of the same dose elicits smaller and smaller responses. This can be demonstrated, for example, in the nictitating membrane of the cat in which the effects of stimulation of the preganglionic nerve are abolished by ganglion blockade.[210] There is often some degree of cross-tolerance between different members of the species. There appears to be less true tolerance to the secondary amine ganglion-blocking drugs than to the quaternary amine type.[211]

The major disadvantage from a clinical point of view is the capacity of the ganglion-blocking drugs to block parasympathetic nerve ganglionic transmission. This induces a reduction in GI motility and interference with both salivary and gastric secretion. Bladder tone is reduced, which may produce retention of urine, and impotence is common in men. Like the effects on the cardiovascular system, the effects on the parasympathetic system are dose related, and the extent of the severity of the parasympathetic blockade depends very much on the sensitivity of the patient to the cardiovascular effects. Patients who achieve large falls of blood pressure with small doses commonly experience little parasympathetic blockade, whereas those patients who require large doses have correspondingly increased parasympathetic effects.

2. Adrenergic Neurone Blocking Drugs

The major drugs of this type which are used in the treatment of hypertension are guanethidine, bethanidine, and desbrisoquine. All of these drugs owe their antihypertensive action to inhibition of the function of the postganglionic sympathetic neurone. All are actively transported into norepinephrine storage granules by the same mechanism which transports catecholamines.[212] During the uptake process, some norepinephrine is released. The major action of guanethidine appears to be the prevention of release of norepinephrine on nerve stimulation. It also prevents the uptake of norepinephrine in a manner similar to that of cocaine. For these reasons, these drugs act on the sympathetic nervous system and not on the parasympathetic. The drugs do not penetrate the brain readily, and their actions appear to be confined to the peripheral autonomic nervous system. When given intravenously in large doses, sufficient norepinephrine may be released to induce a transient pressor reaction, but with oral administration, the release is usually too slow for any physiological effects to be noted. Once taken up by the adrenergic neurone, guanethidine is released slowly, and the effects of a single dose persist for several days. Bethanidine and debrisoquine are released more rapidly and have a much less prolonged action than guanethidine. By virtue of their peripheral sympathetic blocking action, these drugs induce peripheral vasodilatation and venodilatation.Like the ganglion-blocking drugs, the degree of the antihypertensive effect is very variable, some patients having quite marked falls in blood pressure in the recumbent posture with small doses, whereas other patients appear resistant, and the major effect is postural. There is usually some decrease in cardiac output in the standing position. The blood pressure is also decreased during exercise. There is often a fall in glomerular filtration rate and renal blood flow, and these drugs, like the ganglion-blocking drugs, often lead to marked fluid retention, which may lead to false tolerance.

Because they have no effect on parasympathetic activity, there is usually a relative increase in parasympathetic as opposed to sympathetic function, so that there is increased GI motility, usually leading to diarrhea, and there is marked impairment of ejaculation in the male secondary to sympathetic impairment. In rats, guanethidine in prolonged large doses leads to dilatation of the vas deferens.[213] An analogue of guanethidine, guanacline,[214] has been shown to produce persistent postural hypotension in some individuals. Prolonged administration of this drug to rats leads to degeneration of autonomic nerve terminals, with a deposition of heavy deposits of fluorescent material. This syndrome has not yet been described with the other drugs in this class.

Guanethidine is mainly excreted via the kidneys following i.v. administration. About half the dose of guanethidine is excreted rapidly, but continuing excretion occurs for periods up to 10 days. Bethanidine and desbrisoquine have a more rapid onset of action and shorter duration, presumably due to a less firm attachment to the storage vesicles in the peripheral autonomic nervous system.

The actions of guanethidine are blocked by the tricyclic antidepressant drugs such as imipramine and amitriptyline.[212] These block the uptake of guanethidine into the nerve ending and can prevent or reverse the action of the drug. Phenothiazines also interfere with the uptake. Guanethidine, bethanidine, and debrisoquine all lead to supersensitivity to norepinephrine, but not to the indirectly acting sympathomimetic drugs such as tyramine and ephedrine. The administration of adrenergic blocking drugs to patients with pheochromocytoma may lead to markedly exaggerated rises in blood pressure.

3. Monoamine Oxidase Inhibitors

These drugs are used predominantly as antidepressants, but pargyline (*n*-benzyl-*n*-methyl 2 propynylamine) has a significant antihypertensive action. Although there is no doubt that this drug is capable of inhibiting the actions of monoamine oxidase within the sympathetic neurone, the mechanism by which it induces its hypotensive effect is far from clear. It does not appear to reduce release of norepinephrine during nerve stimulation. Inhibition of monoamine oxidase allows the accumulation of octopamine and dopamine, and it has been suggested that by incorporation of these substances with adrenergic stores, they could act as weak false transmitters.[215]

Pargyline has clinical effects similar to the adrenergic blocking drugs, but is slower in onset. Postural hypotension is common. This drug is seldom used in clinical practice.

4. α-Adrenergic Blocking Agents

a. Phenoxybenzamine

Phenoxybenzamine is a potent α-adrenoceptor antagonist which blocks both prejunctional and postjunctional α-receptors. It also blocks the reuptake of norepinephrine following its release into the synaptic cleft. It is capable of blocking the α-agonist effects of infused norepinephrine and epinephrine and for this reason is useful in the treatment of patients with pheochromocytoma who have elevated circulatory levels of catecholamines. Its effectiveness in patients with hypertension, other than those with pheochromocytoma, is very limited. The falls induced in blood pressure are small and inconstant and are associated with a marked tachycardia, elevation of plasma renin activity, and often postural falls in blood pressure. Rand et al.[46] suggested that the reason that phenoxybenzamine and other α-adrenoceptor antagonists have been so unsuccessful in hypertension is a consequence of the fact that they block prejunctional as well as postsynaptic α-receptors. The loss of this important feedback inhibitory loop whereby norepinephrine regulates its own release by a negative feedback mechanism would lead to an increased release of norepinephrine, and there is evidence that the administration of phenoxybenzamine is associated with an increase in plasma catecholamines and urinary catecholamine excretion.

Phenoxybenzamine suffers from the same disadvantages as most of the vasodilator drugs, namely, that it induces sodium retention, tachycardia, and a rise in plasma renin levels. Its use in hypertension is now confined to patients with pheochromocytoma.

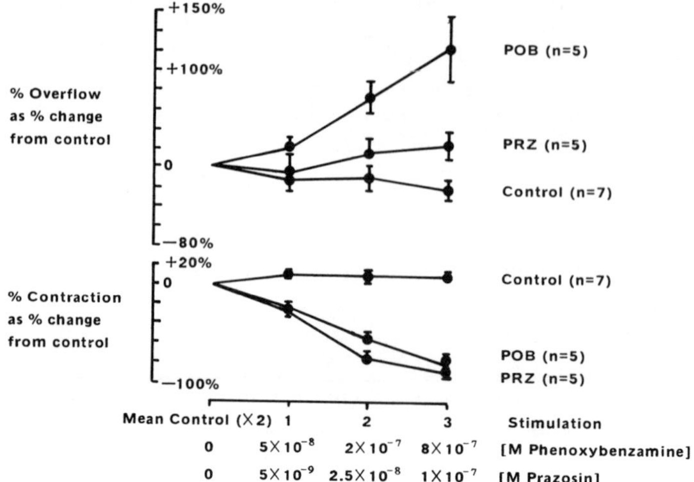

FIGURE 42.   Effect of prazosin and phenoxybenzamine on contraction and ^{3}H-norepinephrine overflow in rabbit pulmonary artery. (From Cambridge, D., Davey, M. J., and Massingham, R., *Med. J. Aust.*, (Suppl. 2), 2, 2, 1977. With permission.)

b. Prazosin

This interesting compound was synthesized in the belief that effective inhibitors of phosphodiesterase would be likely to be potent vasodilating agents by an action on vascular smooth muscle. Initial pharmacological studies suggested that prazosin was a powerful phosphodiesterase inhibitor and that it acted predominantly on vascular smooth muscle.[216] Radioactive prazosin was shown to localize to blood vessel walls. The mode of action of prazosin has recently been reassessed, and it is now claimed[217,218] that the major action of prazosin is as an α-adrenoceptor-blocking drug with a specific effect on postjunctional receptors and no affinity for the presynaptic α-receptors. This is based on the fact that it appears to reverse the pressor effect of intravenously administered norepinephrine, being approximately ten times more potent on a molar basis than phentolamine in this respect.

Responsiveness to angiotensin II, 5-hydroxytryptamine, and vasopressin is said to be unimpaired.[218] The affinity of prazosin and phenoxybenzamine for presynaptic receptors was estimated by measuring the stimulation-induced overflow of tritiated norepinephrine. Whereas phenoxybenzamine markedly increased the outflow of tritiated norepinephrine during nerve stimulation, prazosin had no effect on this (Figure 42). Both drugs appeared to block postsynaptic α-adrenoceptors as judged by measurements of the effects on muscle contraction induced by nerve stimulation in rabbit pulmonary artery preparations. This apparently unique specificity for postsynaptic receptors is the first demonstration that the structure of the two receptors differs.[217] Prazosin produces no rise in plasma renin levels and appears, in fact, to produce a small fall in plasma renin activity, both in dogs and in man.[219] It has not been noted to evoke the expected baroreceptor-mediated compensatory rise in cardiac output, and there is usually little, of any, tachycardia following its oral administration. Both the failure of plasma renin levels to rise and the absence of tachycardia are attributed to the selective affinity of prazosin for postjunctional receptors.

Doubt has been cast as to whether prazosin has any direct vasodilating action. Simpson[220] reported that in the perfused hind limb of the rat, prazosin only reduced perfusion pressure when the limb was innervated and had no effect in denervated limbs

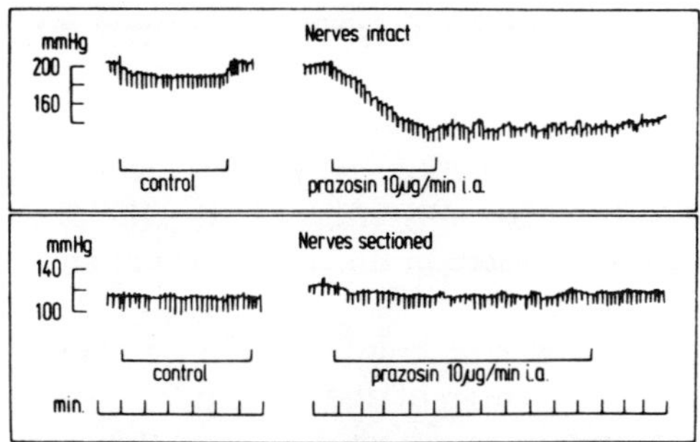

FIGURE 43. Perfusion pressure in hind limb of genetically hypertensive rat, perfused with the rat's own blood at constant rate. Prazosin added to perfusing blood. Upper trace: nerves to limb intact. Lower trace: nerves to limb sectioned. (From Simpson, F. O., *Med. J. Aust.* (Suppl. 2), 7, 1977. With permission.)

(Figure 43), whereas sodium nitroprusside induced a substantial fall in perfusion pressure in the denervated limbs.

Distribution studies indicate that the drug is taken up rapidly in tissues and disappears from the plasma, with a half-life of approximately 3 to 4 hr. Prazosin is rapidly transformed, mainly by acetylation and glucuronidase formation, and 90% of the dose is eliminated by the fecal route. Although the mean plasma half-life is between 3 and 4 hr, the antihypertensive action persists considerably longer.[216] The drug appears to induce falls of blood pressure in both the recumbent and erect postures without, as a rule, much compensatory tachycardia. It is claimed that it dilates veins as well as arteries. A number of controlled clinical studies have been performed, all of which suggest that there is only a slightly greater fall in blood pressure in the standing position than in the supine.[221] The majority of studies have suggested that between 60 and 70% of patients obtain useful falls in blood pressure. The antihypertensive effects of prazosin are enhanced by coincident diuretic therapy.[218]

The major adverse reaction to prazosin appears to be the rather frequent occurrence of what has been called the "first dose phenomenon".[222] There are now many reports of an acute syndrome, the features of which are transient faintness, dizziness, and palpitations occurring almost immediately after the initial dose of prazosin or as a response to an increase in dose. It appears that this syndrome is usually due to postural hypotension which is exaggerated after exercise and which may be due to dilatation of the veins. Its occurrence seems to be related, in part, to the dosage used, it being less common with initial doses of 0.5 mg than with doses of 2 mg. Stokes[222] has claimed that it is related also to dietary sodium intake and is enhanced by diuretic therapy.

Although prazosin seldom induces reflex cardiac effects, an increase in the frequency or severity of anginal attacks has been observed in some patients. An interaction between prazosin and trinitrin leading to syncope has also been reported. A few patients experience persistent postural hypotension and tachycardia, but these appear to be in the minority. In a small number of patients, fluid retention, headache, and nasal congestion have been reported. There usually appears to be little interference with male sexual function.

III. β-ADRENOCEPTOR-BLOCKING DRUGS

A. Introduction

Cellular receptors are those structures which by virtue of their chemical structure and shape bind biologically active substances to alter the physiological process of the cell. In general, receptors are present in finite numbers in any given cell and bind small quantities of ligands with both chemical specificity and high affinity in a reversible and saturable manner. The order of binding affinities between ligands and receptors parallels the biological effectiveness of the ligand. The β-adrenoceptor is classically defined as that receptor present on effector cells of the sympathetic nervous system which responds better to 1-isoproterenol than either 1-epinephrine or 1-norepinephrine.

The diverse physiological responses associated with β-adrenoceptor stimulation are well defined, as are the intracellular biochemical events which correlate with these responses. The membrane events however, which translate receptor occupation to the generation of an intracellular biochemical signal are not well understood.

In 1948, Ahlquist[223] investigated the ability of a series of catecholamines to produce inhibitory or excitatory responses in a range of tissues and found that the order of potency of these compounds was characteristic in all tissues examined, depending on whether an excitatory or inhibitory response was generated. He therefore postulated the existence of two separate classes of adrenoceptor, namely, α-receptors, which are activated best by norepinephrine and least effectively by isoproterenol to produce generally excitatory responses, and β-receptors, which were markedly activated by the synthetic catecholamine, isoproterenol, and only moderately stimulated by the naturally occurring catecholamines, epinephrine and norepinephrine, to produce generally inhibitory responses.

In 1946, von Euler[224] demonstrated that norepinephrine was the neurotransmitter released locally at the sympathetic neuroeffector junction and that epinephrine was confined primarily to the adrenal medulla, which released this compound into the general circulation.

In 1957, Sutherland and Rall[225] isolated a heat-stable factor which was produced from ATP by the action of glucagon and epinephrine in liver homogenates. This factor was identified as adenosine cyclic 3′,5′-monophosphate. It has subsequently been identified in a wide variety of biological tissues. In mammalian tissues and cells, hormone-dependent elevations of cyclic AMP were found to correlate with the time and concentration of specific hormones producing specific responses. Moreover, it could be demonstrated that exogenously added cyclic AMP or dibutyryl cyclic AMP (a less easily hydrolyzed analogue) mimicked the physiological response elicited by the hormone. In 1965, Sutherland and associates [226] proposed the second messenger hypothesis in which cyclic AMP functions as an intracellular mediator for catecholamines and a number of polypeptide hormones. The latter react specifically with the cell membrane at receptor sites, but do not enter the cell. Once the appropriate response has been mediated, intracellular cyclic AMP is converted by phosphodiesterase to the inactive 5′-AMP.[227]

The enzyme, adenylate cyclase, which is present on the plasma membrane of cells, is thought to be responsible for the synthesis of cyclic AMP from ATP. Assays for this enzyme in membrane preparations indicate that adenylate cyclase is stimulated by a wide variety of agents including peptide hormones and catecholamines. Isoproterenol is a potent stimulator of the enzyme in a wide variety of tissues such as cardiac muscle, liver, fat cells, and bronchial and uterine smooth muscle. β-Antagonists, but not α-antagonists, specifically inhibit isoproterenol-induced enzyme activity.

In 1958, Powell and Slater[228] classified the pharmacological properties of dichloro-isoproterenol as being due to a β-receptor-blocking action in terms of Ahlquist's hypothesis. Since that time, a large number of β-adrenoceptor-blocking drugs have been synthesized and their clinical use in angina and hypertension has become very widespread. The present section attempts to classify these drugs on the basis of their various properties and provide a pharmacological background to the understanding of their clinical use.

B. Pharmacology

1. β-Blockade

β-Adrenoceptor-blocking drugs reduce or abolish β-adrenoceptor stimulation, regardless of whether it is due to catecholamines released from sympathetic nerve endings, the adrenal medulla, or injected sympathomimetic agents. It appears that most β-blocking drugs block the effects of endogenous or exogenous catecholamines equally well. Chemically, the β-adrenoceptor-blocking drugs are closely related to the synthetic catecholamine isoproterenol with which they have the hydroxyethylamino group in common (Figure 44).

This class of drugs appears to have a very high degree of specificity for the receptor. Thus, while they block the positive inotropic and positive chronotropic effects of catecholamines on the heart, they do not inhibit the cardiac-stimulating effects of calcium, digitalis glycosides, or theophylline. Furthermore, in general they have little or no effect on responses to α-adrenoceptor stimulation. Likewise, although they can abolish the vasodilatation in response to isoproterenol, the response to acetylcholine is not affected. These compounds are competitive antagonists, which means that they combine reversibly with the receptor and can be displaced by increasing the concentration of the agonist. Put in another way, they shift the dose-response curve to the right without affecting either the slope of the curve or the height of the maximum response (Figure 45). The extent to which individual drugs possess potency in competitive antagonism varies considerably from one agent to the next. The potency of β-blocking drugs is usually assessed in experimental animals by calculating the dose necessary to inhibit a response to a β-adrenergic stimulant such as isoproterenol. This usually has to be done by making a comparison between the drug under investigation and a reference compound, usually propranolol. Potencies may be expressed in relation to such responses as the inhibition of increase in heart rate in response to isoproterenol or may be studied in isolated tissue preparations, which have the advantage that many of the complicating factors such as the pharmacodynamic and pharmacokinetic effects which are encountered in intact animals are not important. Potency is sometimes expressed in terms of PA_2.[229] This value is the negative logarithm of the concentration of antagonist which just doubles the amount of agonist required to achieve a given effect.

Drugs which interact with β-adrenoceptors either to stimulate or to block show structural similarities. The side chain of the antagonist is similar or identical to the agonist isoproterenol, and it is presumably the side chain with an isopropyl or tertiary butyl substituted secondary amine which determines interaction with β-adrenoceptors. The asymmetric carbon atom gives rise to two optically active isomers, and as with the catecholamines, the l-isomer of an antagonist has greater activity than the d-isomer.

Whether the effect of a compound will be to mainly induce activation or blockade depends on the nature of the substitutes on the aromatic ring. Hydroxyl groups in the 3-4 positions of the aromatic ring are optimal for stimulating activity. β-Blocking potency is increased by the insertion of a methylene-oxy bridge (O-CH$_2$) between the aromatic ring and the asymmetric carbon atom and is found in most β-blocking drugs which have been recently synthesized (see Figure 44).

Selective blockade of only a few of the pharmacological effects of β-adrenoceptors can be achieved by specific structural alterations. A number of compounds have a

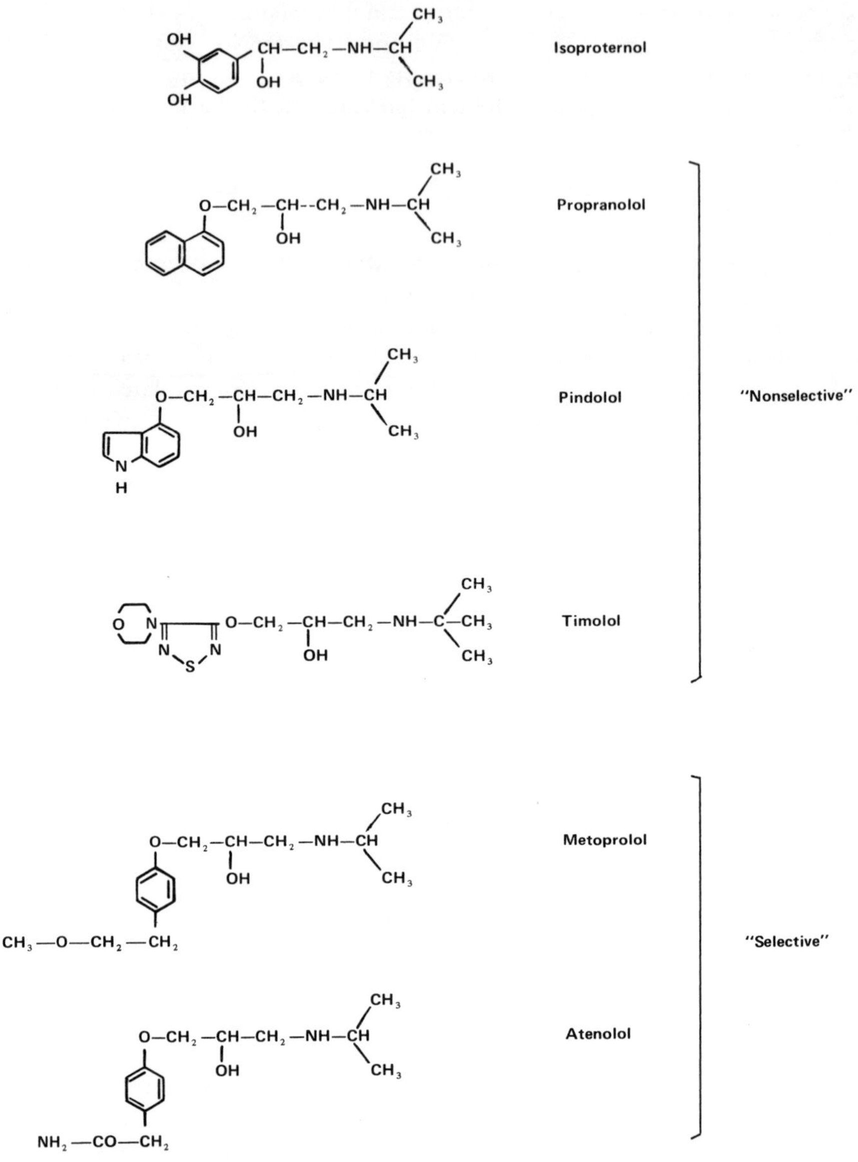

FIGURE 44.   Structural relationship of various β-adrenoceptor-blocking drugs to Isoproterenol.

greater affinity for cardiac receptors than for those in other smooth muscle tissues such as the bronchial smooth muscle. Most of these compounds have a substituent group in the para position of the aromatic ring, whereas similar substitution in the meta and ortho positions leads to a loss of selectivity.[230] This is consistent with the work of Lands and colleagues,[231,232] who suggested that β-adrenoceptors could be divided into two distinct groups, namely, those concerned in cardiac stimulation and intestinal relaxation (β_1) and those concerned in smooth muscle relaxation in the trachea and blood vessels (β_2). It seems probable that this is an oversimplification, and it has been suggested that there may be three or more types of β-adrenoceptors.[233] Whether this proves to be so or not will depend on further study, but it appears to be

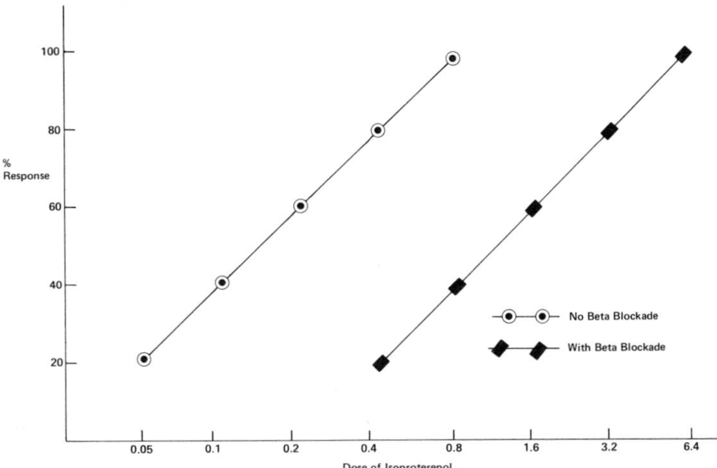

FIGURE 45.   Diagram to illustrate the competitive inhibitory effect of β-adrenoceptor blockade. In the presence of blockade, any given response requires a larger dose of Isoproterenol.

clear at present that adrenoceptors in bronchial smooth muscle have different properties from those in the heart or blood vessels.[234]

It needs to be emphasized that selectivity for one or the other type of receptor is relative rather than absolute. Selectivity is demonstrated by relative potency in reducing the effects of isoproterenol-induced stimulation of various tissues and showing dissociation of the dose-response curves in different tissues (Figure 46).

2. Membrane Stabilizing Activity

Propranolol is a powerful local anesthetic with about double the activity of procaine in depressing the action potential in frog sciatic nerve,[235] and like many other local anesthetics, shows even greater specificity for cardiac membranes than for nerves. It is stated that the concentration influencing myocardial excitability is approximately 200 times less than that which is effective on nerves. This action, which is termed a "membrane stabilization effect", results from the inhibition of the transfer of sodium across the membrane. Not all β-blocking agents have detectable effects on nerve membranes, but most have been shown to have some action on heart muscle resembling that of quinidine, in that they diminish both the rates of rise and the magnitude of the action potentials. Resting potentials and repolarization time are not significantly altered. It is of interest that d-propranolol possesses the same local anesthetic activity and is almost as potent as the l-isomer in its effects on cardiac action potentials,[236] whereas as has been previously stated, the l-isomer has much more marked β-adrenoceptor-blocking potency. There is therefore no correlation between the two activities. The ratio of the β-blocking activity and membrane effect varies from compound to compound. There is some evidence that the local anesthetic membrane-stabilizing effect may be one component of the action of the β-blocking drugs on arrhythmias. Thus, arrhythmias produced by injected catecholamines can be reversed by very small doses of β-blocking agents, whereas in contrast, restoration of sinus rhythm in arrhythmias induced by experimental ischemia or ouabain[236-239] can only be achieved with very high doses of β-blocking drugs. Drugs which possess relatively little membrane-stabilizing effects such as pindolol or practolol are ineffective.

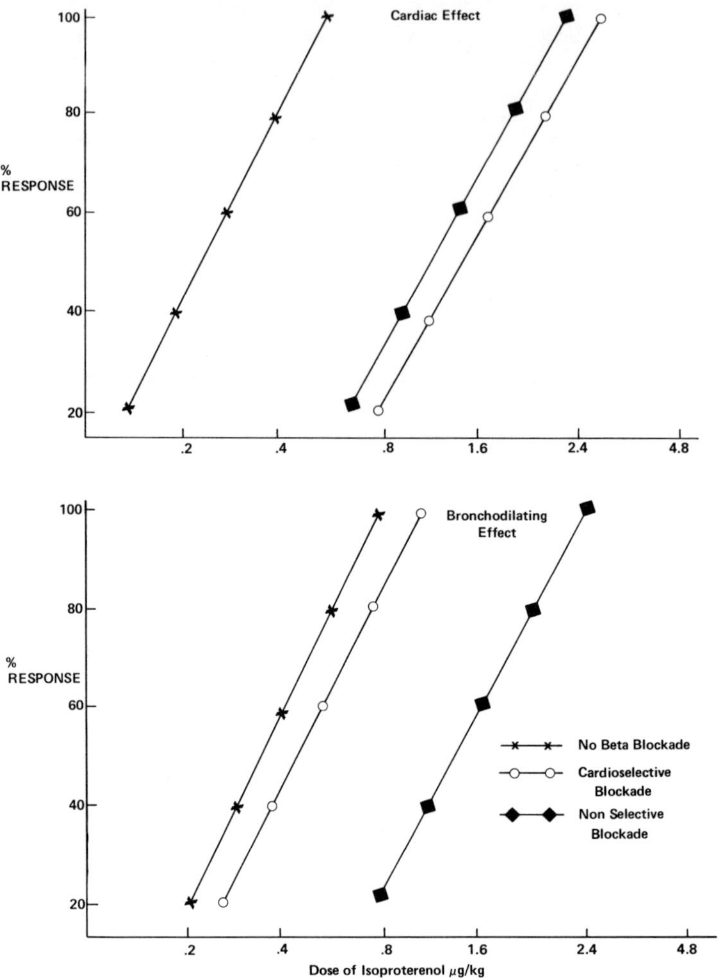

FIGURE 46. Diagram to illustrate the nature of cardioselective blockade. In the upper panel, a cardioselective and a nonselective drug have similar potency on the cardiac effect of Isoproterenol. The lower panel illustrates the smaller potency of the cardioselective agent in blocking the dilating action of isoproterenol on bronchial smooth muscle.

3. Cardiac Effects

Most β-blocking drugs have depressant actions on heart rate, contractile force, and cardiac output. These changes occur mainly as a result of inhibition of the stimulant effect of norepinephrine released from cardiac sympathetic nerve endings. With larger doses (in excess of 1 mg/kg), direct myocardial depression may be due also to membrane-stabilizing activity. Drugs which have intrinsic sympathomimetic activity or partial agonistic properties probably produce less effect on heart rate and possibly on myocardial contractile force and cardiac output. Almost all β-blocking drugs decrease the rate at which the myocardium uses oxygen. Regardless of whether the blockade is accompanied by a reduction in myocardial blood flow or not, there are again small differences between drugs with intrinsic sympathomimetic activity and those without. Drugs without intrinsic sympathomimetic activity, such as propranolol, decrease the ability of the left ventricle to perform useful mechanical work, but increase the efficiency with which the work is performed. On the other hand, pindolol and practolol, which have the same effects on oxygen requirements and efficiency, may actually increase the amount of work done.[240] It is not certain whether these actions are related to their β-blocking activity. β-Blocking agents have little action on coronary blood vessels. When coronary blood flow is reduced by these drugs, it is usually the consequence of a decrease in cardiac work and oxygen demand rather than of an active vasoconstriction. Moreover, these drugs do not prevent the coronary vessels from dilating in response to metabolic demands. Vasodilator responses to hypoxia or carbon dioxide accumulation are not affected. It is of some interest that in animals with experimental occlusion of the coronary arteries, β-blocking drugs induce a greater reduction in blood flow to nonischemic than to the ischemic areas of the myocardium.[241-243] This is probably due to the fact that cells in the ischemic areas remain hypoxic and the vessels consequently remain fully dilated in response to local release of vasodilator metabolites.

The administration of almost all β-adrenergic blocking drugs, whether cardioselective or with intrinsic agonist activity, leads to an acute rise in total peripheral resistance.[244-246] It is likely that these increases in total peripheral resistance occur as secondary responses to the reductions in cardiac output induced by these drugs. It has to be emphasized that these increases in peripheral resistance refer only to the acute changes following a single injection. The changes in regional vascular resistance during chronic administration may be quite different, particularly in hypertensive animals or man, as will be discussed later.

Catecholamines acting on β-adrenoceptors induce a number of significant metabolic actions which are blocked by β-blocking agents. Thus, catecholamines stimulate breakdown of glycogen both in vivo and in vitro, resulting in rises of blood glucose and lactic acid levels, as well as depletion of stores of glycogen in the liver and skeletal muscle, and lypolysis results in the release of free fatty acids from fat. All these actions are suppressed by β-blockade, presumably by preventing the action of catecholamines on the adenyl cyclase system.

4. Pharmacokinetics

β-Blocking agents differ not only in their pharmacological properties such as the possession of intrinsic agonistic activity, cardiac specificity, and membrane-stabilizing action, but also differ in pharmacokinetic characteristics. These characteristics determine the time course of the effect of drugs and contribute to individual differences between drugs. It is of critical importance in the clinical use of these drugs to have an idea of the rate of absorption and distribution and elimination if the drug is to be used adequately.

Almost all β-blockers, when given by mouth, are rapidly and almost completely absorbed. Maximal plasma levels after oral administration are usually obtained between ½ and 2 hr for most drugs. Absorption takes place from the gut as is to be expected with drugs with pK_a values of about 9. Following absorption, the drugs pass into the portal circulation and then to the liver where biotransformation may occur. Many β-blocking drugs, notably propranolol, alprenolol, and oxprenolol, are rapidly metabolized in the liver. Some, notably practolol, do not undergo biotransformation and other compounds such as timolol or pindolol are not rapidly metabolized.

If a large percentage of a drug is cleared from hepatic blood, the systemic availability after oral administration will be low due to extensive removal from portal blood during the first pass through the liver. The magnitude of the first-pass effect can be estimated by a comparison of the total plasma levels of drugs following both i.v. and oral administration. In drugs which are predominantly cleared by the liver on the first-pass through that organ, both the peak levels and the duration of plasma levels are considerably lower after oral administration than after i.v. administration, whereas in drugs

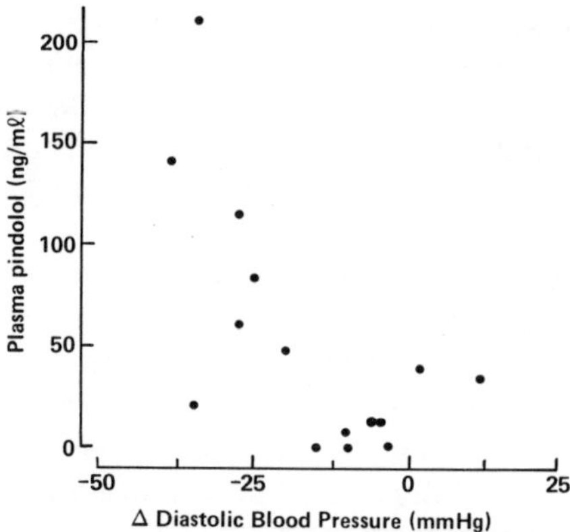

FIGURE 47.   Relationship between peak concentration of pindolol in plasma and maximal fall in diastolic blood pressure after the oral administration of pindolol (20 mg). The correlation coefficient (r) = 0.648 and the Spearman rank correlation coefficient (r,) = 0.764. (From Anavekar, S. N., Louis, W. J., Morgan, T. O., Doyle, A. E., and Johnston, C. I., *Clin. Exp. Pharmacol. Physiol.*, 2, 203, 1975. With permission.)

in which the first-pass metabolism is low, the two plasma level curves for the two routes of administration do not differ very greatly. Using such a technique, the availability of propranolol following an oral administration is between 15 and 25% of that following an i.v. dose,[247] while that of alprenolol is 1 to 15%,[248] and metoprolol is 30 to 50%.[249] By contrast, pindolol[250] and practolol[251] give similar plasma levels from oral and i.v. doses. A further factor which has to be taken into account is the variation in plasma levels achieved between different individuals. In general, the greater the removal during the first pass through the liver, the greater will be the variation between individuals in plasma levels following oral administration, since the magnitude of the first-pass effect varies from one individual to the next. The first-pass effect is seen predominantly following acute administration and may be due in part to binding within hepatic tissue as well as metabolism. There is some evidence that chronic administration changes the pharmacokinetic parameters of these drugs. This may be due to saturation of slowly equilibrating tissue compartments or to the induction of drug metabolism. Thus, although after a single initial dose, plasma levels of propranolol may be very low, with continued administration, plasma levels rise, reaching therapeutic levels within 72 hr to 7 days.[252] By contrast, plasma levels of pindolol, which is not extensively metabolized in the liver, can be demonstrated to reach much the same levels after a single dose or after chronic administration[253] (Figure 47).

It may be assumed that the effect of β-blocking drugs as competitive inhibitors is directly related to the concentration at the receptor site. While the concentration at the receptor site is not necessarily in equilibrium with the plasma concentration, in general it would be to be expected that higher plasma levels would lead to higher levels at the receptor site. It is certainly true that in patients in whom plasma levels are persistently low, biological effects are usually correspondingly weak.[253,254] The half-life of the plasma concentration of β-blocking drugs depends on the dose and peak level reached, the extent of first-pass metabolism, and the apparent volume of distribution

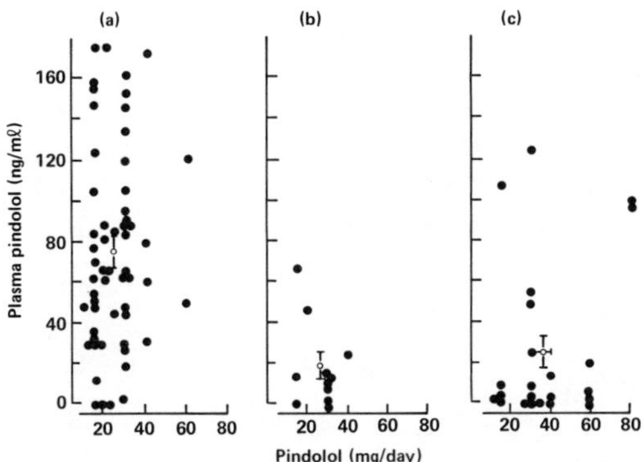

FIGURE 48. Relationship between plasma pindolol concentrations and daily intake of pindolol (mg/day) in patients on chronic treatment with pindolol plus other antihypertensive drugs. (a) Good responders: diastolic blood pressure (DBP) fell by at least 15 mmHg to below 100 mmHg; (b) fair responders: DBP fell by at least 15 mmHg to below 110 mmHg; (c) nonresponders: DBP fell less than 15 mmHg and remained above 110 mmHg. The open symbol in each panel represents the group mean with standard errors (which fell inside the symbol in some cases). (From Anavekar, S. N., Louis, W. J., Morgan, T. O., Doyle, A. E., and Johnston, C. I., *Clin. Exp. Pharmacol. Physiol.*, 2, 203, 1975. With permission.)

into which the drug is diluted. The major determinant of the volume of distribution with most drugs is the extent of plasma protein binding. This is usually more obvious with larger doses than with small. Although the plasma half-life of most β-blockers is relatively short, pharmacological activity of most drugs can be demonstrated for a much longer period than would be suggested by their plasma half-lives. This may be due to time taken for the drug to dissociate from tissue receptors or may merely be due to deficiencies in the biochemical assays. In some instances, it may be due also to the occurrence of active metabolites. A time lag has been reported after the oral administration of several β-blockers between the maximum blood levels and the development of an antihypertensive effect. This may reflect time for the drug to reach tissue receptors and may explain why there have been dissimilar reports on the correlation between the antihypertensive effect of drugs and their plasma levels. It has been reported[255] that there is no correlation between the plasma levels and β-blocking effects of metoprolol, either in the acute situation or during the steady state, and Brunner[256] could find no clear relationship between plasma oxprenolol concentration and the blockade of exercise-induced hypertension. On the other hand, with pindolol there was a significant relationship between the peak concentration of pindolol in the plasma and the maximum change in blood pressure in previously untreated hypertensive patients[253] (Figures 47 and 48).

Plasma half-lives and peak blood levels of drugs which are largely metabolized by the liver, such as propranolol or alprenolol, increase with the age of the subject.[257] Likewise, in patients with liver disease, peak plasma levels tend to be higher and of longer duration when propranolol is used,[258] presumably because in this situation the hepatic first-pass metabolism of oral propranolol is decreased, with a consequent increase in circulating plasma levels of unchanged drug. In advanced kidney disease also, hepatic first-pass metabolism may be reduced, so that propranolol again may have longer duration of effect in such patients. In patients with chronic renal failure, drugs mainly eliminated by the kidney, such as practolol[259] and sotalol,[260] certainly exhibit a prolonged duration of half-life. On the other hand, it appears that the half-life of pindolol, which is normally mainly excreted unchanged in the urine, does not become prolonged in uremic patients.[260] This is attributed to an increased biotransformation of the drug following the loss of the capacity to excrete the drug in the kidney and may be due in part to reduced protein binding. Some of the major properties of different drugs are shown in Table 1.

C. Antihypertensive Activity

Although there is convincing evidence concerning the antihypertensive properties of β-adrenoceptor-blocking drugs in man, these drugs do not always produce a satisfactory antihypertensive action in experimental animals, which may well be one of the reasons why the mechanism of their antihypertensive action is still in doubt. Models of renal hypertension in the rat and dog have failed to respond either to propranolol or to timolol. On the other hand, it has been reported that pindolol produces a substantial fall in blood pressure in the renal hypertensive dog. Fernandes et al.[262] studied the relationship between antihypertensive effect and effect on plasma renin levels in rats with aortic ligations. They reported that in this model, propranolol at doses of either 3 or 60 mg/kg daily had hardly any discernible antihypertensive action, although at both dose levels plasma renin levels were markedly reduced (Figure 49). By contrast, treatment in the same animal model with either hydrallazine or frusemide led to a substantial fall in blood pressure and also to a fall in plasma renin. In the DOCA salt-treated rat, Dusting and Rand[263] showed that the dose of propranolol used is critical for an antihypertensive action. They reported that s.c. administration of propranolol at a dose of 0.2 mg/kg twice daily for a period of 7 weeks reduced blood pressure to normotensive levels, whereas a dose of 0.5 mg/kg twice daily was ineffective. In the adult spontaneously hypertensive rat, propranolol and timolol both appeared to be effective antihypertensive agents. With both these drugs, Sweet[264] reported that the greatest antihypertensive effect at any dose level was not evident until the second or third day of treatment. There was also a tendency for arterial pressure to return toward pretreatment values when treatment was discontinued. Sweet further reported that timolol acted more rapidly than did propranolol in this model. It is also stated that if treatment is begun with β-blockers in very young animals and continued throughout the development stage of hypertension, there is a reduction in the level to which the blood pressure rises.[265,266] These experimental findings have done little to elucidate the mechanism of antihypertensive action of these drugs which is still not yet completely clear in spite of a considerable amount of work. A number of hypotheses to explain the antihypertensive action of these drugs have been advanced. These include:

1.   Reduction of cardiac output
2.   Suppression of renin secretion
3.   Inhibition of sympathetic neuronal activity
4.   A central inhibition of sympathetic activity
5.   An interaction with prostaglandins

D. Mechanisms of Antihypertensive Action

1. Effects on Cardiac Output

There is general agreement that almost all β-blocking drugs seem to have the acute effects of producing both a reduction in heart rate and cardiac output, with a rise in total peripheral resistance. With many drugs such as propranolol and oxprenolol, there

TABLE 1

Characteristics of Some β-Adrenoceptor-Blocking Drugs

Drug	Synonyms	Beta-block-ade potency ratio (pro-pranolol = 1)	Cardioselec-tivity	Partial agonist activity	Mem-brane-sta-bilizing activity	Elimination half-life (hr)	Relative oral bioavailabil-ity	Variation in plasma level	β-Blocking plasma concen-tration
Acebutolol	Sectral M & B 17,803A	0.3	+	+	+	About 8(po)	Fair		0.2—2 μg/ml
Alprenolol	H56/26 Aptin Betaptin Betacard	0.3	0	+ +	+	2—3 (i.v., po)	Low	10—20-fold	50—100 ng/ml
Atenolol	ICI66082 Tenormin	1	+	0	0	6/9(oral)	Fair	Low	0.2—0.5 μg/ml
Metoprolol	H93/26 Lopresor Betaloc	1	+	0	±	3—4(i.v., po)	Fair	7-fold	50—100 ng/ml
Oxprenolol	Ciba39089 BaTrasicor	0.5—1	0	+ +	+	2(po)	Fair	5-fold	80—100 ng/ml
Pindolol	LB46 Visken	6	0	+ + +	+	3—4(i.v.) 3—4(i.v.)	Good	4-fold	50—150 ng/ml
Practolol	ICI50172 Eraldin	0.3	+	+ +	0	9—12(i.v.) 6—8(po)	Good		1.5—5 μg/ml
Propranolol	ICI45520 Inderal Aviocardin	1	0	0	+ +	2—4(i.v.) 3.5—6(po)	Low	20-fold	50—100 ng/ml
Sotalol	MJ199 Betacardone Sotacor	0.3	0	0	0	5—13(po)	Good	4-fold	0.5—4 μg/ml
Timolol	MK-950 Blocadren	6	0	±	0	4—5(po)	Good		?5—10 ng/ml

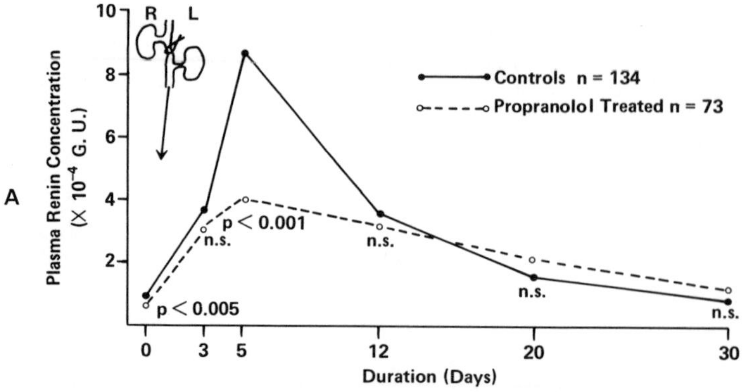

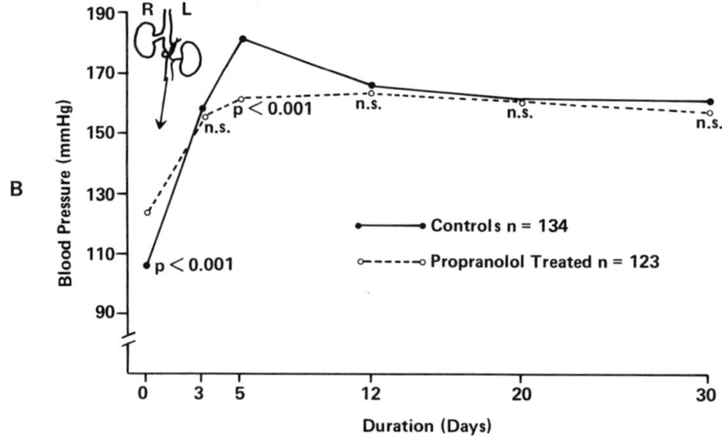

FIGURE 49.   (A) Effect of propranolol (3 mg/kg) on average plasma renin concentration in conscious renal hypertensive rats. (B) Effect of propranolol (60 mg/kg/day) on average mean arterial pressure in conscious renal hypertensive rats. (From Fernandes, M., Onesti, G., Dykyj, R., Gould, A. B., Fiorentini, R., Kwin, K. E., and Swartz, C., *Systemic Effects of Antihypertensive Agents,* Sambhi, M. P., Ed., Stratton Intercontinental, New York, 1976, 287. With permission.)

is usually a delay before the antihypertensive effect develops, even though the changes in heart rate occur rapidly. There is some evidence that after weeks or months on propranolol therapy, the total peripheral resistance seems to decrease, perhaps due to resetting of baroreceptors, but the cardiac output remains low or increases slightly, and the blood pressure remains low or decreases further. The cardiac output continues to be reduced after therapy with propranolol for as long as 20 months.[267] The same authors found that the cardiac index after 20 months was reduced by about 17% at rest in the supine position, compared to the pretreatment cardiac output. On the other hand, Fransciosa and colleagues[268] have suggested that although there is an initial fall in cardiac output using timolol, this had disappeared after 5 weeks continuous treatment, although the antihypertensive action persisted. Lund-Johansen[246] studied the effects of long-term β-blockade, using alprenolol, atenolol, and timolol on the cardiac hemodynamics both at rest and during exercise in patients with essential hypertension (Figures 50, 51, and 52). Previously untreated essential hypertension of mild degree

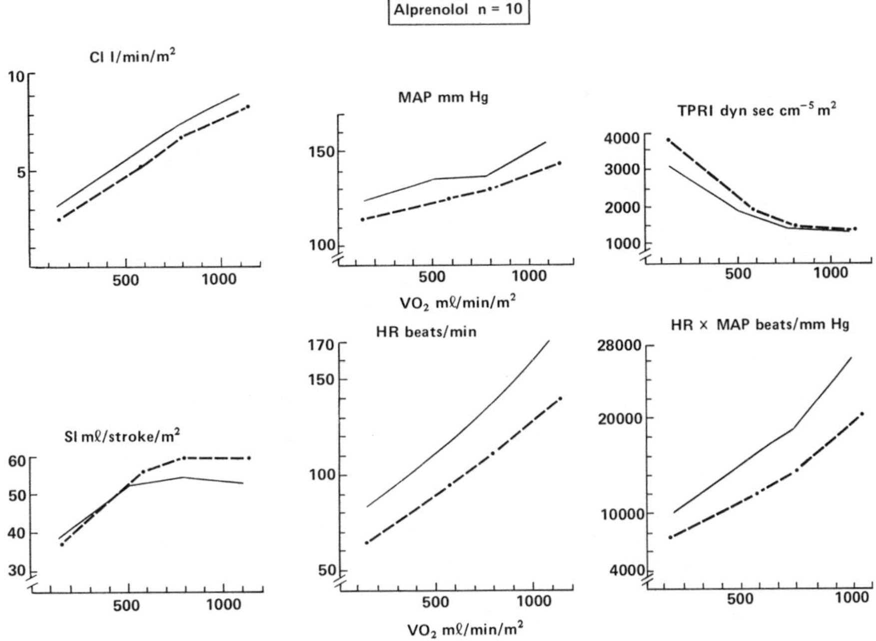

FIGURE 50.   Cardiac index (CI), mean arterial pressure (MAP), total peripheral resistance index (TPRI), stroke index (SI), heart rate (HR), and heart rate-pressure (HR X MAP) in relation to oxygen consumption (VO₂) at rest and during exercise before (—) and during (- - - -) alprenolol therapy, mean values, (From Lund-Johanson, P., *Clin. Exp. Pharmacol. Physiol.* (Suppl. 4), in press. With permission.)

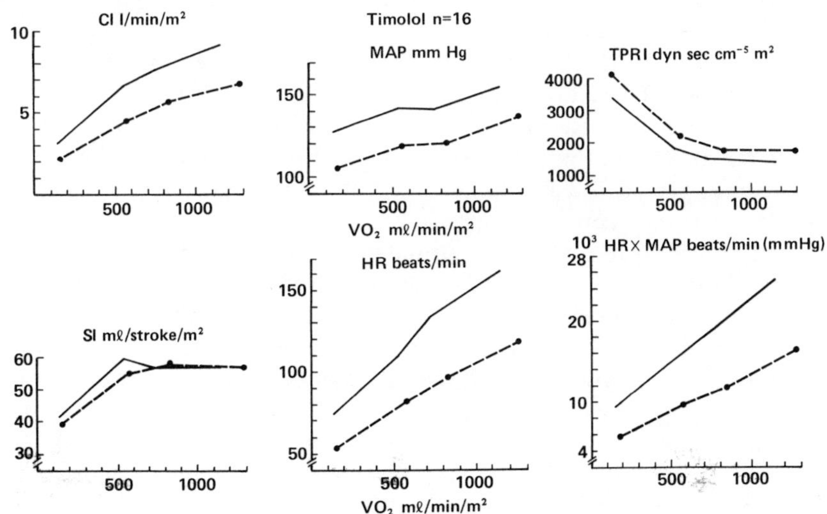

FIGURE 51.   Central hemodynamics before and during timolol therapy. Legend and abbreviations as in Figure 50. (From Lund-Johanson, P., *Clin. Exp. Pharmacol. Physiol.* (Suppl. 4), in press. With permission.)

was studied in 39 men. The subjects were treated during strictly standardized conditions, at rest, supine, and sitting, and during bicycling in a steady state of graded exercise. The studies were made on an outpatient basis, and all subjects received one drug only. The casual blood pressure and heart rate dropped in all subjects during

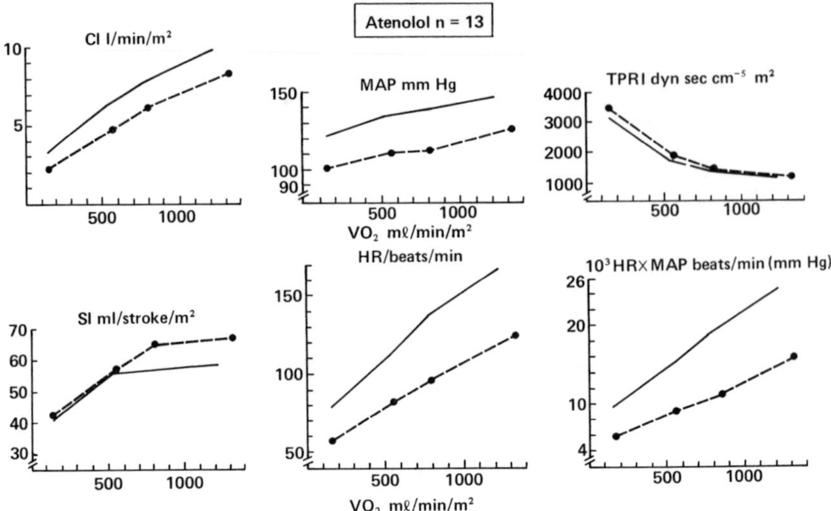

FIGURE 52.   Central hemodynamics before and during atenolol therapy. Legend and abbreviations as in Figure 50. (From Lund-Johanson, P., *Clin. Exp. Pharmacol. Physiol.*, (Suppl. 4), in press. With permission.)

treatment. With only one exception, the cardiac index was lower after treatment in all subjects at rest and during exercise. Reductions in cardiac output were approximately 1.5 to 2 l/min at rest, which represented a fall of about 25%. During exercise, the absolute reductions in cardiac output were greater. All subjects had an increased total peripheral resistance before treatment, which did not decrease significantly in any group, following almost 1 year of treatment and was higher, if anything. Timolol in particular induced a significant increase in total peripheral resistance. Thus, this study suggests that the whole of the fall in blood pressure could be accounted for by reduction in cardiac output. There are, however, several arguments which can be raised in relation to this hypothesis. First, although the cardiac output falls and the total peripheral resistance remains high, there is no dramatic increase in total peripheral resistance such as might be expected if a fall in cardiac output fell for other reasons. There is also the problem that the depressor response with propranolol usually develops slowly, whereas reduction of cardiac output is found immediately without any reduction in blood pressure. Furthermore, the cardiac output is reduced equally, both in patients who have a fall in blood pressure and those who do not, so that in nonresponders, the peripheral resistance rises.[267] An additional factor which has to be taken into account is that effective antihypertensive doses of many β-blocking drugs are far in excess of those required to produce reductions in cardiac output. There is no doubt that reduction in cardiac output is an important mechanism which may be responsible in part for the antihypertensive action, but it seems doubtful whether it is responsible for the whole of the antihypertensive effects.

2. Suppression of Renin Secretion

It has been suggested that one mechanism which might explain the antihypertensive action of these drugs is interference with the renin-angiotensin system. There is reasonable evidence that activation of the autonomic nervous system can result in the release of renin. Increased plasma renin concentrations occur in response to stimulation of the renal nerves, i.v. administration of catecholamines, or the release of endogenous catecholamines. The effects of all these stimuli on renin release appear to be mediated by β-adrenoceptor stimulation, since they can all be blocked by l-propranolol, but not by d-propranolol or α-adrenoceptor-blocking drugs. While β-blocking agents can inhibit renin release evoked by nerve stimulation, they do not always affect the release resulting from other mechanisms. Certainly the rise in plasma renin levels resulting from a reduction in renal perfusion pressure, hemorrhage, or renal artery constriction is not entirely abolished by adrenergic blockade. There is, however, evidence that the renal sympathetic nerves are involved in renin release in response to the upright posture, exercise, or medullary stimulation (Chapter 2, Volume 2). It is not at present clear whether the renin receptor is of β_1 or β_2 type. Weber and colleagues[270] examined the effects of six β-adrenoceptor antagonists on resting and stimulated plasma renin levels in conscious rabbits. Although propranolol, oxprenolol, metoprolol, and practolol all caused a fall in plasma renin activity, only the nonselective antagonists, propranolol, oxprenolol, and pindolol prevented an increase in plasma renin level resulting from the i.v. infusion of isoproterenol. The cardioselective drugs, metoprolol and practolol induced only partial inhibition.

In man, the picture is also confusing. Amery[271] reported that atenolol, a cardioselective agent, did not reduce plasma renin activity, whereas Aberg[272] has reported that atenolol does reduce renin activity, and Esler and Nestel[273] have reported that practolol also does so.

There is no doubt that chronic administration of β-blocking drugs usually decreases plasma renin activity in both normal and hypertensive subjects.[273] The question as to whether this is related to their antihypertensive action is not universally agreed. Bühler[275,276] and colleagues examined the antihypertensive action of propranolol in hypertensive patients subclassified into those having high, normal, and low plasma renin activity in relation to their sodium excretion. They reported that propranolol at a mean dose of 2 mg/kg per day caused a fall of about 30 mmHg in the high renin group with a much smaller fall of only about 5 mmHg in the low renin group. These authors thought that β-blockade might offer a specific form of therapy for the high renin group. These results, however, have not been widely confirmed. Thus, Morgan et al.[274] and Birkenhager et al.,[277] who classified their patients into a similar subgrouping, reported that the falls in diastolic blood pressure were very similar in all three groups and that the numbers of patients responding were approximately equal in each group (Figures 53 and 54). Moreover, there are differences in the time relationships between the effects on plasma renin activity and those on blood pressure. Morgan et al.[274] reported on the acute effects of propranolol and pindolol on both plasma renin activity and blood pressure in hypertensive patients. They found that propranolol produced a sharp fall in plasma renin activity within 2 hr but had no effect on blood pressure at this time, whereas pindolol produced a rapid fall in blood pressure, but had no acute effect on plasma renin activity. It has also been reported that when patients were switched from propranolol to atenolol[278] or pindolol,[279] plasma renin activity rose promptly, although the antihypertensive response was maintained (Figure 55). Dissociation between suppression of plasma renin activity and the falls in blood pressure with propranolol have also been seen in animals with experimental hypertension.[262] The reason for some of these discrepancies have been clarified by the studies of Hollifield and his colleagues and by Leonetti et al.[254] Hollifield[280] reported that low doses of 160 mgm of propranolol both suppressed plasma renin activity and induced a fall in blood pressure in patients with higher plasma renin levels, whereas in patients with low plasma renin levels the same small doses had little effect on blood pressure. With higher doses of propranolol however, up to 460 mgm per day, both high and low renin groups showed a similar reduction in blood pressure (Figure 56). Leonetti[254] has shown that very small doses of propranolol, sufficient to induce blood

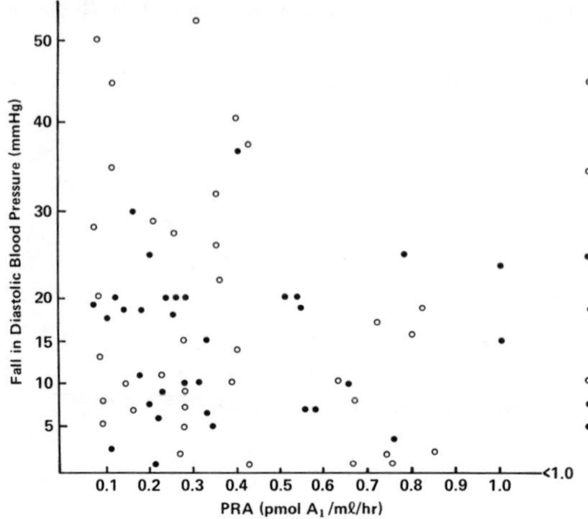

FIGURE 53.   The fall in diastolic blood pressure with propranolol (O) or pindolol (●) is plotted against the basal plasma renin activity (PRA) measured on a high sodium intake diet while in hospital. There was no significant relationship between these variables. (From Morgan, T. O., Roberts, R., Carney, S. L., Louis, W. J., and Doyle, A. E., *Br. J. Clin. Pharmacol.,* 2, 159, 1975. With permission.)

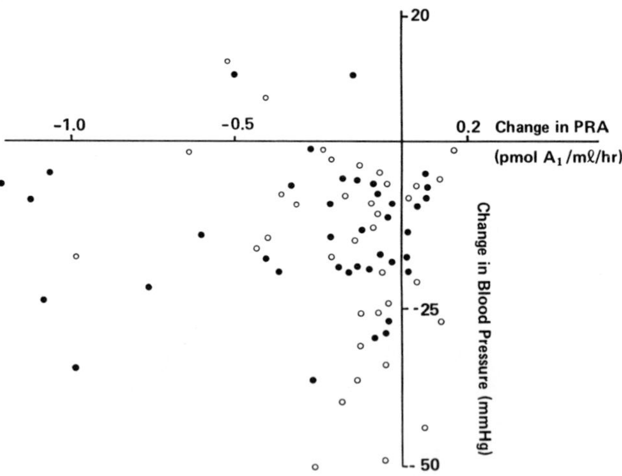

FIGURE 54.   The changes in blood pressure and plasma renin activity (PRA) in ambulant patients treated with propranolol (O) or pindolol (●) are plotted against each other. There was no significant correlation between these variables. (From Morgan, T. O., Roberts, R., Carney, S. L., Louis, W. J., and Doyle, A. E., *Br. J. Clin. Pharmacol.,* 2, 159, 1975. With permission.)

levels of only a few nanograms/ml, are sufficient to reduce both heart rate and plasma renin activity and that in most hypertensive patients these have little effect on blood pressure. It appears from these studies that the effects of propranolol in reducing plasma renin activity may have a contributory effect to its antihypertensive action in a small number of patients whose blood pressures are predominantly maintained by a

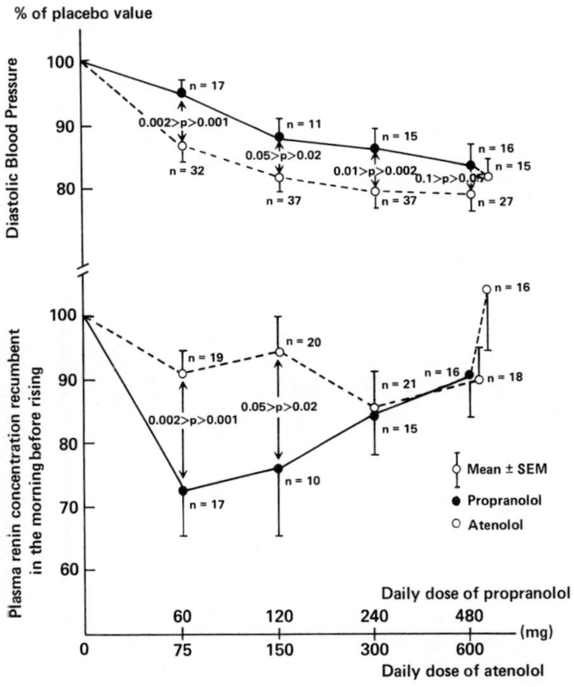

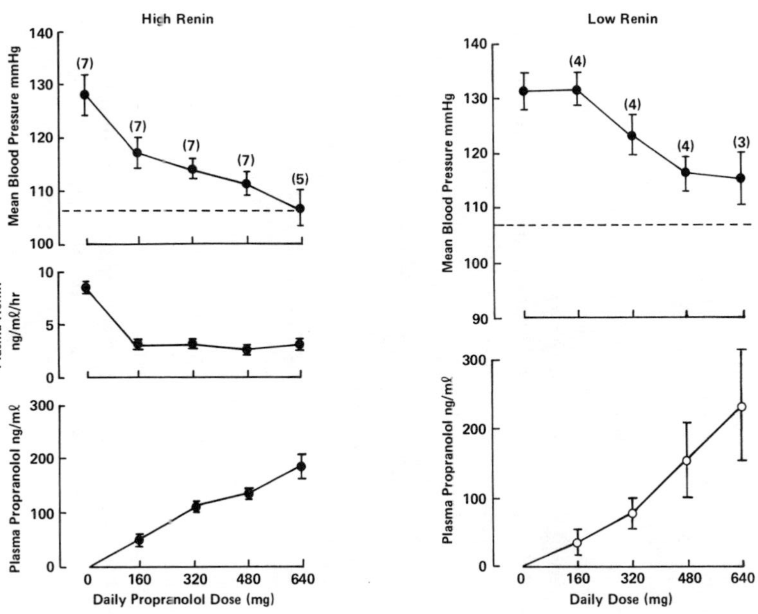

FIGURE 55.   Hypotensive and renin lowering effect of propranolol and atenolol. Values are shown as percent of value obtained during the placebo treatment (O-period) in individual patients. (From Lijnen, P., Amery, A., de Plaen, J. F., Fagard, R., and Reybruck, T., *Beta-Adrenoceptor Blocking Agents,* Saxena, P. R. and Forsyth, R. P., Eds., North-Holland, Amsterdam, 1976, 335. With permission.)

FIGURE 56.   The effects of varying doses of propranolol on the mean blood pressure in patients with high renin and those with low renin levels. The effects on plasma renin are shown for the high renin patients. Plasma levels of propranolol at various doses are shown for each group. (From Hollifield, J. W., *Systemic Effects of Antihypertensive Agents,* Sambhi, M. P., Ed., Stratton Intercontinental, New York, 1976, 201. With permission.)

mechanism related to high plasma renin levels. It is uncertain as to what proportion of patients this constitutes, but it may apply to some with renovascular hypertension, malignant hypertension, or renal failure. The balance of evidence suggests that suppression of plasma renin activity is not a prerequisite for the antihypertensive response to β-blocking drugs. Some patients with higher plasma renin activities may preferentially respond better to β-blockers like propranolol, but it remains possible that even in these patients, plasma and tissue concentrations of propranolol may be higher due to reduced renal elimination, so that the renin-lowering effect may not even in these patients be the antihypertensive mechanism. In the great majority of hypertensive patients, it appears probable that the action of β-blocking drugs in suppressing plasma renin activity contributes little to the overall antihypertensive effects.

3. Inhibition of Peripheral Adrenergic Nerve Function

There have been numerous studies, mainly in animal models, concerning the possible effects of β-adrenoceptor blocking drugs on peripheral adrenergic nerve terminals. Mylecharane and Raper[281,282] have demonstrated that during blockade by low concentrations such as 0.2 µg/ml, propranolol resembles a guanethidine-type of neuronal inhibition in that it has a slow onset, shows resistance to repeated washing, but is readily reversed by amphetamine. By contrast, higher amounts of β-blocking drugs elicited a block which had features of a nonspecific depression of nerve function which could be reversed by washing, but not by amphetamine.

It has been suggested[283,284] that part of the antihypertensive effect of β-adrenergic blocking drugs might be due to an action on presynaptic β-receptors which appear to mediate a positive feedback, facilitating the release of norepinephrine at the neuroeffector junction. It is postulated that a block of these receptors would depress but not completely eliminate norepinephrine release and response to nerve action potentials. Åblad[283] has reported that 6 months treatment with propranolol and metoprolol in spontaneously hypertensive rats reduced blood pressure and decreased the contractions of the portal vein elicited by low frequency transmural stimulation, but did not affect the actions of exogenous norepinephrine. Adler-Graschinsky and Langer[284] found that propranolol produced a significant decrease in the frequency response of guinea pig atria, suggesting that increasing frequency of nerve stimulation facilitated norepinephrine release (Figure 57). Moreover, overflow of tritiated norepinephrine was significantly reduced. It is difficult to determine the precise role of this possible mechanism in the antihypertensive effects in man. The bulk of evidence suggests that there is little fall in total peripheral resistance, but on the other hand, there is a failure to increase peripheral resistance in the face of a fall in cardiac output, so it is possible that this mechanism may have a place in the human antihypertensive action.

4. Inhibition of Central Sympathetic Activity

The relative amount and the speed with which a β-adrenoceptor antagonist enters the brain is determined by its lipid solubility. Propranolol is more lipid soluble than pindolol, sotalol, atenolol, or practolol. It has been shown that propranolol, pindolol, and alprenolol readily enter the brain and achieve high concentrations in brain tissue.[284] It is claimed however that sotalol, atenolol, and practolol do not enter the central nervous system. It is also clear that β-antagonists administered intraventricularly can diffuse from the brain into the plasma, which must lead to caution in interpreting experiments related to the central effects of these drugs.[286,287]

It is probable that norepinephrine has an important inhibitory role in the central control of arterial blood pressure. Although systemic administration raises blood pressure, administration into the ventricular system of the brain decreases both blood pres-

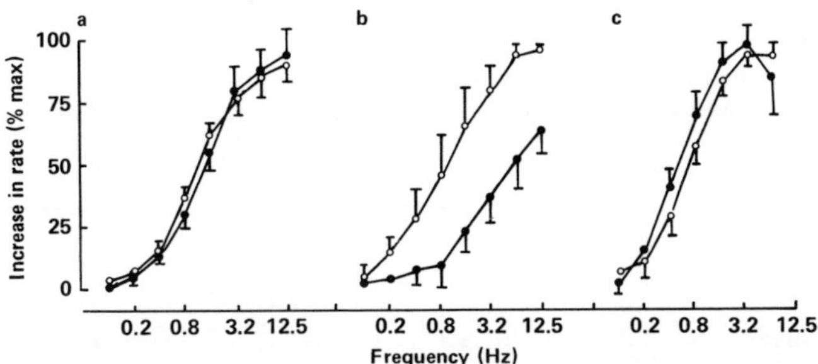

FIGURE 57.   Effects of propranolol and phentolamine on the positive chronotropic effects elicited by accelerans nerve stimulation in guinea pig isolated atria. Ordinates: increase in atrial rate as percent of the maximum of the first (before treatment) frequency-response curve. Abscissae: frequency of nerve stimulation (Hz). Frequency-response curves obtained before (O) and 30 min after (●) treatment in (a) controls (n = 6), atria exposed to propranolol (1.0×10^{-7} M) for 30 min before the second frequency-response curve (n = 3), and (c) atria exposed to phentolamine (3.1×10^{-6} M) for 30 min before the second frequency-response curve (n = 5). Mean values are shown. Vertical bars indicate s.e. mean. n = number of experiments. (From Adler-Graschinsky, E. and Langer, S. Z., *Br. J. Pharmacol.*, 53, 43, 1975. With permission.)

sure and heart rate. de Jong[160] showed that norepinephrine injected bilaterally into the brain stem in the region of the nucleus tractus solitarius decreased arterial blood pressure and the heart rate in anesthetized rats. This effect was prevented by a preceding injection of phentolamine at the same site. It was postulated that this inhibitory mechanism may explain the central hypotensive action observed in patients receiving L3-4 dihydroxyphenylalanine (l-dopa) and clonidine.[288] The fact that α-adrenoceptors in the brain appear to be inhibitory in terms of blood pressure and heart rate has led to speculation that the β-adrenoceptor in the brain might be excitatory, and it has been postulated that central blockade of these receptors by β-adrenoceptor-blocking drugs might be responsible for the antihypertensive effect. This is supported by the fact that the central administration of isoproterenol has been reported to increase blood pressure and induce tachycardia.[288] There have been a number of reports of hypotensive responses after the central administration of β-blocking drugs. Garvey and Ram[290] reported that propranolol and pindolol but not sotalol reduced the blood pressure when injected into the dorsal hippocampus or the septum. Kelliher[291] reported that during perfusion of the lateral ventricle in the cat with propranolol for 1 hr at a concentration of 0.5 mg and 0.1 mℓ of CSF at a rate of 0.1 mℓ per min, both racemic and d-propranolol produced a drop in systemic blood pressure. The racemic form produced a fall of pressure of 30 mmHg, while d-propranolol reduced the blood pressure by 18 mmHg. The magnitude of the effect was not statistically different between the two isomers. The hypotensive response occurred within 1 min and lasted for approximately 4 to 5 min. Intraventricular administration of racemic propranolol reduced heart rate, but d-propranolol given in this way did not. The effects of both forms of propranolol on blood pressure and heart rate were prevented if the spinal cord was previously transsected at the level of C_2, suggesting that the hypotensive response of intraventricular propranolol was not due to a leakage into the peripheral circulation. When the animals were pretreated with reserpine into the lateral ventricle in doses sufficient to cause depletion of 90% in the level of norepinephrine, the blood pressure fell quite markedly. The subsequent perfusion into the ventricles of either racemic propranolol or d-propranolol then led to a sharp rise in blood pressure.

TABLE 2

Effect of Intravenous (+)- and (±)-Propranolol, Sodium Nitroprusside, and Saline on Mean Arterial Pressure (MAP) and Splanchnic Nerve Activity (SNA) in Conscious Rabbits[292]

Infusion	Number of animals	First hour		Second hour	
		MAP	SNA	MAP	SNA
Saline	8	97 ± 2	111 ± 5	99 ± 3	104 ± 16
(+)-Propranolol	8	101 ± 2	122 ± 17	99 ± 4	132 ± 24
(±)-Propranolol	8	94 ± 3	68 ± 11[b]	87 ± 2[a]	52 ± 9[b]
Sodium nitroprusside	8	74 ± 1[a]	178 ± 30[b]	73 ± 2[a]	199 ± 38[b]

Note: Values are the mean ± SEM of the average during 1 hr expressed as a percentage of the average during the hour pretreatment.

Significant differences from saline control group: [a]$P < 0.01$ (student's unpaired t-test); [b]$P < 0.05$.

Direct evidence for a central sympathetic inhibition by propranolol has been obtained by Lewis and Haeusler.[292] These workers recorded blood pressure and integrated activity in the splanchnic nerves from preganglionic sympathetic fibers in conscious rabbits. Neither saline nor d-propranolol given intravenously affected sympathetic nerve activity or arterial pressure, but a 2 hr infusion of l-propranolol decreased both (Table 2).

There seems to be general agreement that the central administration of β-adrenoceptor-blocking drugs almost always induces prolonged hypotension and bradycardia. These are sometimes, but not always, preceded by transient increases in blood pressure and heart rate. The fact that these changes can be prevented by transsection of the spinal cord suggests that they are central in origin and are not due to leakage of the drugs into the general circulation. The question as to whether the dextro isomer is active centrally is as yet uncertain. Lewis et al.,[293] using the conscious rabbit, reported no response to the d-isomer although the l-isomer was effective.

The question as to the importance of the contribution of a central antihypertensive effect in hypertensive patients remains unresolved. The doses administered intraventricularly in animals have in general been rather large, and drugs such as sotalol and practolol, which are said not to enter the central nervous system, seem equally clinically effective as antihypertensive agents as those drugs which are undoubtedly concentrated within the central nervous system. Clinically, the accounts of central nervous system side effects such as nightmares and dreams[294] and the fact that postural control of blood pressure is not interfered with would be consistent with the idea that β-blocking drugs enter the central nervous system in man and may be contributing a significant component by a central action to the antihypertensive effect. It is clear, however, that this is not the only possible effect, and its precise contrbution to the antihypertensive effect in man is currently rather difficult to determine.

5. An Interaction with Prostaglandins

The possibility of an interaction between β-adrenoceptor-blocking drugs and anti-inflammatory drugs such as indomethacin, phenylbutazone, and mefenamic acid has been suggested by the reports that the anti-inflammatory action of these drugs is inhibited or sometimes abolished by the concurrent administration of β-blocking drugs.[295] There is evidence also that indomethacin may interfere with the antihypertensive effect of β-blocking drugs in both the conscious rabbit[296] and hypertensive patients[297] (Figure 58). Prata and Goncalves studied the effects of adding indomethacin on the antihyper-

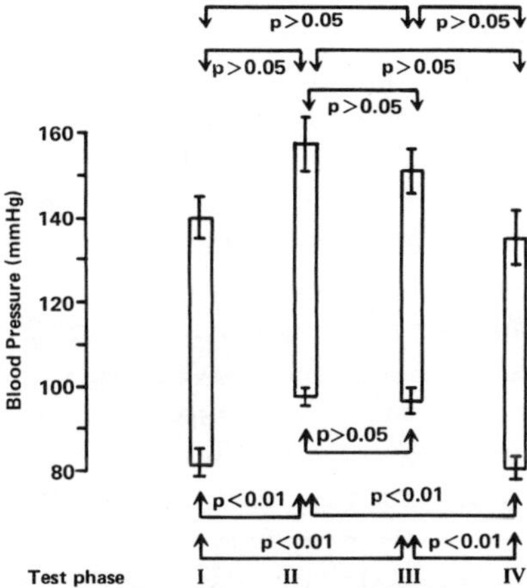

FIGURE 58. Supine systolic and diastolic blood pressure (mean ± S.E.M.) of seven hypertensive patients during the four test phases: phase I, β-blocker only; phase II, placebo; phase III, β-blocker plus indomethacin; phase IV, β-blocker only. P values were calculated using student's *t*-test. (From Duraõ, V., Prata, M. M., and Gonçalves, L. M. P., *Lancet*, 2, 1005, 1977. With permission.)

tensive effects of pindolol and propranolol in seven hypertensive patients. They reported that 100 mg of indomethacin daily almost completely abolished the fall in diastolic blood pressure induced by both propranolol and pindolol, although it had very little effect on pulse rate. They suggested that this effect might be due to the inhibition of prostaglandin synthesis by indomethacin and that the antihypertensive effect of β-blocking drugs might act synergistically with an antihypertensive property of prostaglandins. If this were so, they suggested that β-adrenoceptor-blocking might act synergistically to induce enhancement of the effects of prostaglandins in reducing peripheral resistance. Although this hypothesis is attractive, it is clearly not proven. It remains possible that some other effect of the anti-inflammatory drugs could be involved in the interactions described. However, the hypothesis deserves, and will no doubt gain, further study.

E. Differing Properties of Individual Drugs

1. Intrinsic Sympathomimetic Activity

Propranolol, timolol, atenolol, metoprolol, and sotalol induce no observable effect when they interact with β-receptors in the absence of a primary agonist such as epinephrine or isoproterenol. However, alprenolol, oxprenolol, pindolol, practolol, and acebutolol cause a partial agonistic response, which suggests that they themselves have agonist activity. This property has been called intrinsic sympathomimetic activity. In practice, this property seems to convey no particular clinical advantage or disadvantage in terms of antihypertensive response. It is certainly far less important than bioavailability in determining the effectiveness of the agent. Drugs with marked intrinsic sympathomimetic activity, such as pindolol and alprenolol, induce smaller falls in heart rate than propranolol or timolol, but the antihypertensive response seems to be the same with each group of drugs.[73] Pindolol has been reported to increase plasma renin activity in animals, which is attributed to its intrinsic sympathomimetic activity. In spite of this, it remains a very effective antihypertensive agent.

2. Membrane Stabilizing Actions

The extent to which β-blocking drugs possess membrane-stabilizing or local anesthetic activity varies considerably from one drug to the next in relation to their potency in terms of β-blockade. Propranolol, alprenolol, and oxprenolol have potent membrane-stabilizing activity. Pindolol, which is much more active than propranolol in its β-blocking effects, has only about one tenth of the membrane-stabilizing activity of propranolol, which gives it a large gain in specificity. The cardioselective drug, atenolol, seems to possess no membrane-stabilizing activity, and timolol possesses very little. In spite of these differences, the antihypertensive effects of these various compounds seem very similar. Thus in a double-blind comparison of propranolol, pindolol, alprenolol, and timolol, Morgan et al.[294] found no significant differences in the antihypertensive effect. The dose ratios for the four drugs corresponded with their respective β-blocking potencies as judged by their capacity to inhibit isoproterenol-induced tachycardia. It is unlikely that the possession or otherwise of membrane-stabilizing activity is a relevant factor to be taken into account in clinical usage for hypertension.

3. Cardioselectivity

Practolol, atenolol, metoprolol, and acebutolol possess a greater affinity for cardiac β-adrenoceptors than for those in either bronchial or vascular smooth muscle. Most of the remaining β-blocking drugs are nonselective. There appears to be no important difference between the antihypertensive actions of cardioselective β-blocking drugs as against those with no cardioselectivity. Both appear to be equally effective antihypertensive agents.

4. α-Adrenergic Blocking Properties

As has been previously stated, the great majority of β-adrenoceptor-blocking drugs appear to be highly specific for the β-receptor and do not have any antagonistic activity against α-receptors. However, one drug, labetalol (AH 5158), which is 5,1-hydroxy 2,1 methyl,3 phenyl-propylamino ethyl salicylamide, combines both β- and α-adrenoceptor antagonist properties.[298,299] This drug not only prevents or antagonizes isoproterenol-induced tachycardia, but is also capable of antagonizing norepinephrine-induced vasoconstriction in forearm blood vessels.[300]

Labetalol has been reported[301] to be 16 times as potent in inducing blockade of cardiac β_1-receptors than blockade of vascular α-receptors. The α-blocking properties appear to be about seven times less potent than phentolamine. The action at cardiac β_1-receptors is about 4 times less potent than propranolol, but at bronchial and vascular β_2-receptors, it is reported to be 11 to 17 times less potent than propranolol. The β-adrenoceptor activity therefore appears to be cardioselective. There is a suggestion that the α-blocking properties of this drug may, like those of prazosin, be confined to the postjunctional receptor, since it induced little increase in the overflow of ^{3}H-norepinephrine from the perfused spleen of the cat.[302]

The hemodynamic effects of labetalol differ qualitatively from those of most β-adrenoceptor-blocking drugs. In normotensive and renal hypertensive dogs, labetalol induced a sharp fall in blood pressure. The fall in blood pressure was considerably greater than that induced by propranolol, mainly because of a considerable fall of peripheral resistance, with only a small fall in cardiac output. Similar falls in blood pressure were induced in DOCA salt hypertensive rats.[301]

In man, the hemodynamic effects of labetalol are similar. Lund-Johansen[303] studied the effects of orally administered labetalol on fifteen hypertensive patients treated for 1 year. The blood pressure fell by about 23% both at rest and during exercise. The cardiac index fell by about 7 to 10%, and the peripheral resistance by 12 to 16% (Figure 59). Similar results were noted after 4 weeks treatment by Edwards and Raf-

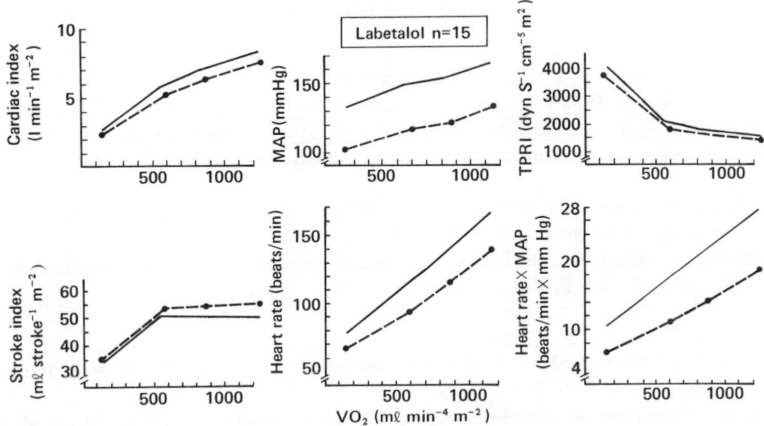

FIGURE 59.   Mean (n = 15) hemodynamic changes at rest (sitting) and during exercise before (———) and during (- - - -) treatment with labetalol. MAP = mean arterial pressure; TPRI = total peripheral resistance index; VO₂ oxygen consumption. (From Lund-Johansen, P. and Bakke, O. M., *Br. J. Clin. Pharmacol.,* in press.)

tery.[304] Systolic pressure fell by 11 to 18% and diastolic blood pressure by 16 to 21%. Changes in cardiac output were not significant, and the fall in blood pressure was entirely due to a fall in total peripheral resistance.

Labetalol is metabolized by glucuronide conjugation in the liver, and less than 5% of the unchanged drug is excreted in the urine.[305]

Louis et al.[306] reported that following oral administration, peak plasma levels occur in about 1 hr. Comparison between plasma concentrations following oral and i.v. administration in seven hypertensive patients suggested a mean bioavailability of 31%, with a range of 11 to 76% after oral doses. Similarly, an oral dose of 100 mg induced about 40% of the depressor response as the same dose given intravenously. Plasma norepinephrine levels showed a small and transient increase 10 min after i.v. administration. Labetalol had no obvious effects on plasma renin activity.

Although the blood pressure falls in the supine position, there is usually an additional fall in blood pressure on standing, which can occasionally be of sufficient magnitude to induce symptoms of faintness or syncope.[303,306]

The capcity of labetalol to induce α- as well as β-adrenoceptor blockade has raised the possibility that other β-adrenoceptor-blocking agents may possess weak α-blocking properties. It has been suggested that some drugs with what has been previously regarded as being intrinsic sympathomimetic activity, such as pindolol and oxprenolol, may in fact have weak α-blocking properties, mainly on the basis of comparatively weak actions on plasma renin and bronchial smooth muscle, as compared to their antihypertensive properties.[307] This hypothesis is interesting and may have implications for the development of new drugs of this class.

REFERENCES

1. **Korner, P. I.**, Integrative neural cardiovascular control, *Physiol. Rev.*, 51, 312, 1971.
2. **Spickler, J W., Kezdi, P., and Geller, E.**, Transfer characteristics of the carotid sinus pressure control system, in *Baroreceptors and Hypertension*, Kedzi, P., Ed., Pergamon Press, Oxford, 1967, 31.
3. **Diamond, J.**, Observations on the excitation by acetylcholine and by pressure of sensory receptors in the cat's carotid sinus, *J. Physiol. (London)*, 130, 513, 1955.
4. **Glick, G. and Braunwald, E.**, Relative roles of the sympathetic and parasympathetic nervous systems in the reflex control of heart rate, *Cir. Res.*, 26, 363, 1965.
5. **Glick, G. and Covell, J. W.**, Relative importance of the carotid and aortic baroreceptors in the reflex control of heart rate, *Am. J. Physiol.*, 214, 955, 1967.
6. **Wang, S. C. and Chai, C. Y.**, Central control of sympathetic cardiacceleration in medulla oblongata of cat, *Am. J. Physiol.*, 202, 31, 1962.
7. **Brender, D. and Webb-Peploe, M. M.**, Influence of carotid baroreceptors on different components of the vascular system, *J. Physiol. (London)*, 205, 257, 1969.
8. **Folkow, B., Johansson, B., and Löfving, B.**, Aspects of functional differentiation of the sympatho-adrenergic control of the cardiovascular system, *Med. Exp.*, 4, 321, 1961.
9. **Malmejac, J.**, Activity of adrenal medulla and its regulation, *Physiol. Rev.*, 44, 186, 1964.
10. **Share, L. and Levy, M. N.**, Carotid sinus pulse pressure — a determinant of plasma antidiuretic hormone, *Am. J. Physiol.*, 211, 721, 1966.
11. **Paintal, A. S.**, Vagal afferent fibres, *Ergeb. Physiol. Biol. Chem. Exp. Pharmakol.*, 52, 75, 1963.
12. **Gauer, O. H. and Henry, J. P.**, Circulatory basis of fluid control, *Physiol. Rev.*, 43, 423, 1963.
13. **Brown, A. M.**, The depressor reflex arising from the left coronary artery of the cat, *J. Physiol. (London)*, 184, 825, 1966.
14. **Eyzaguirre, C. and Lewin, J.**, Effect of different oxygen tensions on the carotid body in vitro, *J. Physiol. (London)*, 159, 238, 1961.
15. **Hornbein, T. F., Griffo, Z. J., and Roos, A.**, Quantitation of chemoreceptor activity: interrelation of hypoxia and hypercapnia, *J. Neurophysiol.*, 24, 561, 1961.
16. **Daly, M. De B. and Scott, M. J.**, The cardiovascular responses to stimulation of the carotid body chemoreceptors in the dog, *J. Physiol. (London)*, 165, 179, 1963.
17. **Crocker, E. F., Johnson, R. O., Korner, P. I., Uther, J. B., and White, S. W.**, Effects of hyperventilation on the circulatory response of the rabbit to arterial hypoxia, *J. Physiol. (London)*, 199, 267, 1968.
18. **Humphrey, D. R.**, Neuronal activity in the medulla oblongata of cat evoked by stimulation of the carotid sinus nerve, in *Baroreceptors and Hypertension*, Kezdi, P., Ed., Pergamon Press, Oxford, 1967, 131.
19. **Muira, M. and Reis, D. J.**, Termination and secondary projections of carotid sinus nerve in the cat brain stem, *Am. J. Physiol.*, 217, 142, 1969.
20. **Fuxe, K.**, Evidence for the existence of monoamine neurons in the central nervous system. IV. Distribution of monoamine nerve terminals in the central nervous system, *Acta Physiol. Scand.*, 64 (Suppl. 247), 1965.
21. **Palkovits, M. and Jacobowitz, D. M.**, Topographic atlas of catecholamine and acetyl- cholinesterase-containing neurons in the rat brain II. Hindbrain (mesencephalon, rhombencephalon), *J. Comp. Neurol.*, 157, 29, 1974.
22. **Versteeg, D. H. G., Van der Gugten, de Jong, W., and Palkovits, M.**, Regional concentration of noradrenaline and dopamine in rat brain, *Brain Res.*, 113, 563, 1976.
23. **Van der Gugten, J., Palkovits, M., Wijnen, H. L. J. M., and Versteeg, D. H. G.**, Regional distribution of adrenaline in rat brain, *Brain Res.*, 107, 171, 1976.
24. **Doba, N. and Reis, D. J.**, Acute fulminating neurogenic hypertension produced by brainstem lesions in the rat, *Circ. Res.*, 32, 584, 1973.
25. **Doba, N. and Reis, D. J.**, Role of central and peripheral mechanisms in hypertension produced by brainstem lesions in the rat, *Circ. Res.*, 34, 293, 1974.
26. **Nathan, M. A. and Reis, D. J.**, Chronic labile hypertension produced by lesions of the nucleus tractus solitarii in the cat, *Circ. Res.*, 40, 72, 1977.
27. **de Jong, W. and Palkovits, M.**, Hypertension after localized transsection of brainstem fibres, *Life Sci*, 18, 61, 1976.
28. **Palkovits, M., de Jong, W., Zandberg, P., Versteeg, D. H. G., Van der Gugten, J. and Leranth, C.**, Central hypertension and nucleus tractus solitarius catecholamines after surgical lesions of the medulla, *Brain Res.*, 127, 307, 1977.
29. **de Jong, W., Nijkamp, F. P., and Bohus, B.**, Role of noradrenaline and serotonin in the central control of blood pressure in normotensive and spontaneously hypertensive rats, *Arch. Int. Pharmacodyn. Ther.*, 213, 272, 1975.

30. **Dahlström, A. and Fuxe, K.**, Evidence for the existence of monoamine neurons in the central nervous system. II. Experimentally induced changes in the intraneuronal amine levels of bulbospinal neuron systems, *Acta Physiol. Scand.*, 64 (Suppl.), 247, 1965.

31. **Chalmers, J. P. and Wurtman, R. J.**, Participation of central noradrenergic neurons in arterial baroreceptor reflexes in the rabbit, *Circ. Res.*, 28, 480, 1971.

32. **Haeusler, G. and Lewis, P. J.**, The relationship of central noradrenergic neurones to the baroreflex arc, in *Central Action of Drugs in Blood Pressure Regulation*, Davies, D. S. and Reid, J. L., Eds., Pitman Medical, Kent, U.K., 1975, 63.

33. **Hilton, S. M.**, Hypothalamic control of the cardiovascular responses in fear and rage, *Lect. Sci. Basis Med.*, 8, 217, 1965.

34. **Wilson, M. F., Clarke, N. P., Smith, D. A., and Rushmer, R. F.**, Interrelation between central and peripheral mechanisms regulating blood pressure, *Circ. Res.*, 9, 491, 1961.

35. **Gebber, G. L. and Snyder, D. W.**, Hypothalamic control of baroreceptor reflexes, *Am. J. Physiol.*, 218, 124, 1970.

36. **Philippu, A., Roensberg, W., and Przuntek, H.**, Effects of adrenergic drugs on pressor responses to hypothalamic stimulation, *Naunyn Schmiedebergs Arch. Pharmakol.*, 278, 373, 1973.

37. **Philippu, A., Demmeler, R., and Roensberg, W.**, Effects of centrally applied drugs on pressor responses to hypothalamic stimulation, *Naunyn Schmiedebergs Arch. Pharmakol.*, 282, 389, 1974.

38. **Folkow, B., Langston, J., Öberg, B., and Prerovsky, I.**, Reactions of the different series-coupled vascular sections upon stimulation of the hypothalamic sympatho-inhibitory area, *Acta Physiol. Scand.*, 61, 476, 1964.

39. **Phillipu, A. and Schartner, P.**, Inhibition by locally applied alpha-adrenoreceptor blocking drugs of the depressor response to stimulation of the anterior hypothalamus, *Naunyn Schmiedebergs Arch. Pharmakol.*, 295, 1, 1976.

40. **Klebens, L. R. and Gebber, G. L.**, Facilitatory forebrain influence on cardiac component of baroreceptor reflexes, *Am. J. Physiol.*, 219, 1235, 1970.

41. **Axelrod, J. and Weinshilboum, R.**, Catecholamines, *N. Engl. J. Med.*, 287, 237, 1972.

42. **Cubeddu, L., Barnes, X. E., and Weiner, N.**, Release of norepinephrine and dopamine-β-hydroxylase by nerve stimulation. IV. An evaluation of a role for cyclic adenosine monophosphate, *J. Pharmacol. Exp. Ther.*, 193, 105, 1974.

43. **Langer, S. Z., Enero, M. A., Adler-Graschinsky, W., Dubocovich, M. L., and Celuch, S. M.**, Presynaptic regulatory mechanisms for noradrenaline release by nerve stimulation, in *Central Action of Drugs in Blood Pressure Regulation*, Davies, D. S. and Reid, J. L., Eds., Pitman Medical, Kent, U.K., 1975, 133.

44. **Zimmerman, B. G. and Gomez, J.**, Increased response to sympathetic stimulation in the cutaneous vasculature in presence of angiotensin, *Int. J. Neuropharmacol.*, 4, 185, 1965.

45. **Boadle, M. C., Hughes, J., and Roth, R. H.**, Angiotensin accelerates catecholamine biosynthesis in sympathetically innervated tissues, *Nature (London)*, 222, 987, 1969.

46. **Rand, M. J., McCulloch, M. W., and Story, D. F.**, Pre-junctional modulation of noradrenergic transmission by noradrenaline, dopamine and acetylcholine in *Central Actions of Drugs in Blood Pressure Regulation*, Davies, D. S. and Reid, J. L., Eds., Pitman Medical, Kent, U.K., 1975, 94.

47. **Celuch, S. M., Dubocovich, M. L., and Langer, S. Z.**, Stimulation of pre-synaptic β-adrenoceptors enhances 3 H-noradrenaline release during nerve stimulation in the perfused cat spleen, *Br. J. Pharmacol.*, 63, 97, 1978.

48. **Dahlof, C., Ablad, B., Borg, K. O., Ek, L., and Waldeck, B.**, Pre-junctional inhibition of adrenergic nervous control due to β-receptor blockade, in *Chemical Tools in Catecholamine Research*, Vol. 2, Almgren, O., Carlsson, A., and Engel, J., Eds., Elsevier, Amsterdam, 1975, 201.

49. **Langer, S. Z.**, The role of α and β-presynaptic receptors in the regulation of noradrenaline release elicited by nerve stimulation, *Clin. Sci. Mol. Med.*, 51, 423S, 1976.

50. **Triner, L., Nahas, G. G., Vulliemoz, Y., Overweg, N. I. A., Verosky, M., Habif, D. V., and Ngai, S. H.**, Cyclic AMP and smooth muscle function, *Ann. N.Y. Acad. Sci.*, 185, 458, 1971.

51. **Shepherd, A. P., Mao, C.C., Jacobson, E. D., and Shanbour, L. L.**, The role of cyclic AMP in mesenteric vasodilatation, *Microvas. Res.*, 6, 332, 1973.

52. **Hamet, P. and Kuchel, O.**, Cyclic nucleotides and control of blood pressure: implication for hypertension, in *Hypertension*, Genest, J., Koiw, E., and Kuchel, O., Eds., McGraw-Hill, New York, 1977, 411.

53. **Burnstock, G.**, Innervation of vascular smooth muscle: histochemistry and electron microscopy, *Clin. Exp. Pharmacol. Physiol.*, 2 (Suppl. 2), 8, 1975.

54. **Furness, J. B.**, Arrangement of blood vessels and their relation with adrenergic nerves in the rat mesentery, *J. Anat.*, 115, 347, 1973.

55. **Dahl, E.**, The innervation of cerebral arteries, *J. Anat.*, 115, 53, 1973.

56. **Brod, J., Fencl, V., Hejl, Z., and Jirka, J.,** Circulatory changes underlying blood pressure elevation during acute emotional stress (mental arithmetic) in normotensive and hypertensive subjects, *Clin. Sci.,* 18, 269, 1959.

57. **Folkow, B., Heymans, C., and Neil, E.,** Integrated aspects of cardiovascular regulation, in *The Handbook of Physiology,* Vol. 3, American Physiological Society, Washington, D.C., 1965, chap. 49, 1787.

58. **Mancia, G., Bacelli, G., and Zanchetti, A.,** Haemodynamic responses to different emotional stimuli in the cat: patterns and mechanisms, *Am. J. Physiol.,* 223, 975, 1972.

59. **Brod, J.,** Haemodynamic patterns of acute pressor reactions and hypertension, *Br. Heart J.,* 25, 227, 1963.

60. **Boyer, J. T., Fraser, J. R. E., and Doyle, A. E.,** The haemodynamic effects of cold immersion, *Clin. Sci.,* 19, 539, 1960.

61. **Hines, E. A. and Brown, G. E.,** The cold pressor test for measuring the reactivity of the blood pressure: data concerning 571 normal and hypertensive subjects, *Am. Heart J.,* 11, 1, 1936.

62. **Pickering, G. W. and Kissin, M.,** The effects of adrenaline and of cold on the blood pressure in human hypertension, *Clin. Sci.,* 2, 201, 1936.

63. **Alam, G. M. and Smirk, F. H.,** Blood pressure raising reflexes in health, essential hypertension and renal hypertension, *Clin. Sci.,* 3, 259, 1938.

64. **Russek, H. I. and Zohman, B. L.,** The influence of age upon blood pressure response to the cold pressor test, *Am. Heart J.,* 29, 113, 1945.

65. **Barath, E.,** Arterial hypertension and physical work, *Arch. Intern. Med.,* 42, 297, 1928.

66. **Wolff, H. H.,** The mechanism and significance of the cold pressor response, *Q. J. Med.,* 20, 261, 1951.

67. **Fowler, P. B. S. and Guz, A.,** Blood pressure during exercise and the effect of hexamethonium, *Br. Heart J.,* 16, 1, 1954.

68. **Brooks, H. and Carrol, J. H.,** A clinical study of the effects of sleep and rest on blood pressure, *Arch. Intern. Med.,* 10, 97, 1912.

69. **Alam, G. M.,** Casual and basal blood pressures. II. In essential hypertension, *Br. Heart J.,* 5, 156, 1943.

70. **Addis, T.,** Blood pressure and pulse rate levels, *Arch. Intern. Med.,* 29, 539, 1922.

71. **Richardson, D. W., Honour, A. J., Fenton, G. W., Stott, F. H., and Pickering, G. W.,** Variation in arterial pressure throughout day and night, *Clin. Sci.,* 26, 445, 1964.

72. **Smirk, F. H.,** Casual, basal and supplemental blood pressures in 519 first-degree relatives of substantial hypertensive patients and in 350 population controls, *Clin. Sci. Mol. Med.,* 51, 13S, 1976.

73. **Smirk, F. H. and Hall, W. H.,** Inherited hypertension in rats, *Nature (London),* 182, 727, 1958.

74. **Okamoto, K. and Aoki, K.,** Development of a strain of spontaneously hypertensive rats, *Jpn. Circ. J.,* 27, 282, 1963.

75. **Henry, J. P., Stephens, P. M., and Santisteban, G. A.,** A model of psychosocial hypertension showing reversibility and progression of cardiovascular complications, *Circ. Res.,* 36, 156, 1975.

76. **Hallbäck, M.,** Consequence of social isolation on blood pressure, cardiovascular reactivity and design in spontaneously hypertensive rats, *Acta Physiol. Scand.,* 93, 455, 1975.

77. **Herd, J. A., Morse, W. H., Kelleher, R. T.,and Jones, L. G.,** Arterial hypertension in the squirrel monkey during behavioural experiments, *Am. J. Physiol.,* 217, 24, 1969.

78. **Benson, H., Herd, J. A., Morse, W. H., and Kelleher, R. T.,** Behaviourally induced hypertension in the squirrel monkey, *Circ. Res.,* 21 (Suppl. 1), 26, 1970.

79. **Graham, J. D. P.,** High blood pressure after battle, *Lancet,* 1, 239, 1945.

80. **Ruskin, A., Beard, O. W., and Shaffer, R. L.,** Blast hypertension: elevated arterial pressure in victims of Texas City disaster, *Am. J. Med.,* 4, 228, 1948.

81. **Wolf, S., Wolff, H. G., Cardon, P. V., Jr., and Shepherd, E. M.,** *Life Stress and Essential Hypertension,* Williams & Wilkins, Baltimore, 1955.

82. **Hambling, J.,** Psychosomatic aspects of essential hypertension, *Br. J. Med. Psychol.,* 25, 39, 1952.

83. **Van der Valk, J. M.,** Blood pressure changes under emotional influences in patients with essential hypertension and control subjects, *J. Psychosom. Res.,* 2, 134, 1957.

84. **Harburg, E., Erfurt, J. C., Hauenstein, L. S., Chape, C., Schull, W. J., and Schork, M. A.,** Socio-ecological stress, suppressed hostility, skin colour, and black-white male blood pressure: Detroit, *Psychosom. Med.,* 35, 276, 1973.

85. **Sokolow, M., Werdegar, D., Perloff, D. B., Cowan, R. M., and Brenenstuhl, H.,** Preliminary studies relating portably recorded blood pressures to daily life events in patients with essential hypertension, *Bibl. Psychiatr.,* 144, 164, 1970.

86. **Bevan, A. T., Honor, A. J., and Scott, F. H.,** Direct arterial pressure recording in unrestricted man, *Clin. jsci.,* 36, 329, 1969.

87. **Chalmers, J. P.,** Brain amines and models of experimental hypertension, *Circ. Res.,* 36, 469, 1975.

88. **Phillipu, A., Przuntek, H., Heyd, G., and Burger, A.**, Central effects of sympathomimetic amines on the blood pressure, *Eur. J. Pharmacol.*, 15, 200, 1971.

89. **Ito, A. and Schanberg, S. M.**, Maintenance of tonic vasomotor activity by alpha and beta adrenergic mechanisms in medullary cardiovascular centres, *J. Pharmacol. Exp. Ther.*, 189, 392, 1974.

90. **Chalmers, J. P. and Wurtman, R. J.**, Participation of central noradrenergic neurons in arterial baroreceptor reflexes in the rabbit, *Circ. Res.*, 28, 480, 1971.

91. **Haeusler, G., Finch, L., and Thoenen, T.**, Cardiovascular effects of 6-hydroxydopamine injected into a lateral brain ventricle of the rat, *Naunyn Schmiedebergs Arch. Pharmakol.*, 274, 211, 1972.

92. **Chalmers, J. P. and Reid, J. L.**, Participation of central noradrenergic neurons in arterial baroreceptor reflexes in the rabbit: a study with intracisternally administered 6 hydroxydopamine, *Circ. Res.*, 31, 789, 1975.

93. **de Champlain, J. and van Ameringen, M. R.**, Regulation of blood pressure by sympathetic fibers and adrenal medulla in normotensive and hypertensive rats, *Circ. Res.*, 31, 617, 1972.

94. **Heymans, C. and Neil, E.**, *Reflexogenic Areas of The Cardiovascular System*, Churchill Livingstone, London, 1958.

95. **Korner, P. I.**, Effect of section of the carotid sinus and aortic nerves on the cardiac output of the rabbit, *J. Physiol. (London)*, 180, 266, 1965.

96. **Wing, L. M. H. and Chalmers, J. P.**, Participation of central serotonergic neurones in the control of the circulation of the unanaesthetized rabbit. A study using 5-6 dihydroxy tryptamine in experimental neurogenic and renal hypertension, *Circ. Res.*, 35, 504, 1974.

97. **McCubbin, J. W., Green, J. H., and Page, I. H.**, Baroreceptor function in chronic renal hypertension, *Circ. Res.*, 4, 205, 1956.

98. **Angell-James, J. E.**, Characteristics of single aortic and right subclavian baroreceptor fibre activity in rabbits with chronic renal hypertension, *Circ. Res.*, 37, 149, 1973.

99. **Bristow, J. D., Honor, A. J., Pickering, G. W., Sleight, P., and Smyth, H. S.**, Diminished baroreceptor sensitivity in high blood pressure, *Circ. Res.*, 29, 48, 1969.

100. **Korner, P. I.**, Central and peripheral resetting of the baroreceptor system, *Clin. Exp. Pharmacol. Physiol.*, 2 (Suppl. 2), 171, 1975.

101. **Kezdi, P.**, Mechanism of altered blood pressure regulation in arterial hypertension, in *Aktuelle Hypertonieprobleme*, Georg Thieme Verlag, Stuttgart, 1973, 16.

102. **Dargie, H. J., Franklin, S. S., and Reid, J. L.**, Plasma noradrenaline concentrations in experimental renovascular hypertension in the rat, *Clin. Sci. Mol. Med.*, 52, 477, 1977.

103. **Lewis, P. J., Reid, J. L., Chalmers, J. P., and Dollery, C. T.**, Importance of central catecholaminergic neurons in the development of renal hypertension, *Clin. Sci.*, 45, 115s, 1973.

104. **Finch, L., Haeusler, G., and Thoenen, H.**, Failure to induce experimental hypertension after intraventricular injection of 6-hydroxydopamine, *Br. J. Pharmacol.*, 44, 356P, 1972.

105. **Ayitey-Smith, E. and Varma, D. R.**, An assessment of the role of the sympathetic nervous system in experimental hypertension using normal and immunosympathectomized rats, *Br. J. Pharmacol.*, 40, 175, 1970.

106. **Axelrod, J.**, Catecholamines and hypertension, *Clin. Sci. Mol. Med.*, 51, 415s, 1976.

107. **Reid, J. L., Zivin, J. A., and Kopin, I. J.**, Central and peripheral adrenergic mechanisms in the development of de-oxycorticosterone-saline hypertension of rats, *Circ. Res.*, 37, 569, 1975.

108. **Nakamura, K., Gerold, M., and Thoenen, H.**, Experimental hypertension in the rat: reciprocal changes of norepinephrine turnover in heart and brain-stem, *Naunyn Schmiedebergs Arch. Exp. Pathol. Pharmakol.*, 268, 125, 1971.

109. **Mueller, R. A., Thoenen, H., and Axelrod, J.**, Adrenal tyrosine hydroxylase: compensatory increase in activity after chemical sympathectomy, *Science*, 163, 468, 1969.

110. **de Champlain, J., Krakoff, L. R., and Axelrod, J.**, The metabolism of norepinephrine in experimental hypertension in rats, *Circ. Res.*, 20, 136, 1967.

111. **Krakoff, L. R., de Champlain, J., and Axelrod, J.**, Abnormal storage of norepinephrine in experimental hypertension in the rat, *Circ. Res.*, 21, 583, 1967.

112. **de Champlain, J., Mueller, R. A., and Axelrod, J.**, Turnover and synthesis of norepinephrine in experimental hypertension, *Circ. Res.*, 25, 285, 1969.

113. **de Champlain, J., Krakoff, L. R., and Axelrod, J.**, Interrelationsip of sodium intake, hypertension and norepinephrine storage in the rat, *Circ. Res.*, 24, Suppl. 1, 75, 1969.

114. **de Champlain, J., Farley, L., Cousineau, D., and van Ameringen, M. R.**, Circulating catecholamine levels in human and experimental hypertension, *Circ. Res.*, 38, 109, 1976.

115. **de Champlain, J., Krakoff, L. R., and Axelrod, J.**, Relationship between sodium intake and norepinephrine storage during the development of experimental hypertension, *Circ. Res.*, 23, 479, 1968.

116. **Finch, L. and Leach, G. D. H.**, The contribution of the sympathetic nervous system to the development and maintenance of experimental hypertension in the rat, *Br. J. Pharmacol.*, 39, 317, 1970.

117. Clarke, D. E., Smookler, H. H., and Barry, H., Sympathetic nerve function and DOCA-NaCl induced hypertension, *Life Sci.*, 9, 1097, 1970.

118. de Champlain, J., Degeneration and regrowth of adrenergic nerve fibers in the rat in peripheral tissues after 6-hydroxydopamine, *Can. J. Physiol. Pharmacol.*, 49, 345, 1971.

119. Hinke, J. A. M., In vitro demonstration of vascular hyper responsiveness in experimental hypertension *Circ. Res.*, 18, 359, 1965.

120. Dusting, G. J., Harris, G. S., and Rand, M. J., Specific increase in cardiovascular reactivity related to sodium retention in DOCA salt treated rats, *Clin. Sci. Mol. Med.*, 45, 571, 1973.

121. Guyton, A. C., Coleman, T. G., Cowley, A. W., Jr., Manning, R. D., Jr., and Norman, R. A., Jr., A systems analysis approach to understanding long range arterial blood pressure control and hypertension, *Circ. Res.*, 35, 159, 1974.

122. de Champlain, J., Hypertension and the sympathetic nervous system, in *Perspectives in Neuropharmacology*, Snyder, S. M., Ed., Oxford University Press, New York, 1972, 215.

123. Volicer, L., Scheer, E., Hilse, H., and Visweswaram, D., Turnover of norepinephrine in the heart during experimental hypertension in rats, *Life Sci.*, 7, 525, 1968.

124. Henning, M., Noradrenaline turnover in renal hypertensive rats, *J. Pharm. Pharmacol.*, 21, 61, 1969.

125. Lefer, L. G. and Ayers, C. R., Norepinephrine metabolism in dogs with chronic renovascular hypertension, *Proc. Soc. Exp. Biol. Med.*, 132, 278, 1969.

126. Wegmann, A., Kako, K., and Bing, R. J., Catecholamine content of various organs in experimental hypertension, *Am. J. Physiol.* 203, 607, 1962.

127. Brodie, M. J., Dorr, L. D., and Schaffer, R. A., Reflex vasodilatation and sympathetic transmission in the renal hypertensive dog, *Am. J. Physiol.*, 219, 1746, 1970.

128. Zimmerman, B. G., Rolewicz, T. F., Dunham, E. W., and Gisslen, J. L., Transmitter release and vascular responses in skin and muscle of hypertensive dogs, *Am. J. Physiol.*, 27, 798, 1969.

129. Zimmerman, B. G., Evaluation of peripheral and central component of action of angiotensin on the sympathetic nervous system, *J. Pharmacol. Exp. Ther.*, 158, 1, 1967.

130. Zimmerman, B. G. and Gisslen, J. L., Pattern of renal vasoconstriction and transmitter release during sympathetic nervous stimulation, *J. Pharmacol. Exp. Ther.*, 163, 320, 1968.

131. Volicer, L. and Visweswaram, D., The effect of angiotensin on the turnover rate of norepinephrine in the heart, *Life Sci.*, 9, 651, 1970.

132. de Champlain, J. and van Ameringen, M. R., Role of sympathetic fibers and of adrenal medulla in the maintenance of cardiovascular homeostasis in normotensive and hypertensive rats, in *Frontiers in Catecholamine Research*, Usdin, E. and Snyder, S., Eds., Pergamon Press, New York, 1973, 951.

133. Smirk, F. H., The neurogenically maintained component in hypertension, in *Hypertension XXVII; Hypertensive Mechanisms*, Reader, R., Ed., *Circ. Res.*, 26 and 27, (Suppl. 2), 55, 1970.

134. Iriuchijima, J., Role of splanchnic nerves in spontaneously hypertensive rats, *Jpn. Circ. J.*, 37, 1251, 1973.

135. Yamori, Y., Ooshima, A., and Okamoto, K., Deviation of central norepinephrine metabolism in the spontaneously hypertensive rat, *Jpn. Heart J.*, 8, 168, 1967.

136. Louis, W. J., Tabei, R., Spector, S., and Sjoerdsma, A., Studies on the spontaneously hypertensive rats: genealogy, effects of varying salt intake and kinetics of catecholamine metabolism, in *Hypertension XVII. Experimental Hypertension*, Mulrow, P. J., Ed., *Circ. Res.*, 24 and 25, (Suppl. 1), 93, 1969.

137. Doyle, A. E. and Smirk, F. H., The neurogenic component in hypertension, *Circulation*, 12, 543, 1955.

138. Korner, P. I., Shaw, J., Uther, J. B., West, M. J., McRitchie, R. J., and Richards, J. G., Autonomic and non-autonomic circulatory components in essential hypertension in man, *Circulation*, 48, 107, 1973.

139. Engelman, K., Portnoy, B., and Lovenberg, W., A sensitive and specific double isotope derivative method for the determination of catecholamines in biological tissues, *Am. J. Sci.*, 225, 259, 1968.

140. Engelman, K., Portnoy, B., and Sjoerdsma, A., Plasma catecholamine concentrations in patients with hypertension, in *Hypertension, XVIII, Circ. Res.*, 27, (Suppl. 1), 141, 1970.

141. De Quattro, V. and Chan, S., Raised plasma-catecholamines in some patients with primary hypertension, *Lancet*, 1, 806, 1972.

142. de Champlain, J., Farley, L., Cousineau, D., and van Ameringen, M. R., Circulating catecholamine levels in human and experimental hypertension, *Circ. Res.*, 38, 109, 1976.

143. Louis, W. J., Doyle, A. E., and Anavekar, S. N., Plasma norepinephrine levels in essential hypertension, *N. Engl. J. Med.*, 288, 599, 1973.

144. Sever, P. S., Birch, M., Osikowska, B., and Tunbridge, R. D. G., Plasma nor-adrenaline in essential hypertension, *Lancet*, 1, 1078, 1977.

145. Ziegler, M. G., Lake, C. R., and Kopin, I. J., Plasma noradrenaline increases with age, *Nature (London)*, 261, 333, 1976.

146. Distler, A., Phillip, T., and Cordes, U., Interrelations between sympathetic responsiveness and blood pressure response to noradrenaline in patients with essential hypertension, in *Circulatory Catecholamines and Blood Pressure,* Birkenhager, W., Ed., in press.

147. Louis, W. J., Doyle, A. E., Anavekar, S. N., and Johnston, C. I., Plasma catecholamine, dopamine beta hydroxylase and renin levels in hypertension, in *Hypertension, Current Problems,* Distler, A. and Wolff, H. P., Eds., Georg Thieme Verlag, Stuttgart, 1973, 269.

148. Geffen, L. B., Rush, R. A., Louis, W. J., and Doyle, A. E., Plasma dopamine β-hydroxylase and noradrenaline amounts in essential hypertension, *Clin. Sci.,* 44, 617, 1973.

149. Horwitz, D., Alexander, R. W., Lovenberg, W., and Keiser, H. R., Human serum dopamine-β-hydroxylase: relationship to hypertension and sympathetic activity, *Circ. Res.,* 32, 594, 1973.

150. Abbey, H., Wetterberg, L., Ross, S. B., and Fröden, O., Dopamine-β-hydroxylase in hypertension, *Acta Med. Scand.,* 196, 17, 1974.

151. Rush, R. A., Thomas, P. E., Nagatsu, T., and Udenfriend, S., Comparison of human serum dopamine-β-hydroxylase levels by radioimmunoassay and enzymatic assay, *Proc. Natl. Acad. Sci. U.S.A.,* 71, 782, 1974.

152. Constantine, J. W. and McShane, W. K., Analysis of the cardiovascular effects of 2-(2,6-dichlorophenylamino)-2-imidazoline hydrochloride (Catapres), *Eur. J. Pharmacol.,* 4, 109, 1968.

153. Hoefke, W. and Kobinger, W., Pharmakologische Wirkungen des 2-(2,6-dichlorophenylamino)-2-imidazolino hydrochlorids, einer neuen antihypertensiven substanz, *Arzneim. Forsch.,* 16, 1038, 1966.

154. Schmitt, H. and Schmitt, H., Localization of the hypotensive effect of 2-(2,6-dichlorophenylamino)-2-imidazoline hydrochloride (St 155, Catapresan), *Eur. J. Pharmacol.,* 6, 8, 1969.

155. Satler, R. W. and Van Zwieten, P. A., Acute hypotensive action of 2-(2-6,dichlorophenylamino)2-imidazoline hydrochloride (St 155) after infusion into cat's vertebral artery, *Eur. J. Pharmacol.,* 2, 9, 1967.

156. Kobinger, W. and Walland, A., Investigations into the mechanism of the hypotensive effect of 2-(2-6,dichlorophenylamino)-2-imidazoline-HCl, *Eur. J. Pharmacol.,* 2, 155, 1967.

157. Reid, J. L., Clonidine and central noradrenaline turnover, in *Central Actions of Drugs in Blood Pressure Regulation,* Davies, D. L. and Reid, J. L., Eds., Pitman Medical, Kent, U.K., 1975, 194.

158. Kobinger, W. and Pilcher, L., Evidence for direct α-adrenoceptor stimulation of effector neurones in cardiovascular centres by clonidine, *Eur. J. Pharmacol.,* 27, 151, 1974.

159. Sinha, J. N., Tangi, K. K., Bhargava, K. P., and Schmitt, H., Central sites of sympatho-inhibitory effects of clonidine and l-dopa, in *Recent Advances in Hypertension,* Milliez, P. and Safar, M., Eds., Boehringer Ingelheim, Reims, 1975, 97.

160. de Jong, W., Noradrenaline: central inhibitory control of blood pressure and heart rate, *Eur. J. Pharmacol.,* 29, 179, 1974.

161. Struyker-Boudier, H. A. J., Clinidine induced cardiovascular effects following stereotaxic application in the hypothalamus of rats, *J. Pharm. Pharmacol.,* 24, 410, 1972.

162. Zaimis, E., On the pharmacology of Catapres (St 155), in *Catapres in Hypertension,* Connolly, E. M., Ed., Butterworths, London, 1970, 9.

163. Fügner, A. and Hoefke, W., A sleeplike state in chicks caused by biogenic amines and other compounds: quantitative evaluation, *Arzneim. Forsch.,* 21, 1243, 1971.

164. Fügner, A., Antagonism of the drug-induced behavioural sleep in chicks, *Arzneim. Forsch.,* 21, 1350, 1971.

165. Rand, M. J., Rush, M., and Wilson, J., Some observations on the inhibition of salivation by St 155, 2-(2-6 dichlorophenylamino) 2-imidazoline hydrochloride, Catapres®, Catapresan®, *Eur. J. Pharmacol.,* 5, 169, 1969.

166. Rand, M. J. and Wilson, J., Mechanisms of the pressor and depressor actions of St 155; Catapres, *Eur. J. Pharmacol.,* 3, 27, 1968.

167. Nayler, W. G. and Stone, J., An effect of St 155 (clonidine) 2-(2,-6 dichlorophenylamino) 2-imidazoline hydrochloride, Catapres, on relationship between blood pressure and heart rate in dogs, *Eur. J. Pharmacol.,* 10, 161, 1970.

168. Finnerty, F. A., Onesti, G., and Schwartz, A. G., Antihypertensive effects of clonidine, *Circ. Res.,* 28 and 29, (Suppl. 2), 69, 1971.

169. Barnett, A. J. and Cantor, S., Observations on the hypotensive actions of "Catapres", St 155 in man, *Med. J. Aust.,* 1, 87, 1968.

170. Doyle, A. E., Anavekar, S. N., Louis, W. J., and Morgan, T. O., Antihypertensive drug treatment and plasma renin, in *Systemic Effects of Antihypertensive Agents,* Sambhi, M. P., Ed., Stratton Intercontinental, New York, 1976, 185.

171. Zanchetti, A., Leonetti, G., Morganti, A., Terzoli, L., Schwartz, E., Manfrin, M., and Bernasconi, M., Longitudinal study of plasma renin activity in hypertensive patients under antihypertensive treatment including diuretics, in *Systemic Effects of Antihypertensive Agents,* Sambhi, M. P., Ed., Stratton Intercontinental, N.Y., 1976, 251.

172. Brod, J., Horbach, J., Just, H., Rosenthal, J., and Nicolescu, R., Acute effects of clonidine on central and peripheral haemodynamics and on plasma renin activity, *Eur. J. Clin. Pharmacol.,* 4, 107, 1972.

173. Hunyor, S. N., Hansson, L., Harrison, T. S., and Hoobler, S. W., Effects of clonidine withdrawal: possible mechanisms and suggestions for management, *Br. Med. J.,* 2, 209, 1973.

174. Wilkins, R. W., New drug therapies in arterial hypertension, *Am. Intern. Med.,* 37, 1144, 1952.

175. Doyle, A. E. and Smirk, F. H., Hypotensive action of reserpine, *Lancet,* 1, 1096, 1954.

176. Doyle, A. E., McQueen, E. G., and Smirk, F. H., Treatment of hypertension with reserpine, with reserpine in combination with pentapyrollidinium, and with reserpine in combination with veratrum alkaloids, *Circulation,* 11, 170, 1955.

177. Freis, E. D. and Ari, R., Clinical and experimental effects of reserpine in patients with essential hypertension, *Ann. N.Y. Acad. Sci.,* 59, 45, 1954.

178. Wilkins, R. W. and Judson, W. E., The use of rauwolfia serpentina in hypertensive patients, *N. Engl. J. Med.,* 248, 48, 1953.

179. Carlsson, A., Pharmacology of the sympathetic nervous system, in *Antihypertensive Therapy, Principles and Practice, International Symposium,* Gross, F., Ed., Springer-Verlag, New York, 1966, 5.

180. Häggendahl, J. and Dahlström, A., The recovery of the capacity for uptake retention of [H^3]noradrenaline in rat adrenergic nerves after reserpine, *J. Pharm. Pharmacol.,* 24, 565, 1972.

181. Trendelenburg, U., Supersensitivity and sub-sensitivity to sympathomimetic amines, *Pharmacol. Rev.,* 15, 225, 1963.

182. Freis, E. D., Mental depression in hypertensive patients treated for long periods with large doses of reserpine, *N. Engl. J. Med.,* 251, 1006, 1954.

183. Boston Collaboration Drug Surveillance Program, Reserpine and breast cancer, *Lancet,* 2, 669, 1974.

184. Armstong, B., Stevens, N., and Doll, R., Retrospective study of the association between use of rauwolfia derivatives and breast cancer in English women, *Lancet,* 2, 672, 1974.

185. Heinonen, O. P., Shapiro, S., Tuominen, L., and Turunen, M. I., Reserpine use in relation to breast cancer, *Lancet,* 2, 675, 1974.

186. Sjoerdsma, A., Oates, J. A., and Zaltzman, P., Serotonin synthesis in carcinoid patients: its inhibition by alphamethyl dopa, with measurement of associated increases in urinary 5-hydroxytryptophan, *N. Engl. J. Med.,* 263, 585, 1960.

187. Oates, J. A., Gillespie, L., Udenfriend, S., and Sjoerdsma, A., Decarboxylase inhibition and blood pressure reduction by alphamethyl 3,4-dihydroxy dl phenylalanine, *Science,* 131, 1890, 1960.

188. Gillespie, L., Oates, J. A., Crout, J. R., and Sjoerdsma, A., Clnical and chemical studies with alphamethyl dopa in patients with hypertension, *Circulation,* 25, 281, 1962.

189. Carlsson, A. and Lindqvist, M., In vivo decarboxylation of alphamethyl dopa and alphamethyl metatyrosine in vivo, *Acta Physiol. Scand.,* 54, 87, 1962.

190. Day, M. D. and Rand, M. J., A hypothesis for the mode of action of alpha-methyl dopa in relieving hypertension, *J. Pharm. Pharmacol.,* 15, 221, 1963.

191. Trinker, F. R., The significance of the relative potencies of noradrenaline and alphamethyl noradrenaline for the mode of action of alphamethyl dopa, *J. Pharm. Pharmacol.,* 23, 306, 1971.

192. Heise, A. and Kroneberg, G., α Sympathetic stimulation in the brain and hypotensive activity of α methyldopa, *Eur. J. Pharmacol.,* 17, 315, 1972.

193. Heise, A. and Kroneberg, G., Central nervous adrenergic receptors and the mode of action of alpha methyl dopa, *Naunyn Schmiedelbergs Arch. Pharmakol.,* 268, 348, 1973

194. Heise, A., Hypotensive action by central α-adrenergic and dopaminergic receptor stimulation, in *New Antihypertensive Drugs,* Scriabine, A. and Sweet, C. S., Eds., Spectrum Publications, New York, 1976, 135.

195. Finch, L., Hersom, A., and Hicks, P., The central regulation of blood pressure by sympathomimetics, in *Recent Advances in Hypertension,* Milliez, P. and Safar, M., Eds., Boehringer Ingelheim, Reims, 1975, 73.

196. Kersting, F., Reid, J. L., and Dollery, C. T., Site of action of methyl dopa in lowering the blood pressure in man, *Clin. Exp. Pharmacol. Physiol.* (Suppl. 4), in press.

197. Louis, W. J., Vajda, F. J. E., McNeil, J. J., and Doyle, A. E., The combined use of L-alphamethyl dopa hydrazine and methyldopa in the treatment of hypertension, *Clin. Exp. Pharmacol. Physiol.* (Suppl. 4), in press.

198. Sjoerdsma, A., Vendsalu, A., and Engelman, K., Studies on the metabolism and mechanism of action of methyl dopa, *Circulation,* 28, 492, 1963.

199. **Sannerstedt, R., Varnauskas, E., and Werko, L.**, Hemodynamic effects of methyl dopa (Aldomet) at rest and during exercise in patients with hypertension, *Acta Med. Scand.*, 171, 75, 1961.

200. **Lund-Johansen, P.**, Haemodynamic changes in long term alpha-methyl dopa therapy of essential hypertension, *Acta Med. Scand.*, 192, 221, 1972.

201. **Chai, C. Y. and Wang, S. C.**, Cardiovascular actions of diazepam in the cat, *J. Pharmacol. Exp. Ther.*, 154, 271, 1966.

202. **Sigg, E. B. and Sigg, T. D.**, Hypothalamic stimulation of preganglionic autonomic activity and its modification by chlorpromazine, diazepam and pentobarbital, *Neuropharmacology*, 8, 567, 1969.

203. **Antonaccio, M. J. and Halley, J.**, Physiological and pharmacological aspects of the central regulation of blood pressure, in *New Antihypertensive Drugs*, Scriabine, A. and Sweet, C. S., Eds., Spectrum Publications, New York, 1976, 147.

204. **Scholtysik, G. and Jerie, P.**, Pharmacological and clinical effects of BS 100-141, a new antihypertensive agent, in *New Antihypertensive Drugs*, Scriabine, A. and Sweet, C. S., Eds., Spectrum Publications, New York, 1976, 359.

205. **Royds, R. B.**, Initial clinical experience with indoramin, a new antihypertensive agent, *Br. J. Pharmacol.*, 44, 379P, 1972.

206. **Royds, R. B., Coltart, D. J., and Lockhart, J. D. F.**, Pharmacological studies of indoramin in man, *Clin. Pharmacol. Ther.*, 13, 380, 1972.

207. **Alps, B. J., Burrows, E. T., Johnson, E. S., Staniforth, M. W., and Wilson, A. B.**, A comparison of the cardiovascular actions of indoramin, propranolol, lignocaine, and quinidine, *Cardiovasc. Res.*, 6, 226, 1972.

208. **Bohme, P., Corrodi, H., and Fuxe, K.**, Possible mechanism for the hypotensive action of 2-6-dichlorobenzylidene aminoguanidine: evidence for central noradrenaline stimulation, *Eur. J. Pharmacol.*, 23, 175, 1973.

209. **Nash, D. T.**, Clinical trial with guanbenz, a new antihypertensive agent, *J. Clin. Pharmacol.*, 13, 416, 1973.

210. **Paton, W. D. M. and Zaimis, E. J.**, The pharmacological actions of polymethylene bis-trimethylammonium salts, *Br. J. Pharmacol. Chemother.*, 4, 381, 1949.

211. **Stone, C. A., Torchiana, M. L., Navaro, A., and Beyer, K. H.**, Ganglionic blocking properties of 3-methylaminoisocamphane hydrochloride (Mecamylamine), a secondary amine, *J. Pharmacol. Exp. Ther.*, 117, 169, 1956.

212. **Boura, A. L. A. and Green, A. L.**, Adrenergic neuron blocking agents, *Ann. Rev. Pharmacol.*, 5, 183, 1965.

213. **Gannon, B. J., Iwayama, T., Burnstock, G., Gerkens, J. F., and Mashford, M. L.**, Prolonged effects of chronic guanethidine treatment on sympathetic innervation of the genitalia of male rats, *Med. J. Aust.*, 2, 207, 1971.

214. **Burnstock, G., Doyle, A. E., Gannon, B. J., Gerkens, J. F., Iwayama, T., and Mashford, M. L.**, Prolonged hypotension and ultrastructural changes in sympathetic neurones following guanacline treatment, *Eur. J. Pharmacol.*, 13, 175, 1971.

215. **Kopin, I. J., Fischer, J. E., Musacchio, J. M., Horst, W. D., and Weise, V. K.**, "False neurochemical transmitter" and the mechanism of sympathetic blockade by monoamine oxidase inhibitors, *J. Pharmacol. Exp. Ther.*, 147, 186, 1965.

216. **Hess, H. J.**, Biochemistry and structure activity studies with prazosin, in *Prazosin: Evaluation of a New Antihypertensive Agent*, Colton, D. W. K., Ed., Excerpta Medica, New York, 1974, 3.

217. **Cambridge, D., Davey, M. J., and Massingham, R.**, The pharmacology of antihypertensive drugs with special reference to vasodilators, α adrenergic blocking agents and prazosin, *Med. J. Aust.*, 2 (Suppl. 2), 2, 1977.

218. **Stokes, G. S. and Oates, H. F.**, Prazosin: new alpha-adrenergic blocking agent in treatment of hypertension, *Cardiovasc. Med.*, 3, 41, 1978.

219. **Hayes, J. M., Graham, R. M., O'Connell, B. P., Speers, E., and Humphrey, T. J.**, Effect of prazosin on plasma renin activity, *Aust. N. Z. J. Med.*, 6, 82, 1976.

220. **Simpson, F. O.**, Some aspects of the pharmacology of prazosin and their clinical implications, *Med. J. Aust.*, 2 (Suppl. 2), 7, 1977.

221. **Bolli, P., Wood, A. J., and Simpson, F. O.**, Effects of prazosin in patients with hypertension, *Clin. Pharmacol. Ther.*, 20, 138, 1976.

222. **Stokes, G. S., Graham, R. M., Gain, J. M., and Davis, P. R.**, Influence of dosage and dietary sodium of the first-dose effects of prazosin, *Br. Med. J.*, 1, 1507, 1977.

223. **Ahlquist, R. P.** A study of the adrenotropic receptors, *Am. J. Physiol.*, 153, 586, 1948.

224. **von Euler, U. S.**, A specific sympathomimetic ergone in adrenergic nerve fibres (sympathin) and its relations to adrenaline and noradrenaline, *Acta Physiol. Scand.*, 12, 73, 1946.

225. **Sutherland, E. W. and Rall, T. W.**, The properties of an adenine ribonucleotide produced with cellular particles ATP, Mg^{++} and epinephrine and glucagon, *J. Am. Chem. Soc.*, 79, 3608, 1957.

226. **Sutherland, E. W., Øye, I., and Butcher, R. W.,** The action of epinephrine and the role of the adenyl cyclase system in hormone action, *Rec. Prog. Horm. Res.,* 21, 623, 1965.

227. **Sutherland, E. W. and Rall, T. W.,** Fractionation and characterization of a cyclic adenine ribonucleotide formed by tissue particles, *J. Biol. Chem.,* 232, 1077, 1958.

228. **Powell, C. E. and Slater, I. H.,** Blocking of inhibitory adrenergic receptors by a dichloro analog of isoproterenol., *J. Pharmacol. Exp. Ther.,* 122, 480, 1958.

229. **Schild, H. O.,** PA₂: a new scale for the measurement of drug antagonism, *Br. J. Pharmacol.,* 2, 189, 1947.

230. **Åblad, B., Brogard, M., Carlsson, E., and Ek, L.,** Beta-adrenergic receptor blocking properties of three allyl-substituted phenoxypropranolamines, *Eur. J. Pharmacol.,* 13, 59, 1970.

231. **Lands, A. M., Arnold, A., McAuliff, J. P., Luduena, F. P., and Brown, T. G.,** Differentiation of receptor systems activated by sympathomimetic amines, *Nature (London),* 214, 597, 1967.

232. **Lands, A. M., Luduena, F. P., and Buzzo, H. J.,** Differentiation of receptors responsive to isoproterenol, *Life Sci.,* 6, 2241, 1967.

233. **Bristow, M., Sherrod, T. R., and Green, R. D.,** Analysis of beta-receptor drug interactions in isolated rabbit atrium, aorta, stomach and trachea, *J. Pharmacol. Exp. Ther.,* 171, 52, 1970.

234. **Boiaaiwe, J. -F., Advenier, C., Gindicelli, J. -F., and Viars, P.,** Studies on the nature of bronchial adrenoceptors, *Eur. J. Pharmacol.,* 15, 101, 1971.

235. **Morales-Aguilera and Vaughan Williams, E. M.,** The effects on cardiac muscle of β receptor antagonists in relation to their activity as local anaesthetics, *Br. J. Pharmacol. Chemother.,* 24, 332, 1965.

236. **Dobadwaka, A. N., Freedburg, A. S., and Vaughn Williams, E. M.,** The relevance of beta-receptor blockade to ouabain induced cardiac arrhythmias, *Br. J. Pharmacol.,* 36, 257, 1969.

237. **Barrett, A. M. and Cullum, V. A.,** The biological properties of the optical isomers of propranolol and their effects in cardiac arrhythmias, *Br. J. Pharmacol.,* 34, 43, 1968.

238. **Howes, R. and Shanks, R. G.,** The optical isomers of propranolol, *Nature (London),* 210, 336, 1966.

239. **Raper, C. and Jowett, A.,** Antifibrillary and anti-adrenaline activity of β-receptor blockade, *Eur. J. Pharmacol.,* 1, 353, 1967.

240. **Somani, P., Laddu, A. R., and Hardman, H. F.,** Nutritional circulation in the heart. III. Effect of isoproterenol and beta-adrenergic blockade on myocardial hemodynamics and nibidium-86 extraction in the isolated supported heart preparation, *J. Pharmacol. Exp. Ther.,* 175, 577, 1970.

241. **Ledingham, I. McA., Parratt, J. R., and Vance, J. P.,** Effect of propranolol on hypoxia-induced myocardial vasodilatation, *Br. J. Pharmacol.,* 41, 387, 1971.

242. **Pitt, B. and Graven, P.,** Effect of propranolol on regional myocardial blood flow in acute ischaemia, *Cardiovasc. Res.,* 4, 176, 1970.

243. **Becker, L. C., Fortium, N. J., and Pitt, B.,** Effect of ischaemia and anti-anginal drugs on radioactive microspheres in the canine left ventricle, *Circ. Res.,* 28, 263, 1971.

244. **Hansson, L.,** Beta-adrenergic blockade in hypertension, *Acta Med. Scand., (Suppl.),* 50, 1973.

245. **Lund-Johansen, P.,** Hemodynamic changes at rest and during exercise in long term β blocker therapy of essential hypertension, *Acta Med. Scand.,* 195, 117, 1974.

246. **Lund-Johansen, P.,** Alpha-methyl dopa and beta-blockers in hypertension — a comparison of their haemodynamic effects, *Clin. Exp. Pharmacol. Physiol.,* (Suppl. 4), in press.

247. **Shand, D. G. and Rango, R. E.,** The disposition of propranolol. I. Elimination during oral absorption in man, *Pharmacology,* 7, 159, 1972.

248. **Åblad, B., Borg, K. O., Johnsson, G., Regardh, C. G., and Sölvell, L.,** Combined pharmacokinetic and pharmacodynamic studies on alprenolol and 4-hydroxyalprenolol in man, *Life Sci.,* 14, 693, 1974.

249. **Regårdh, C. G., Borg, K. O., Johansson, R., Johnsson, G., and Palmer, L.,** Pharmacokinetic studies on the selective beta-1 receptor antagonist metoprolol, in man, *J. Pharmacokinet. Biopharm.,* 2, 347, 1974.

250. **Gugler, R., Harold, W., and Dengler, H. J.,** Pharmacokinetics of pindolol in man, *Eur. J. Clin. Pharmacol.,* 7, 17, 1974.

251. **Carruthers, S. G., Kelly, J. G., McDevitt, D. G., and Shanks, R. G.,** Blood levels of practolol after oral and parenteral administration and their relationship to exercise heart rate, *Clin. Pharmacol. Ther.,* 15, 497, 1974.

252. **Evans, G. H. and Shand, D. G.,** Disposition of propranolol. V. Drug accumulation and steady-state concentrations during chronic oral administration in man, *Clin. Pharmacol. Ther.,* 14, 487, 1973.

253. **Anavekar, S. N., Louis, W. J., Morgan, T. O., Doyle, A. E., and Johnston, C. I.,** The relationship of plasma levels of pindolol in hypertensive patients to effects on blood pressure, plasma renin, and plasma noradrenaline levels, *Clin. Exp. Pharmacol. Physiol.,* 2, 203, 1975.

254. **Leonetti, G., Mayer, G., Morganti, A., Tergoli, L., Zanchetti, A., Bianchetti, G., Di Salle, E., Morselli, P. L., and Chidsey, D. A.,** Hypotensive and renin-suppressing activities of propranolol in hypertensive patients, *Clin. Sci. Mol. Med.,* 48, 491, 1975.

255. **Bengtsson, C., Johnsson, G., and Regårdh, C. G.**, Plasma levels and effects of metoprolol on blood pressure and heart rate in hypertensive patients after an acute dose and between doses during long term treatment, *Clin. Pharmacol. Ther.,* 17, 400, 1975.

256. **Brunner, L., Imhof, P., and Jack, D.**, Relation between plasma concentrations and cardiovascular effects of oral oxprenolol in man, *Eur. J. Clin. Pharmacol.,* 8, 3, 1975.

257. **Castleden, C. M., Kaye, C. M., and Parsons, R. L.**, The effect of age on plasma levels of propranolol and practolol in man, *Br. J. Clin. Pharmacol.,* 2, 303, 1975.

258. **Branch, R. A., James, J., and Read, A. E.**, The pharmacokinetics of ± propranolol in normal subjects and patients with chronic liver disease, *Br. J. Clin. Pharmacol.,* 2, 183P, 1975.

259. **Bodens, G. and Chidsey, C. A.**, Pharmacokinetic studies of practolol, a beta-adrenergic antagonist, in man, *Clin. Pharmacol. Ther.,* 14, 26, 1973.

260. **Tjandramaga, T. B., Nerbedck, R., Verbessett, R., Verberckmoes, R., and de Schepper, P. J.**, *Beta-Adrenoceptor Blocking Agents,* Saxena, P. R. and Forsyth, R. P., Eds., American Elsevier, New York, 1976, 323.

261. **Ohnhans, E. E., Nuesch, E., Meier, J., and Kalbera, F.**, Pharmacokinetics of unlabelled and ^{14}C labelled pindolol in uremia, *Eur. J. Clin. Pharmacol.,* 7, 25, 1974.

262. **Fernandes, M., Onesti, G., Dykyj, R., Gould, A. B., Fiorentini, R., Kwim, K. E., and Swartz, C.**, Effects of antihypertensive agents on blood pressure and renin in severe experimental renal hypertension, in *Systemic Effects of Antihypertensive Agents,* Sambhi, M. P., Ed., Stratton Intercontinental, New York, 1976, 287.

263. **Dusting, G. J. and Rand, M. J.**, An antihypertensive action of propranolol in DOCA/salt treated rats, *Clin. Exp. Pharmacol. Physiol.,* 1, 87, 1974.

264. **Sweet, C. S., Scriabine, A., Wenger, H. C., Ludden, C. T., and Stone, C. A.**, Comparative antihypertensive effects of intracerebroventricular injection vs. oral administration of β-adrenergic blocking drugs in the spontaneously hypertensive rat, in *Central Regulation of Arterial Pressure,* Onesti, G., Kim, K., and Fernandes, M., Eds., Grune and Stratton, New York, 1975, 123.

265. **Vavra, I. H. T. and Greslin, E.**, Chronic propranolol treatment in young spontaneously hypertensive and normotensive rats, *Can. J. Physiol. Pharmacol.,* 51, 727, 1973.

266. **Weiss, L., Lundgren, Y., and Folkow, B.**, Effects of prolonged treatment with adrenergic β-receptor antagonists on blood pressure, cardiovascular design and reactivity in spontaneously hypertensive rats (SHR), *Acta Physiol. Scand.,* 91, 447, 1974.

267. **Tarazi, R. C. and Dustan, H. P.**, Beta-adrenergic blockade in hypertension, *Am. J. Cardiol.,* 29, 633, 1972.

268. **Franciosa, J. A., Freis, F. D., and Conway, J.**, Antihypertensive and hemodynamic properties of the new beta adrenergic blocking agent, timolol, *Circulation,* 43, 118, 1973.

269. **Davis, J. O.**, The control of renin release, *Am. J. Med.,* 55, 333, 1973.

270. **Weber, M. A., Thomett, I. R., and Stokes, G. S.**, Effects of β-adrenergic blocking agents on plasma renin activity in the conscious rabbit, *J. Pharmacol. Exp. Ther.,* 188, 234, 1974.

271. **Amery, A., Billiet, L., and Fagard, R.**, Beta-receptors and renin release, *N. Engl. J. Med.,* 31, 284, 1974.

272. **Aberg, H.**, Plasma renin activity after the use of a new beta-adrenergic blocking agent (I.C.I. 66082), *Int. J. Clin. Pharmacol.,* 9, 98, 1974.

273. **Esler, M. D. and Nestel, P. J.**, Evaluation of practolol in hypertension; effects on sympathetic nervous system and renin responsiveness, *Br. Heart J.,* 35, 469, 1973.

274. **Morgan, T. O., Roberts, R., Carney, S. L., Louis, W. J., and Doyle, A. E.**, β-Adrenergic receptor blocking drugs, hypertension and plasma renin, *Br. J. Clin. Pharmacol.,* 2, 159, 1975.

275. **Bühler, F. R., Laragh, J. H., Baer, L., Vaughan E. D., and Brunner, H. R.**, Propranolol inhibition of renin secretion, a specific approach to diagnosis and treatment of renin-dependent hypertensive diseases, *N. Engl. J. Med.,* 287, 1209, 1972.

276. **Bühler, F. R., Laragh, J. H., Vaughan, E. D., Brunner, H. R., Gavras, H., and Baer, L.**, Antihypertensive action of propranolol. Specific anti-renin responses in high and normal renin forms of essential, renal, renovascular and malignant hypertension, *Am. J. Cardiol.,* 32, 511, 1972.

277. **Birkenhäger, W. H., Wester, A., Kho, T. L., Schalekamp, M. A. D. H., Zaal, G. A., and de Leeuw, P. W.**, Use of β-adrenoreceptor blockers in relation to the pathophysiology of hypertension, in *Beta-Adrenoceptor Blocking Agents,* Saxena, P. R. and Forsyth, R. P., Eds., North-Holland, Amsterdam, 1976, 229.

278. **Lijnen, P., Amery, A., de Plane, J. F., Fagard, R., and Reybruck, T.**, Hyporeninaemic and hypotensive effect of a cardioselective and a non cardioselective Beta blocker, in *Beta-Adrenoceptor Blocking Agents,* Saxena, P. R. and Forsyth, R. P., Eds., North-Holland, Amsterdam, 1976, 335.

279. **Stokes, G. S., Weber, M. A., and Thornell, I. R.**, β-Blockers and plasma renin activity in hypertension, *Br. Med. J.,* 1, 60, 1974.

280. **Hollifield, J. W.**, In discussion, in *Systemic Effects of Antihypertensive Agents* Sambhi, M. P., Ed., Stratton Intercontinental, New York, 1976, 201.

281. **Mylecharane, E. J. and Raper, C.**, Prejunctional actions of some beta-adrenoceptor antagonists in the vas deferens of the guinea-pig, *Br. J. Pharmacol.*, 39, 128, 1970.

282. **Mylecharane, E. J. and Raper, C.**, Further studies on the adrenergic neurone blocking action of some beta-adrenoceptor antagonists, and guanethidine, *J. Pharm. Pharmacol.*, 25, 213, 1973.

283. **Åblad, B., Ek, L., Johanssen, B., and Waldeck, B.**, Inhibitory effect of propranolol on the vasoconstrictor response to sympathetic nerve stimulation, *J. Pharm. Pharmacol.*, 22, 627, 1970.

284. **Adler-Graschinsky, E. and Langer, S. Z.**, The possible role of a beta-adrenoceptor in the regulation of noradrenaline release by nerve stimulation through a positive feed-back mechanism, *Br. J. Pharmacol.*, 53, 43, 1975.

285. **Garvey, H. L. and Ram, N.**, Comparative antihypertensive effects of tissue distribution of beta-adrenergic blocking drugs, *J. Pharmacol. Exp. Ther.*, 194, 220, 1975.

286. **Offerhans, L. and van Zwieten, P. A.**, Comparative studies on central factors contributing to the hypotensive actions of propranolol, alprenolol and their enantiomers, *Cardiovasc. Res.*, 8, 488, 1974.

287. **Anderson, W., Korner, P. I., Bobik, A., and Chalmers, J. P.**, Leakage of d-l propranolol from cerebro-spinal fluid to the blood stream in the rabbit, *J. Pharmacol. Exp. Ther.*, 202, 320, 1977.

288. **Finch, L.**, The cardiovascular effects of intraventricular clonidine and BAY 1470 in conscious hypertensive cats, *Br. J. Pharmacol.*, 52, 333, 1974.

289. **Day, M. D. and Roach, A. G.**, Central adrenoceptors and the control of arterial blood pressure, *Clin. Exp. Pharmacol. Physiol.*, 1, 347, 1974.

290. **Garvey, H. L. and Ram, N.**, Centrally induced hypotensive effects of β-adrenergic blocking drugs, *Eur. J. Pharmacol.*, 33, 283, 1975.

291. **Kelliher, G. J.**, Evidence for a central site of action in the hypertensive response to propranolol, in *New Antihypertensive Drugs*, Scriabine, A. and Sweet, C. S., Eds., Spectrum Publishing, New York, 1976, 257.

292. **Lewis, P. J. and Haeusler, G.**, Reduction in sympathetic nervous activity as a mechanism for hypotensive effect of propranolol, *Nature (London)*, 256, 440, 1975.

293. **Lewis, P. J., Reid, J. L., Myers, M. G., and Dollery, C. T.**, Cardiovascular effects of intracerebroventricular d,l, and d-l propranolol in the conscious rabbit, *J. Pharmacol. Exp. Ther.*, 188, 394, 1974.

294. **Morgan, T., Sabto, J., Anavekar, S. N., Louis, W. J., and Doyle, A. E.**, A comparison of beta-adrenergic blocking drugs in the treatment of hypertension, *Postgrad. Med. J.*, 50, 253, 1974.

295. **Riesterer, L. and Jaques, R.**, The local anti inflammatory action of non steroidal compounds on the paw oedema caused by kaolin in the rat, *Helv. Physiol. Pharmacol. Acta*, 26, 287, 1968.

296. **Durão, V. and Gião, T. Rico, J. M.**, Modification by indomethacin of the blood pressure lowering effect of pindolol and propranolol in conscious rabbits, *Eur. J. Pharmacol.*, 43, 377, 1977.

297. **Durão, V., Prata, M. M., and Gonçalves, L. M. P.**, Modification of antihypertensive effect of β-receptor-blocking agents by inhibition of endogenous prostaglandin synthesis, *Lancet*, 2, 1005, 1977.

298. **Farmer, J. B., Kennedy, I., Levy, G. P., and Marshall, R. J.**, Pharmacology of AH 5158, a drug which blocks both α and β receptors, *Br. J. Pharmacol.*, 44, 660, 1972.

299. **Kennedy, I. and Levy, G. P.**, Combined α and β-adrenoreceptor blocking drug AH 5158: further studies on α-adrenoreceptor blockade in anaesthetized animals, *Br. J. Pharmacol.*, 53, 585, 1975.

300. **Collier, J. G., Dauney, N. A. H., Nachev, C. H., and Robinson, B. F.**, Clinical investigation of an antagonist of α and β receptors — AH 5158, *Br. J.Pharmacol.*, 44, 286, 1972.

301. **Brittain, R. T. and Levy, G. P.**, A review of the animal pharmacology of labetalol, a combined α- and β-adrenoceptor blocking drug, *Br. J. Clin. Pharmacol.*, 3 (Suppl. 3), 681, 1976.

302. **Blakely, A. G. H. and Summers, R. J.**, The effects of AH 5158 on the overflow of transmitter and the uptake of (^{3}H) (−) noradrenaline in the cat spleen, *Br. J. Pharmacol.*, 56, 264, 1976.

303. **Lund-Johansen, P. and Bakke, O. M.**, Haemodynamic effects and plasma concentrations of labetalol during long-term treatment of essential hypertension, *Br. J. Clin. Pharmacol.*, in press.

304. **Edwards, R. C. and Raftery, E. B.**, Haemodynamic effects of long term oral labetalol, *Br. J. Clin. Pharmacol.*, 3 (Suppl. 3), 733, 1976.

305. **Martin, L. E., Hopkins, R., and Bland, R.**, Metabolism of labetalol by animals and man, *Br. J. Clin. Pharmacol.*, 3 (Suppl. 3), 695, 1976.

306. **Louis, W. J., Christophidis, N., Brignell, M., Vijayasekaran, V., McNeil, J., and Vajda, F. J. E.**, Labetalol: bioavailability, drug plasma levels, plasma renin and catecholamines in acute and chronic treatment of resistant hypertension, *Aust. N.Z. J. Med.*, in press.

307. **Cocco, G., Burkart, F., Chu, D., and Follath, F.**, Intrinsic sympathomimetic activity of β-adrenoceptor blocking agents, *Eur. J. Clin. Pharmacol.*, 13, 1, 1978.

Chapter 2

VASCULAR SMOOTH MUSCLE, VASCULAR REACTIVITY AND DRUGS WHICH AFFECT VASCULAR SMOOTH MUSCLE

I. VASCULAR SMOOTH MUSCLE AND VASCULAR REACTIVITY

The function of the circulation is to carry oxygenated blood and nutrients to cells in various areas of the body and to return metabolic products from these cells for disposal in the lungs, kidneys, and other sites.

The arterial side of the system consists of a reticulation of elastic and muscular vessels capable of transmitting blood rapidly to the periphery, using the pressure generated by the left ventricle. As the arteries divide, their structure changes, so that the smallest arteries, or arterioles, which are vessels with an internal diameter of 20 to 90 μm have medial layers consisting of smooth muscle cells arranged concentrically with supporting connective tissue. Contraction, or relaxation, of the vascular smooth muscle cells gives rise to corresponding changes in internal diameter, with the result that resistance to flow is altered. Various physiological stimuli affect the state of contraction of vascular smooth muscle cells. These stimuli may be local and due to local anoxia or local accumulation of metabolic products or may be controlled by transmitter release from sympathetic nerve endings or may be due to hormonal substances such as angiotensin. These mechanisms permit regional alterations to blood flow to occur in response to local requirements or to central circulatory control mechanisms.

Because resistance to flow is inversely proportional to the fourth power of the radius, the smaller arteries provide the main peripheral resistance vessels within the circulation, so that the major energy loss occurs as the blood passes along these small vessels, with the result that the pressure at the arterial end of the capillaries has been adjusted to a very stable level, almost irrespective of the central arterial pressure.[1] The capillaries, which are the site of gaseous and metabolic exchange, pass into collecting venules, and these to veins, which return blood to the heart to enter the pulmonary circulation. The venous side of the circulation has an important capacitance function.

II. CONTRACTILE MECHANISMS

Vascular smooth muscle depends for its contractile properties on the same kind of machinery for contraction as skeletal and cardiac muscle, namely, two sets of interdigitating filaments, containing myosin on the one hand and actin on the other. It is now widely accepted that muscle contraction is based on the relative sliding of these two sets of filaments one upon the other, either to produce shortening or where this is prevented, to increase tension.[2,3] Actin filaments are thin (50 to 80 Å) in diameter, while myosin filaments are thicker (155 Å).[4] The average ratio in smooth muscle of thin to thick filaments is about 16:1.[4] The actin filaments in vascular smooth muscle are attached to dense bodies, analogous to the Z-lines in striated muscle. The myosin molecules are asymmetrical and consist of long rod-like sections to which two globular heads are attached which appear to be the sites which combine with actin. Thick filaments consist of strands of myosin molecules from which the myosin heads project. The thin filaments contain not only actin but also a regulatory protein, tropomyosin, which in skeletal muscle is associated with additional proteins called troponins. Although tropomyosin has been identified in smooth muscle, there is some doubt as to whether troponins are present in vascular smooth muscle.[5] The function of the regulatory proteins appears to be to bind intracellular calcium. The trigger for activation of the contractile process is a rise in intracellular free calcium (activator calcium) which binds the regulatory protein tropomyosin, thus allowing interaction between actin and myosin. At ionic calcium concentrations of between 10^{-5} and 10^{-7} M of activator calcium,[6] the actin-activated myosin releases energy from ATP by inactivation of the troponin-tropomyosin system which inhibits the ATPase activity of actomyosin.

An increase in activator calcium with subsequent contraction can be induced in vascular smooth muscle by a variety of mechanisms. Calcium concentration within the cell cytoplasm may be increased either from intracellular or extracellular sources.

Intracellular stores of calcium appear to be present in the sarcoplasmic reticulum, mitochondria, and plasma membrane, which contains surface vesicles. The sarcoplasmic reticulum is a system of tubules which lies close to the surface membrane at some sites only 10 to 12 nm from the membrane. It has been suggested that action potentials at these sites may release calcium[7] from extracellular sources which then passes into the cell. In support of this is the fact that incubation of vascular muscle with strontium is followed by accumulation of electron-dense strontium in the lumen of the sarcoplasmic reticulum. The size of the sarcoplasmic reticulum appears to vary in different types of smooth muscle and in those with extensive systems, such as large elastic arteries, drugs appear able to elicit contractions in calcium-free media.[8] These observations suggest that calcium contained in the sarcoplasmic reticulum may be an important intracellular site from which activator calcium is released in a free form within the cell. They also suggest that the stores of calcium within the sarcoplasmic reticulum may be derived from extracellular sources by passage across the adjacent surface membrane. The mitochondria also make close contact with surface vesicles and likewise accumulate strontium, and it has been reported that angiotensin in physiological amounts accelerates the release of bound calcium from the microsomal fraction,[9] suggesting that the mitochondria may also function as a calcium storage site.

Somlyo and Somlyo[10] have summarized two possible modes of action for drugs on smooth muscle. They assume that excitatory drugs act by a common mechanism of increasing the ion permeability of vascular smooth muscle plasma membrane, and that the quantititatively most important source of activator calcium is external to the plasma membrane. Pharmacomechanical coupling (the action of compounds on the contractile system independent of the membrane potential) is suggested by the fact that electrical and mechanical events in smooth muscle can be dissociated under some circumstances and that drugs may induce contraction or relaxation after depolarization of the plasma membrane by high potassium concentration.

The effects of drugs such as verapamil, which reduce the permeability of the membrane to calcium have been used to study the source of activator calcium.[11] These studies have suggested that various constrictor agents such as angiotensin and histamine are capable of initiating contraction independently of passage of extracellular calcium through the plasma membrane, therefore suggesting that they can mobilize calcium from an intracellular source. Whether they do so under physiological circumstances has not been demonstrated. Devine, Somlyo, and Somlyo[8] have suggested that vasoactive drugs induce a change in permeability at the site of coupling, which is then propagated along the sarcoplasmic reticulum membrane as a local circuit Ca^{++} current.

Excitation-contraction coupling is the process during which depolarization of the plasma membrane leads to an intracellular increase in calcium ion permeability and which has been demonstrated experimentally by measuring both action potentials and radioisotopic ionic fluxes. There is some correlation between the maximal contraction and the maximum permeability changes produced by different drugs.[12] Under physiological circumstances, it is suggested that either excitation coupling, or pharmacomechanical coupling could function.

The role which cyclic nucleotides play in the contractile process in vascular smooth muscle is uncertain. In rabbit colonic smooth muscle,[13] a microsomal fraction has been isolated which accumulated calcium in the presence of ATP and magnesium. This effect was stimulated by both isoproterenol and by cyclic AMP. It was suggested that relaxation induced by β-adrenergic stimulation was mediated via cyclic AMP, which caused a shift from free intracellular calcium into a bound form in the mitochondria. In the mesenteric artery, similar findings were obtained.[14] In the same study, stimulation of α-receptors caused a fall in cyclic AMP. Both norepinephrine and angiotensin decrease the incorporation of labeled adenosine into cyclic AMP.[15] A reduction of the cyclic AMP content of smooth muscle seems therefore to be an initial event associated with contraction. However, there is evidence that the mechanical events and changes in cyclic AMP can be dissociated under some circumstances. In the rabbit endometrium, isoproterenol in low doses induced relaxation with no increase in cyclic AMP. Propranolol blocked the increase in cyclic AMP, but not the relaxation.[16] If these results can be translated to vascular tissue, it appears that while cyclic AMP may be a mediator of the contractile process, there does not seem to be an essential link between the contractile process and cyclic AMP. The situation is further complicated by the fact that calcium is able to modulate vascular phosphodiesterase activity, which also probably influences cyclic nucleotide concentrations.

The recent discovery of prostacyclin and thromboxane[17,18] has given further impetus to the possibility that the vascular contractile process may be in part mediated via cyclic nucleotides. Platelets contain a cyclo-oxygenase and a peroxidase which leads to the formation of an endoperoxide (PGH_2). The platelet contains an enzyme, thromboxane synthetase, which converts PGH_2 to thromboxane, which induces platelet aggregation and contracts vascular smooth muscle. Blood vessel walls contain the enzyme prostacyclin synthetase, which can convert PGH_2, which migrates from the platelet, to prostacyclin. Prostacyclin has a relaxing action on vascular smooth muscle and can disaggregate platelets.[19] It appears that the two compounds have opposite effects on cyclic AMP, probably by an effect on calcium migration. There is currently insufficient information to determine whether any of these possible mechanisms for the control of vascular smooth muscle contraction are deranged in coronary disease, strokes, or hypertension. Prostaglandins have been proposed as being locally active in controlling the contractile states of vascular smooth muscle in response to local stimuli.[20] Evidence for their relevance to the overall problem of hypertension is not convincing, although there is evidence that prostaglandin mechanisms are abnormal in the New Zealand strain of genetic hypertensive rats,[21] which may contribute to a disturbance in vascular responses.[22]

Of particular relevance to hypertension is the relationship between changes in intracellular concentrations of monovalent cations, such as sodium and potassium. Sitrin and Bohr[23] have reported that an increase in sodium concentration appears to enhance contractions caused by intracellular calcium mobilization, but to diminish contractions caused by an inflow of extracellular calcium.

Although there have been considerable advances in understanding of the mechanisms of vascular smooth muscle contraction, it is not yet evident whether, and if so in what way, there are disturbances in these mechanisms in hypertension which might be underlying mechanisms of the rise in peripheral resistance or of a change in vascular reactivity.

III. VASCULAR REACTIVITY IN HYPERTENSION

Although there is general agreement that the rise in blood pressure in hypertension is due to constriction of the small arteries and arterioles, the nature of the process which causes the peripheral resistance to increase is obscure. One possibility is that in hypertension the resistance vessels themselves respond to stimuli of normal magnitude by an excessive constriction, either as a primary defect or as a secondary sustaining mechanism, so causing hypertension.

Direct comparison of changes in blood pressure between hypertensive patients and normotensives is complicated by the fact that the starting levels of blood pressure and the state of vasoconstriction are different in the two groups, so that if other factors remain constant, any increase in cardiac output or rises in peripheral resistance could be expected to induce proportionately larger blood pressure changes in the hypertensives in relation to the initial blood pressure. The situation is further complicated by the fact that in both hypertensive and normotensive patients, changes in blood pressure are moderated by the baroreceptor mechanisms,[24-27] although the responses of these are changed in hypertension (Volume 2, Chapter 1).

Before alterations in vascular responsiveness to pressor stimuli can be accepted as being of importance in the pathogenesis of hypertension, it is important to discover whether the resistance vessels respond to pressor stimuli by a greater contraction in hypertension than in normotension. If this is established, it has then to be shown whether the greater response in hypertension applies to pressor agents in general or only to some particular stimulus and also whether it precedes the hypertension or results from vascular or other changes induced by the high blood pressure. These questions as to the presence or absence of vascular hyperreactivity are obviously important not only in essential hypertension, but also in the pathogenesis of secondary hypertension; for no matter what kind of initiating vasoconstrictor stimulus is present, the extent of the blood pressure response would be dependent on the vascular reactivity.

Early studies attempted to solve this problem by the use of either reflex pressor responses or by the infusion of vasoconstrictor agents. These studies did not distinguish between the peripheral vascular response and changes in cardiac output or homeostatic regulatory changes induced by the stimulus.

It became clear that to study the reactions of resistance vessels, agonists needed to be introduced into local vascular beds in amounts sufficient to act locally, but inadequate to induce homeostatic responses. Most of these studies in man have been carried out in the peripheral circulation.

IV. VASCULAR REACTIVITY IN MAN

Duff[29] studied the effects of intra-arterial administration of epinephrine and norepinephrine on hand blood flow in normotensive and hypertensive individuals. He reported a marked increase in sensitivity in the hypertensive group to epinephrine, but found little or no change in responsiveness to norepinephrine. He found that the increased epinephrine sensitivity was in general related to the severity of the hypertension, being on the average more marked in malignant hypertension. These results are open to criticism, for his two groups were ill matched, the hypertensives being mostly elderly females, while the control group were healthy young men. Since epinephrine constricts skin vessels and may dilate muscle vessels, and since the proportion of skin to muscle in the hand might well be greater in elderly hypertensive women than in young men, the question of epinephrine hyperresponsiveness cannot be regarded as having been entirely resolved.

Doyle, Fraser, and Marshall[30] studied the response of the forearm circulation to norepinephrine, angiotensin, and 5-hydroxytryptamine, infused into the brachial artery. They found that the hypertensive patients responded with greater constriction both to norepinephrine and 5-hydroxytryptamine than age- and sex-matched normotensives, the differences being highly significant (Figures 1 through 5). For norepineph-

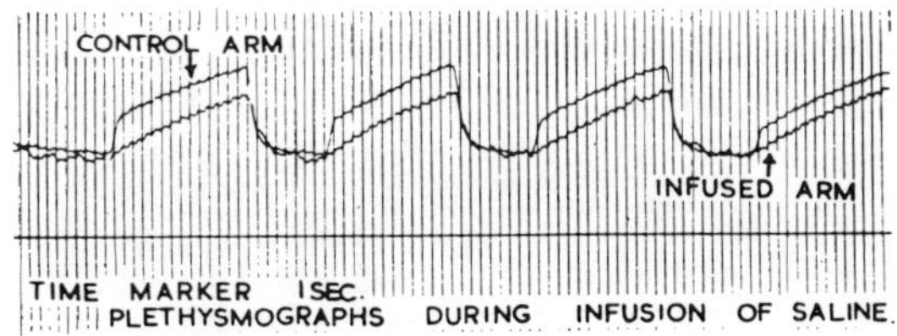

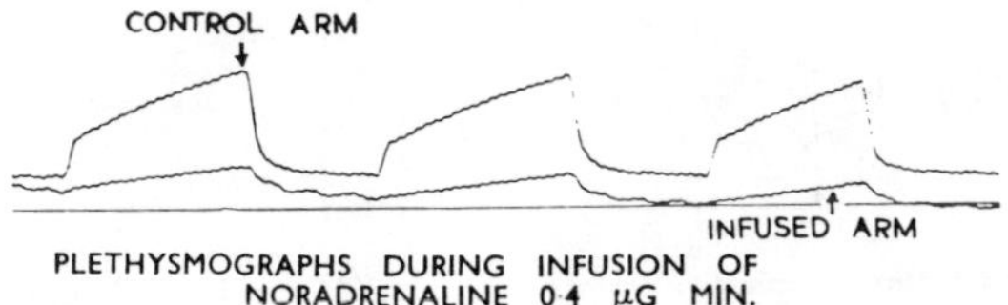

FIGURE 1. Plethysmograph illustrating the effect of norepinephrine. The upper record was taken during the infusion of saline into the left arm; the lower record was taken during the infusion of norepinephrine (0.4 μg/min) into the left arm. In both records, the lower tracing is from the left arm. (From Doyle, A. E., Fraser, J. R. E., and Marshall, R. J., *Clin. Sci.*, 18, 441, 1959. With permission.)

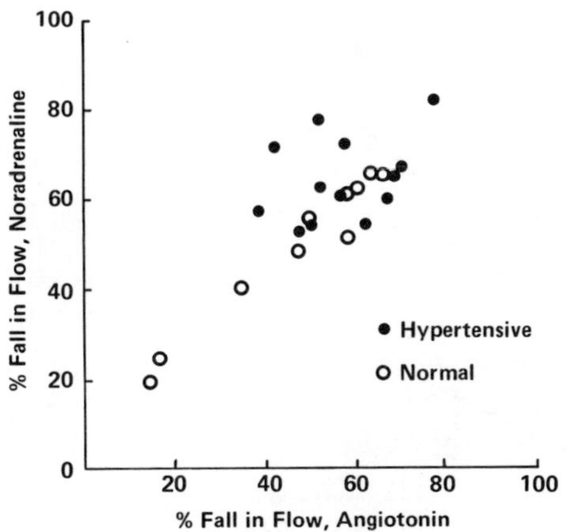

FIGURE 2. The relationship between responses in individual subjects to norepinephrine and angiotonin. (From Doyle, A. E., Fraser, J. R. E., and Marshall, R. J., *Clin. Sci.*, 18, 441, 1959. With permission.)

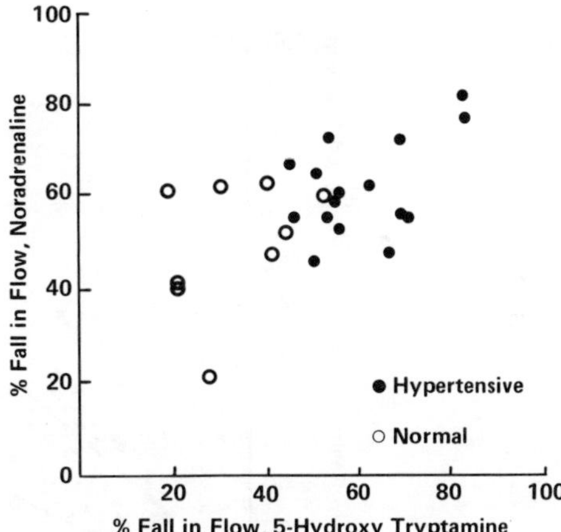

FIGURE 3. The relationship between responses in individual subjects to norepinephrine and 5-hydroxytryptamine. (From Doyle, A. E., Fraser, J. R. E., and Marshall, R. J., *Clin. Sci.*, 18, 441, 1959. With permission.)

rine, the hypertensive patients achieved a given constriction with about half the dose required for normotensives. With angiotensin, the response of the hypertensives was slightly, but not significantly, greater than those of the normotensive subjects. Commenting as to the effect of the initial state of vasoconstriction on the response to norepinephrine, Doyle et al. found that in both hypertensive and normotensive subjects the rise in resistance induced by norepinephrine increased as the initial peripheral resistance rose (Figure 6). Because of the variation in forearm blood flow, there was substantial overlap of initial forearm resistance in the two groups. An analysis of

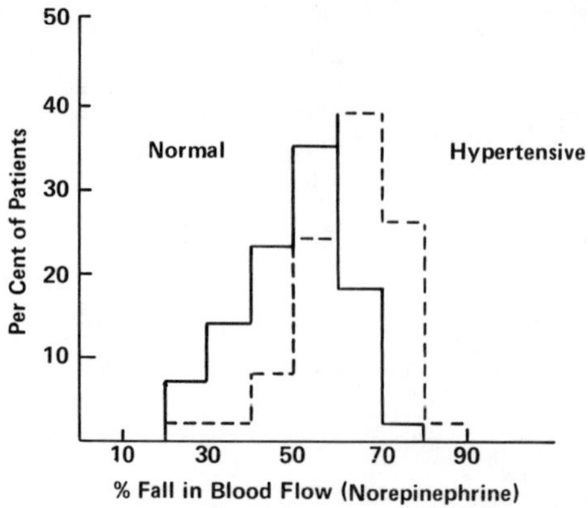

FIGURE 4.   Histogram showing the responses of 50 hypertensives and 48 normal subjects to the infusion of norepinephrine (0.4 μg/min). The normal subjects are indicated by continuous lines; the hypertensives by interrupted lines. (From Doyle, A. E. and Fraser, J. R. E., *Lancet,* 2, 509, 1961. With permission.)

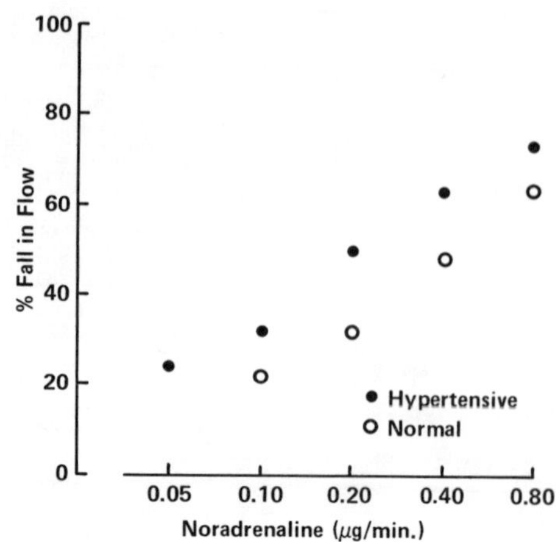

FIGURE 5.   The relationship between the rate of infusion of norepinephrine and the percentage fall in blood flow. The solid circles represent the mean responses for ten hypertensive subjects; the open circles refer to the mean responses of ten normal subjects. (From Doyle, A. E., Fraser, J. R. E., and Marshall, R. J., *Clin. Sci.,* 18, 441, 1959. With permission.)

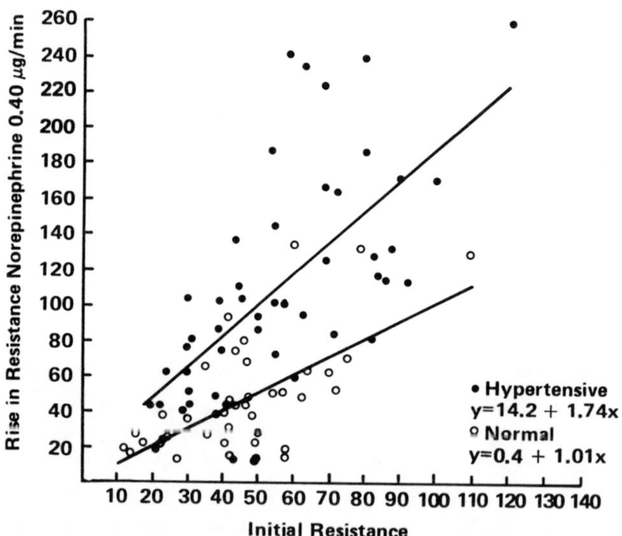

FIGURE 6.   The relationship between initial forearm resistance and the rise in forearm resistance caused by the intra-arterial infusion of 0.4 μg of norepinephrine per minute. (From Doyle, A. E. and Fraser, J. R. E., *Lancet,* 2, 509, 1961. With permission.)

regression between the rise in resistance indicated that at all levels of initial resistance the response of the hypertensives was larger than that of the normotensives and that the increase in resistance induced by norepinephrine was steeper for hypertensives than for normotensives for given changes in initial forearm resistance. This study appears to indicate that in hypertension, vascular reactivity to pressor agents is increased, even allowing for differences in the initial state of vasoconstriction. The fact that the response to angiotensin was not significantly greater in hypertensive patients than in normal subjects might be because some hypertensive patients have a specific lack of sensitivity to angiotensin. More detailed study is necessary to elucidate this further.

Other studies on the reactivity of the peripheral circulation have been carried out using i.v. administered pressor agents. Fatheree and Brown[31] studied the effects on heat elimination from the hand of i.v. administered epinephrine and noted no distinct difference between hypertensive and normotensive subjects. Greisman[32] observed increased reactivity to the arterial segments of the terminal capillary loops of the nail beds of hypertensive patients to epinephrine and norepinephrine. Mendlowitz and associates[33-35] have studied the response of blood flow in the finger after sympathetic blockade by indirect heat and a ganglion-blocking drug. With such a technique, they demonstrated that in primary hypertension there was increased reactivity to norepinephrine and to angiotensin, whereas in renal hypertension the reactivity was normal or only slightly elevated. Moulton, Spencer, and Willoughby,[36] using a radioactive sodium technique to measure muscle blood flow, noted an increased constrictor response to norepinephrine in hypertensive subjects, and Lee and Holze[37] noted increased sensitivity of the metarterioles and precapillaries to topically applied epinephrine in the conjunctivae. This was also observed by Jackson.[38] Barany and James[39] reported that greater reduction of heat elimination of the nerve-blocked heel occurred in response to norepinephrine in hypertensive than in normotensive patients.

There thus appears to be almost general agreement among different workers that in essential hypertension, various parts of the peripheral arterial system display increased reactivity to pressor agents, in particular, to norepinephrine, epinephrine and 5-hydroxytryptamine. The evidence about differences between renal hypertension and essential hypertension seem less clear-cut, but the balance of evidence suggests that in renal hypertension, there may also be a heightened vascular responsiveness to these agents. The question as to whether there is also an increased sensitivity to angiotensin remains unsettled. It appears that a more detailed study of the effects of various types of pressor agents in more clearly defined types of hypertension is still needed.

The question as to whether the increased constrictor responses to pressor agents is due to an abnormality of contractile response or merely reflects a structural abnormality, with an increase in the wall to lumen ratio, is not entirely resolved. Sivertsson[40] and Folkow[41] believe that the whole difference can be attributed to structural change secondary to hypertension. They base this on the fact that using plethysmographic techniques, resistance in the hand vessels at maximal dilatation was greater in the hypertensives than in the normotensives and that the threshold dose of norepinephrine needed to induce vasoconstriction was not markedly reduced in the hypertensives. However, hand plethysmography is difficult to use in the situation of maximal vasodilatation such as is induced by reactive hyperemia, because maximal dilatation is very transient, and a few seconds discrepancy in the time of measurement can induce very large errors. Moreover, the hypertensives in their series had a small but definite (13%) decrease in threshold dose of norepinephrine.

While it seems very probable that structural changes in the arterial wall are in part responsible for the increase in vascular reactivity, it is by no means certain that such changes are the only mechanism operating. The question is of importance, for if an increased vascular reactivity is the result rather than a cause of hypertension, a search for contributing factors in smooth muscle or receptors is not likely to be fruitful.

There is some evidence to suggest that in some instances increases in vascular reactivity may precede hypertension. Doyle and Fraser[42] measured forearm vascular responses to norepinephrine in normotensive children, one or both of whose parents had essential hypertension, and compared them with similar measurements made in nor-

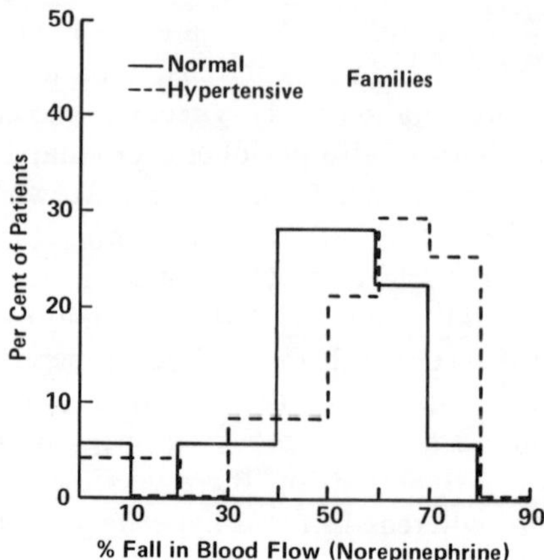

FIGURE 7. Histogram showing the responses of 23 sons of hypertensive parents and 17 sons of normal parents. The continuous lines indicate the normal families; the interrupted lines the hypertensive families. (From Doyle, A. E. and Fraser, J. R. E., *Lancet*, 2, 509, 1961. With permission.)

motensive students of similar age, both of whose parents had normal blood pressures. They found clear evidence of increased vascular responses (Figure 7) in the children of the hypertensive parents. This was less marked than in established hypertensives.

Other evidence that increased vascular reactivity may be due to a functional rather than a structural change has been provided by Mendlowitz and colleagues.[34] These workers studied the work done in the digital vascular bed during vasoconstriction induced by norepinephrine and angiotensin. They found increased responses in the digital vessels in essential hypertensive patients, with more work being performed per unit of agonist. Moreover, these changes were not found in patients with renal vascular hypertension in whom structural change should have been evident.

These data suggest that in essential hypertension there is an intrinsically increased vascular responsiveness which can precede the development of hypertension and is undoubtedly reinforced by structural vascular changes which follow the development of hypertension.

V. VASCULAR REACTIVITY IN EXPERIMENTAL HYPERTENSION

In experimental animals, as in man, there is evidence suggesting that constrictor responses of arterial smooth muscle are enhanced in hypertensive animals, whether the hypertension is spontaneous or genetic or induced by a variety of techniques.

Studies in perfused vascular beds have generally shown increased reactivity to a variety of pressor agents. McQueen[43] studied vascular responses in the perfused hindquarters of renoprival and renal hypertensive rats and found exaggerated responses in both groups. Hinke[44,45] studied the ventral tail artery of the DCA hypertensive rat. He showed enhanced responsiveness to norepinephrine and pitressin, but not to angiotensin II. The basal resistance was also increased, and the muscle was capable of generating a greater contractile force. McGregor and Smirk[46] demonstrated increased reactivity to both norepinephrine and angiotensin II in the isolated mesenteric arteries of both genetically hypertensive rats and renal hypertensive rats. In a later study,[47] the same workers found an even more exaggerated response to 5-hydroxytryptamine in the mesenteric arteries of both genetic and renal hypertensive rats, with little difference between the two agents in control animals. Haeusler and Finch[48] confirmed these latter findings, and also found the perfusion of the isolated renal artery from the same rats did not exhibit the same responsiveness to 5-hydroxytryptamine.

Folkow et al.[49] studied dose-response curves to vasoconstrictor agents in hindquarter preparations from 7-month-old spontaneously hypertensive rats and normotensive control rats in paired experiments. They found that even at maximal dilatation, resistance was higher in the hypertensive preparation than in the normotensive, that the two preparations showed the same threshold sensitivity, but the dose-response curves were steeper in the hypertensive preparations than in the normotensive controls. Folkow et al. propose that these findings are consistent with the theoretical curves which would be expected if there was no smooth muscle hypersensitivity, but merely an increased wall to lumen ratio caused by a relative medial hypertrophy.

The problem as to whether functional changes in vascular reactivity precede structural change has been studied by several workers. Collis and Alps[50] studied the responses to norepinephrine, angiotensin, and KCl in the mesenteric vascular bed of the one-kidney Goldblatt hypertensive model in the rat. They found exaggerated responses to norepinephrine and angiotensin at 1 week, but no change in response to KCl. With time, the responses to both norepinephrine and angiotensin increased further and hyperresponsiveness to KCl also appeared (Figures 8 and 9). These authors also noted that infusion of angiotensin enhanced the response to norepinephrine but not KCl in normotensive rat preparations (Figure 10).

More recently, Berecek and Bohr[51] have described enhanced vasoconstrictor responses in the hind limb of the DOCA salt hypertensive pig. These authors also reported that enhanced responses also occurred in hind limbs which had been protected from the high arterial pressure by ligation of the external iliac artery (Figures 11 and 12).

Numerous studies have been undertaken using helical strips of blood vessels. While these avoid the problems of wall to lumen ratio and permit a more direct assessment of smooth muscle sensitivity, they bring their own problems in that preparation of strips leads to severe disruption of structure, with a possible consequent change in function.[52] Many of these studies have employed strips of rat aorta, which have the disadvantage of having relatively high proportions of elastic tissue. Most studies have not demonstrated a capacity of the aorta to generate a greater contractile force in response to constrictor agents. Thus, Redleaf and Tobian,[53] Mallov,[54] and Spector et al.[55] found either no difference or a lower contractile force in strips from hypertensive animals than from normotensives. On the other hand, Bohr and Sitrin[56] and Holloway and Bohr,[57] using strips from femoral arteries of rats reported that smooth muscle from hypertensive animals responded to lower concentrations of epinephrine or potassium chloride, but developed less contractile force at maximum shortening. Shibata and Kurahishi[58] reported that manganese, strontium, and lanthanum cause contractions of aortic smooth muscle in spontaneously hypertensive but not in normotensive rats, while barium produced a greater response in normotensive than in hypertensive rats. These findings have been confirmed by Bohr,[6] who also found similar responses to barium and strontium in DCA hypertensive rats.

There seems to be very general agreement that the reaction of resistance vessels in experimental hypertension is such that a wide variety of constrictor agents evokes a larger degree of lumen reduction in most hypertensive models than in normal. There is no doubt that much, if not all, of the increased vascular reactivity can be attributed to the greater wall to lumen ratio found in established hypertension. There are some

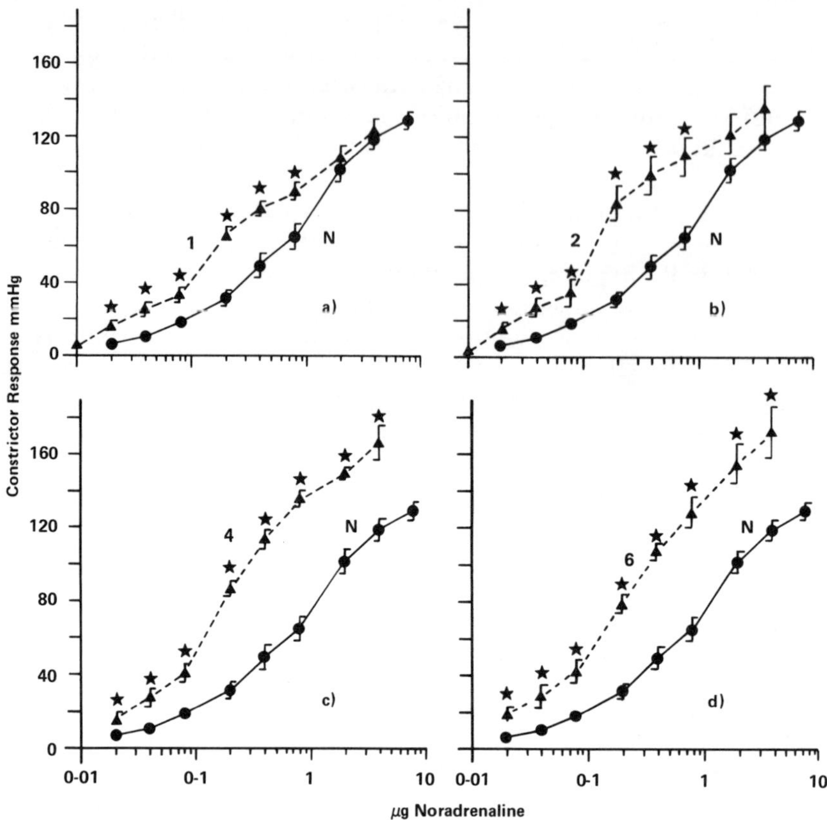

FIGURE 8.   Mean constrictor responses to norepinephrine of mesenteric arterioles from normotensive (N) rats (n = 9-19) ●—● and renal hypertensive rats ▲—▲ at (a) 1 week, (b) 2 weeks, (c) 4 weeks, and (d) 6 weeks after nephrectomy. Mean responses of hypertensive preparations significantly different from normotensives are denoted by asterisks. (From Collis, M. G. and Alps, B. J., *Cardiovasc. Res.*, 9, 118, 1975. With permission.)

difficulties in accepting this as the entire mechanism, however, and the demonstration that an increased wall to lumen ratio is always due to structural change is far from proven. Structural change would not readily account for the excessive response of some vessels to 5-hydroxytryptamine nor to the often found lack of increased responsiveness to angiotensin. Neither would it explain differences in response to nonphysiological agonists such as strontium barium or manganese.

While medial hypertrophy is one obvious cause of increased wall thickness, giving a larger wall to lumen ratio, it is not the only possibility. Decreased lumen might be due to an increase in nonmuscular components of the vessel wall or perhaps to an intrinsic change in the conformation of smooth muscle, leading to a decreased compliance of the actin and myosin cross bridges or an increased cooperativity which might provide a background of minor reduction in lumen.

There have been a number of studies on the changes which occur in arteries following the induction of hypertension. Bevan et al.[59] studied the changes in reactivity of rabbit arteries 2 week after hypertension had been induced by experimental coarctation of the abdominal aorta. They found that the maximum active tension produced by norepinephrine and the thickness of rings from the rabbit ear arteries were increased. The internal diameter of the arteries was unchanged. These authors attributed these changes to muscle hypertrophy or hyperplasia. Subsequent studies by Bevan et al.[60]

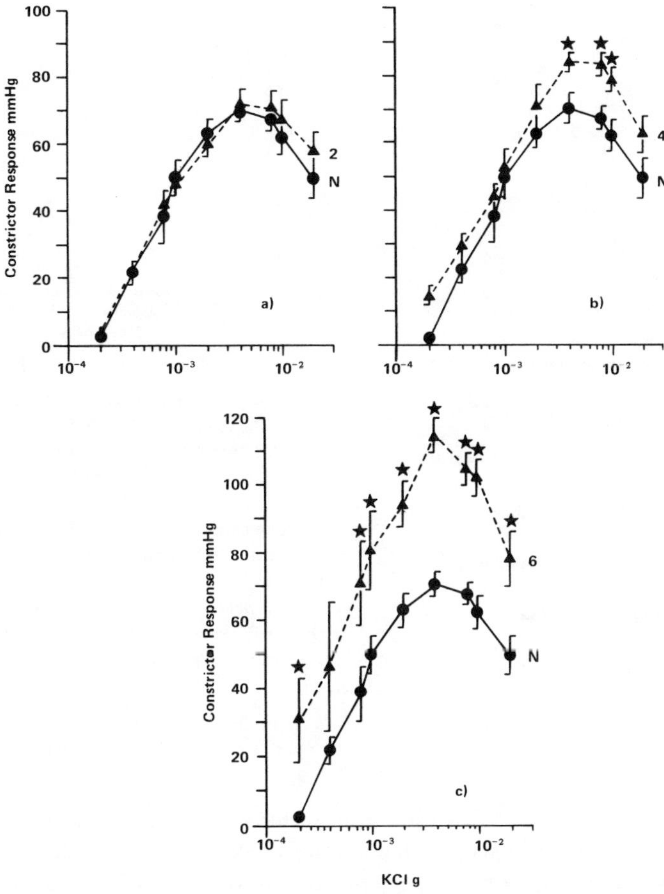

FIGURE 9.   Mean constrictor responses to KCl of mesenteric arterioles from normotensive (N) rats (n = 9-19) •—•, and renal hypertensive rats ▲—▲ at (a) 2 weeks, (b) 4 weeks, and (c) 6 weeks after nephrectomy. Mean responses of hypertensive preparations significantly different from normotensives are denoted by asterisks. (From Collis, M. G. and Alps, B. J., *Cardiovasc. Res.,* 9, 118, 1975. With permission.)

involving mitotic counts and the incorporation of tritiated thymidine revealed considerable muscle cell proliferation, although whether this was due to an increased number of muscle cells or to replacement as a result of injury was not clearly established. In a later study, the same group showed that DNA content of arteries was not increased. Busse et al.[61] found that wall cross-sectional area was the same for tail arteries from spontaneously hypertensive and normotensive rats with no evidence of muscle hypertrophy, although the arteries from hypertensives were much smaller than from normotensive rats at all transmural pressures in the fully relaxed state. Similar changes were noted by Friedman et al.[62] in the DOCA salt hypertensive rat model. In human hypertension, Short[63] found a reduction in the size of mesenteric arteries with no change in wall cross-sectional area, which he attributed to shortening of the circular elements of the arterial wall.

The balance of evidence suggests that changes in smooth muscle responsiveness to pressor stimuli precede or cause the development of established hypertension and that structural change, due to medial muscle hypertrophy or to other mechanisms, might further reinforce preexisting vascular responses. One such possible mechanism relates to electrolyte changes within blood vessels.

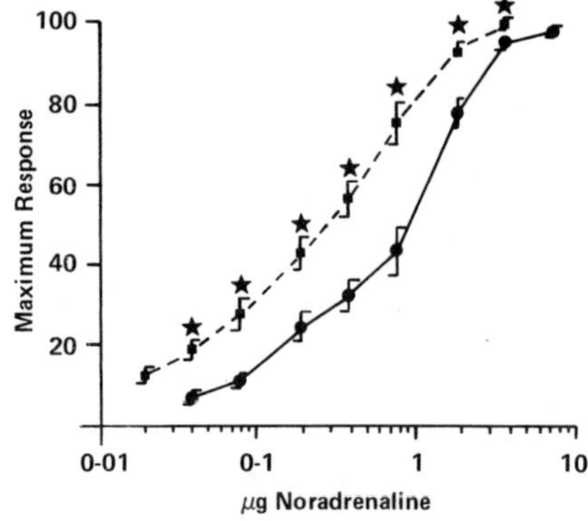

FIGURE 10. Mean % responses (n = 11) to norepinephrine, injected into the perfused isolated mesenteric vasculature of normotensive rats, in the absence (●—●) and presence (■—■) of angiotensin II amide (10^{-7} M). Mean responses to norepinephrine were significantly greater (indicated by asterisks) in the presence of angiotensin than in its absence. (From Collis, M. G. and Alps, B. J., *Cardiovasc. Res.*, 9, 118, 1975. With permission.)

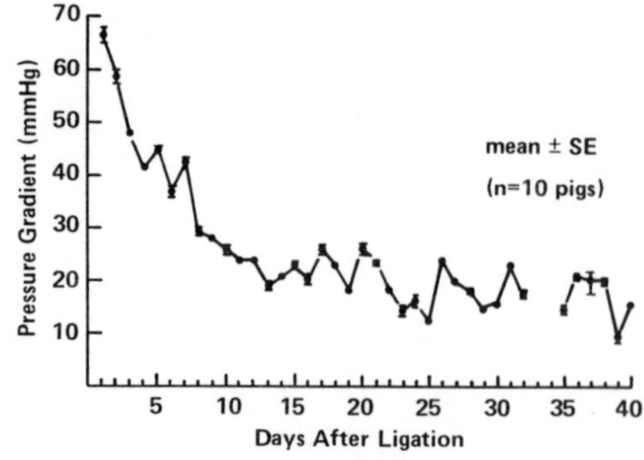

FIGURE 11. Mean arterial pressure gradient between the aorta and left femoral artery after left external iliac artery ligation. Pressures are direct measurements from arterial catheters. Data from DOCA and control pigs are displayed together. Results are expressed as mean ± SE. The high initial pressure gradient diminished rapidly as collateral blood supply developed. A pressure gradient of 15 to 20 mmHg persisted throughout the observation period. (From Berecek, K. H. and Bohr, D. F., *Circ. Res.*, 20(Suppl. 2), 147, 1977. With permission.)

VI. CATIONS AND BLOOD VESSELS IN HYPERTENSION

In 1952, Tobian and Binion[64] studied the sodium and water content of renal arteries and psoas muscle in hypertensive patients at autopsy and reported an increase in both. They suggested that an increase in sodium and water might lead to expansion of the arterial wall, due to waterlogging, so reducing lumen size and hence increasing peripheral resistance. The same group later reported[65] an increased sodium ion content in arteries from renal and DOCA salt-treated rats. Raab et al.[66] noted potentiation of pressor effects in man by desoxycorticosterone using epinephrine and norepinephrine, and Raab later suggested[67] that pressor sensitivity depends on the membrane potential of the muscle cell, which is influenced by the relative intracellular and extracellular electrolyte concentration.

The arterial wall contains mucopolysaccharides in considerable amounts,[68,69] which have a high affinity for cations,[70] whereas nonvascular smooth muscle tissue contains little or no mucopolysaccharides. In experimental hypertension, sulfate utilization and mucopolysaccharide synthesis is increased.[71] Arterial wall mucopolysaccharide is increased in the aorta above, but not below, an experimentally induced coarctation,[72] suggesting that it may be a response to increased intravascular pressure.

The sodium content in arterial tissue is considerably higher than in skeletal muscle, the concentration being 250 to 350 mol/g of dry tissue.[73] The sodium content is higher in small vessels than larger, which has been attributed to the relatively increased amount of connective tissue in smaller arteries. Arterial connective tissues, as has been noted earlier, contains mucopolysaccharides which have a high affinity for cations, presumably because of the negatively charged sulfate and phosphate groups.

Headings[74] concluded that most arterial sodium was extracellular. Friedman et al.[75] found that approximately 93% was extracellular, of which about 13% was bound to the matrix. Jones and Swain[76] found the extracellular component to be approximately

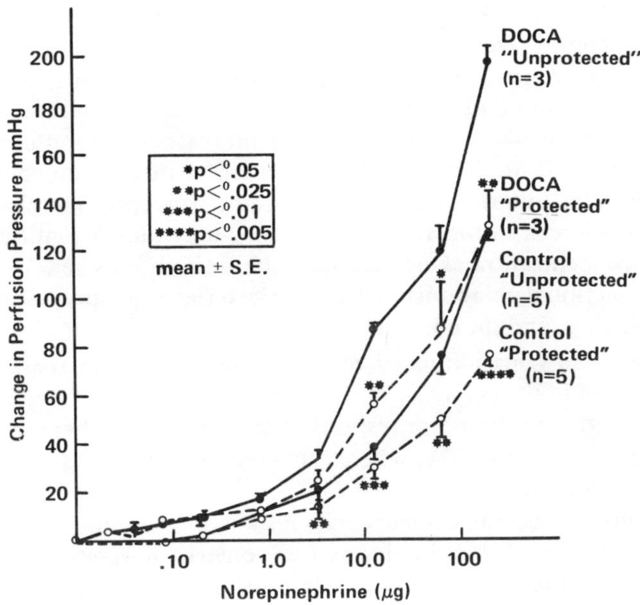

FIGURE 12. "Unprotected" and "protected" hind limb vascular reactivity to norepinephrine in control and DOCA-hypertensive pigs. Data are expressed as mean perfusion pressure changes ± SE in response to intra-arterial injections of norepinephrine. The threshold concentration of norepinephrine required for vasoconstriction in the hind limbs of the hypertensive pigs was only 1/10 that required in the hind limbs of the normotensive pigs. This indicates that vascular smooth muscle sensitivity is increased in both the "protected" and "unprotected" vascular beds in DOCA hypertension. The magnitude of the constrictor response to large doses of norepinephrine is less in the "protected" than in the "unprotected" vascular beds. This difference is thought to reflect a diminished arteriolar wall thickness in the "protected" leg. (From Berecek, K. H. and Bohr, D. F., *Circ. Res.*, 40(Suppl. 1), 1, 1977. With permission.)

93% of which approximately 80% was in the ^{60}Co EDTA space and the remainder associated with the connective tissue. Both had a rapid turnover.

Increased arterial wall sodium has been noted in most types of experimental hypertension studied, including single- kidney clip hypertension in rats and dogs, two-kidney hypertension in rats, DOCA salt hypertension, and in the spontaneously hypertensive rat. However, most of the studies were made in established hypertension. Constantopoulos et al.[77] studied arterial sodium content in the single-kidney renal clipped dog at 7 days and after 60 days. No increase in sodium content was found after 7 days, but arterial sodium content was increased after 60 days. Halpern et al.[78] noted similar changes in the rabbit. In the early phase of hypertension in the spontaneously hypertensive rat, Nagoaka et al.[79] noticed no sodium ion increase, whereas it was present in the later stages.

The effects of changing sodium content on the response of vascular preparations to constrictor stimuli has also been studied. A rise in sodium concentration was reported to increase responses in rat aortic strips.[80] Other studies[81] suggested that large increases in sodium concentrations reduced, while reductions in sodium concentrations increased, vascular responses.

More recently, Harris and Palmer[82] studied the effect of enzymatic depolymerization of arterial wall mucopolysaccharides, using testicular hyaluronidase and ascorbic acid. Using the rabbit ear artery, they found that hyaluronidase reduced both the sodium content of the arterial wall and the responses to electrical stimulation and norepinephrine. In control experiments using a number of nonvascular smooth muscle preparations, hyaluronidase had no demonstrable effect either on sodium content or on contractile response. The authors suggested that since mucopolysaccharide molecules surround each muscle cell in the arterial wall, they may play a significant role in any changes in ionic concentration associated with the smooth muscle cell. They proposed that there is a functional relationship between arterial mucopolysaccharides, cation binding, water binding, and the contractile response.

In a later study, the same authors[83] reported that a small increase (8 mmol/ℓ) of sodium concentration in the perfusing medium of an isolated perfused rabbit ear artery preparation increased the constrictor responses. It is of interest that the sodium content of the perfused artery rose by 20%, whereas in control tissues a much smaller increase in sodium content occurred.

There thus seems to be some evidence which links the sodium and water content of arterial wall to reactivity of the blood vessel to constrictor agents. It may be that the dominant effect is an altered geometrical relationship between wall and lumen, which would be favored by wall thickening or waterlogging. On the other hand, it remains possible that ionic changes may have effects on the muscle cell plasma membrane.[76] Permeability to potassium, sodium, and chloride, acting with concentration gradients, controls membrane potential, and most constrictor agents have a major effect on ionic permeabilities at the cell surface membrane. It is possible that changes in the gradient of sodium ions from extracellular to intracellular may have important effects on vascular contractile mechanisms. There is certainly good evidence that when smooth muscle contracts, there is a shift of sodium into the cell. Friedman and Friedman[84] point out that sodium enters the cell whether constriction is induced by catecholamines or angiotensin and also relate this to the effects of intravascular pressure, which also shifts sodium into the cell. They suggest that this process may lead to increased protein synthesis within the cell, leading to hypertrophy of smooth muscle and an increase in polyanion sodium-binding sites, leading to hyperreactivity because of altered geometry and possibly also by an alteration in either membrane potential or calcium and sodium relationships (Figure 13). Such a mechanism, or series of mechanisms, might well be responsible as a sustaining mechanism for hypertension. Whether it is capable of an initiating role is much more difficult to evaluate.

There is some evidence that ion transport is altered in vascular smooth muscle during the prehypertension phase of DOCA hypertension in the rat. Jones and Hart[85] suggested that the changes in hypertension might result from a reduced capacity of calcium to stabilize the vascular muscle cell membrane. Similarly, Friedman and Friedman[84] have reported that in the tail artery of the spontaneously hypertensive rat and in DOCA hypertension sodium, lithium and sodium and potassium exchanges are enhanced at an early stage and are associated with increased sodium transport.

To summarize, considerable advances have been made in the understanding of the contractile process of vascular smooth muscle and its possible disturbance in hypertension. There is almost general agreement that in hypertension, vascular responses are exaggerated. This is due in part to structural change, but evidence is accumulating that early changes in ion transport may lead initially to hypersensitivity to constrictor stimuli and subsequently to structural changes which reinforce the exaggerated reactivity further. Such changes might go far towards explaining how initiating factors and sustaining factors in the pathogenesis of hypertension may interact.

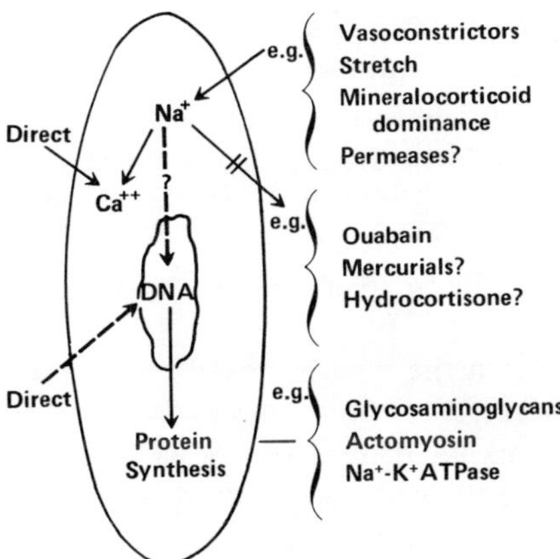

FIGURE 13. Schema of the interrelation between factors tending to increase cell Na⁺ pool, acute vasoconstriction, and increase in the synthesis of contractile, transport, and export protein. (From Friedman, S. M. and Friedman, C. L., *Circ. Res.*, 39, 433, 1976. With permission.)

VII. ANTIHYPERTENSIVE DRUGS WHICH DILATE VASCULAR SMOOTH MUSCLE

In all forms of hypertension, there is increased resistance to blood flow in the peripheral arteriolar bed, due to narrowing of the small resistance vessels. While many factors are relevant to the majority of hypertensive situations, the final common pathway through which they operate is the contractile process in arteriolar smooth muscle. Even in the severest forms of hypertension, very marked vasodilatation can be induced in all vascular beds, as for example in reactive hyperemia, during which blood flow may be increased up to tenfold from resting levels. For these reasons, the use of agents acting to induce relaxation of vascular smooth muscle would appear to be a logical procedure in the control of hypertension. Although drugs are available which can indeed cause vasodilatation, these have so far attained only a limited role in the practical therapeutic situation. The reasons for their lack of success relate predominantly to the fact that when circulatory mechanisms are intact, any reduction in blood pressure induced by peripheral vasodilatation immediately sets in train circulatory responses designed to buffer the hypotensive effect. These include autonomic responses and responses related to circulatory volume.

Autonomic responses presumably operate via the baroreceptor mechanisms whose sensory receptors are located in the aortic arch and carotid sinus. Most vasodilators given systemically lead to a fall in blood pressure which provokes a reflex tachycardia, and an increase in cardiac output. This latter response is particularly noticeable when drugs are used which selectively relax arterial rather than venous vascular smooth muscle. Such drugs include minoxidil, hydralazine, and diazoxide. These agents almost certainly induce reflex venoconstriction, leading to a consequent increase in cardiac output. The reflex response of tachycardia and increased cardiac output induces palpitations, flushing of the face, headache, and sometimes anginal pain.

The administration of vasodilatory drugs also induces longer term effects, which lead to an increased circulating blood volume. These include a sharp increase in renin release, so that plasma renin activity rises rapidly, with a secondary increase in aldosterone production, diminished sodium excretion, and an increase in extracellular fluid and plasma volume. It should be noted that these latter changes, while developing more dramatically with vasodilator drugs, also occur in response to some drugs which act via the autonomic nervous system such as guanethidine, α-methyldopa, and the ganglion-blocking drugs.[86] They also occur when α-adrenergic blocking drugs lke phenoxybenzamine, which act at the postsynaptic and presynaptic receptors, are administered.[87]

These disadvantages have in the past imposed severe limitations on the clinical use of vasodilator drugs. However, the situation has been strikingly altered by the availability of β-adenoceptor-blocking drugs, which when given concurrently, effectively block the capacity to achieve the reflex responses to the fall in blood pressure induced by vasodilator drugs, presumably by inducing β blockade at cardiac receptors, so preventing reflex tachycardia and increases in cardiac output. Moreover, by blocking the presumably reflexly induced increase in renin release, β-adenoceptor drugs partly prevent the rise in plasma renin levels and the volume changes induced by vasodilator drugs. Fluid retention can be further prevented by the concurrent use of diuretics.

The availability of β-adrenoceptor-blocking drugs and diuretics has thus allowed the practical use of vasodilator drugs to develop and has led to a renewed clinical interest in the use of these drugs.

VIII. MECHANISMS OF ACTION

Drugs which act directly on vascular smooth muscle almost certainly operate by reducing activator calcium within smooth muscle cells, hence inhibiting the contractile process. They may exert their effects either by reducing calcium influx across the plasma membrane or by intracellular actions which alter the binding mechanisms for free calcium ions within the cell. Somlyo and Somlyo[10] have emphasized, however, that ionized calcium may not be the sole modulator of contractile activity, since actomyosin ATPase activity at a given calcium concentration can vary depending on such factors as pH, temperature, and the concentration of magnesium or phosphate ions. It is not established whether drugs can affect the contractile process in vascular smooth muscle by a process independent of intracellular calcium ion concentration.

A possibly important mechanism of action of vasodilator drugs is inhibition of phosphodiesterase activity, which leads to an accumulation of cyclic AMP. Andersson[14] reported that the relaxant action of papaverine, nitroglycerin, and diazoxide correlated with an increase in cyclic AMP content of smooth muscle. All these drugs reduced ATP content, and the magnitude of the effect of this reduction correlated with the degree of relaxation. No fall in ATP content was found in a calcium-free solution. Andersson further reported that papaverine reduced phosphodiesterase activity of smooth muscle, mainly in a subcellular fraction which bound calcium ions under utilization of ATP in smooth muscle. Inhibition of phosphodiesterase activity has also been reported with the benzothiadiazine diuretics and diazoxide and minoxidil.

The vasodilating action of sodium nitroprusside on the other hand seemed to be independent of phosphodiesterase activity, since prior incubation of smooth muscle strips with 3-isobutyl-1-methyxanthine did not affect the depressant action of nitroprusside.[88] The suggestion has been made that the drug may prevent, or reverse, mobilization of calcium from intracellular stores. Since nitroprusside relaxes both arterial and venous smooth muscle, whereas the phosphodiesterase inhibitors, diazoxide and minoxidil, affect arterial muscle predominantly, it seems possible that cyclic AMP accumulation may be a less significant mechanism for vasodilatation in venous than in arterial muscle, but this is speculative.

The point has been made earlier that information concerning abnormalities of the contractile mechanism of vascular smooth muscle in hypertension is far from complete and it is therefore not surprising that vasodilating drugs so far developed are apparently somewhat nonspecific, and their use is mainly empirical. Nevertheless individual drugs do differ in potency, duration of effect, and in the possession of other actions. A detailed consideration of properties of individual drugs allows their therapeutic indications to be more clearly establisbed.

A. Hydralazine

The pharmacology of hydralazine (1-hydrazine-phthalazine) was described in 1950[89] and the mechanism of the hemodynamic effect was studied extensively by Ablad and colleagues.[90-92] Its site of action appears to be predominantly on smooth muscle in arterial wall, where an isotopic derivative has been shown by autoradiography to concentrate.[93] Dilatation occurs more in the renal, coronary, and splanchnic circulations than in the brain, skin, or muscle.[94]

Following an i.v. injection of 12.5 mg, the antihypertensive effect is delayed for about 5 to 10 min, after which time the mean arterial pressure decreases, with an increase in heart rate. Intra-arterial infusion of hydralazine leads to an increase in forearm and hand blood flow.[90]

After oral administration, the antihypertensive action is noticeable within an hour, and peak plasma levels occur in 3 to 4 hr.

Postural hypotension is not prominent, presumably because relaxation of venous smooth muscle is less marked than that in arterial vessels. Orthostatic hypotension may occur with larger doses. Hydralazine commonly induces headache, facial flushing, and tachycardia with the fall in blood pressure, and nausea and vomiting sometimes occur.

Hydralazine is metabolized in the liver, partly by ring hydroxylation and partly by N-acetylation.[95] The latter mode of degradation is important because of the genetic variation in the rate of acetylation between different individuals. Slow acetylators metabolize the drug less rapidly than fast acetylators, and hence slow acetylators tend to have higher plasma levels and more prolonged responses than do those who metabolize the drug more rapidly.[95]

Prolonged administration of hydralazine in doses above 200 mg/day may lead to a syndrome consisting of joint pain, myalgia, and fever, which is accompanied by a raised erythrocyte sedimentation rate, positive antinuclear reaction, abnormalities in DNA binding, and sometimes a positive lupus erythematosus cell reaction.[96] The syndrome is usually reversible, but symptoms may persist for several months after the hydralazine has been discontinued.

B. Prazosin

Prazosin is a comparatively recently introduced drug, whose precise mode of action has not yet been fully elucidated. Its most important action seems related to interference with α-adrenoceptor blockade, but it may also have some action in arterial smooth muscle, possibly related to inhibition of phosphodiesterase activity. Prazosin inhibits both the low affinity high K_m phosphodiesterases with a potency approximately 20 times that of theophylline and inhibits the hydrolysis of both cyclic GMP and cyclic AMP.[97] Infused intra-arterially in dogs, it induced a fall in perfusion pressure and arteriolar resistance, with, however, an increase in pressure in the venous segments. In aortic strips, it antagonized the effects of both norepinephrine and barium. The vasodilatation induced by the intra-arterial infusion of prazosin could be partially prevented by the preceding i.v. administration of the ganglion-blocking drug, hexamethonium, suggesting that part of the vasodilating action might be due to interference with sympathetic function, and the remainder to a direct action on smooth muscle. Prazosin, like phentolamine, exerts a protective effect against the irreversible effect of phenoxybenzamine on the α-receptor. Prazosin appears to reduce the effect of sympathetic nerve stimulation to a greater extent than it does the effects of norepinephrine.[98] The suggestion has been made that prazosin is taken up into catecholamine stores at the peripheral nerve ending and released during sympathetic nerve activity, together with norepinephrine, whose effects on the adrenergic receptor it inhibits competitively.[99]

Prazosin appears to have a long duration of action. The antihypertensive effect of large doses is maximal at 2 to 4 hr after oral administration and persists to some extent for 24 to 48 hr. There are usually few effects on heart rate, and postural effects are generally not conspicuous, although severe postural hypotension has been reported in some clinical studies.

Intravenous administration reduced blood pressure in normotensive rats, rats with spontaneous hypertension, and the one-kidney renal hypertensive rat.

In four patients with essential hypertension, the acute i.v. administration of prazosin produced a fall in mean arterial pressure, with a corresponding fall in peripheral vascular resistance.[100]

The long-term hemodynamic effects of oral prazosin have been studied by Lund-Johnsen.[101] He reported a fall in mean arterial pressure at rest and during exercise. Total peripheral resistance was reduced, and the effects on cardiac output were trivial at rest, but there was an increased cardiac output during exercise. Heart rate did not change significantly. Prazosin has been reported to decrease plasma renin activity, both in the anesthetized dog[102] and patients with hypertension.[103] In another study, prazosin was found to have no consistent effect on plasma renin activity in conscious renal hypertensive dogs, although in the same animals, hydralazine induced a rise in renin.[104]

Prazosin appears to differ in its effects from most other vasodilating drugs in that it often induces a substantial fall in peripheral vascular resistance without obvious tachycardia, postural effects, fluid retention, or rise in PRA.

These factors probably render it superior in clinical use to most other peripherally acting drugs currently available. The adrenergic blocking effects of prazosin are discussed in Volume 1, Chapter 2.

C. Minoxidil

Minoxidil is an extremely potent vasodilator drug, which, like hydralazine, is effective by mouth, and which also resembles hydralazine in producing greater relaxation in arterial than in the venous smooth muscle.[105] It is considerably more potent than hydralazine and reduces blood pressure in a dose range of from 3 to 30 mg. It has a prolonged duration of action and can usually be administered in a single daily dose. Given alone, it induces hypotension, tachycardia, increased cardiac output, increase in plasma renin activity, urinary aldosterone excretion, and considerable sodium retention.[106]

Almost all reports agree that minoxidil needs to be given in conjunction both with a β-adrenoceptor-blocking drug and a diuretic.[106,107] When used in this way, minoxidil appears to be considerably more effective than hydralazine. It has been used successfully in patients with intractable malignant hypertension and renal failure, as an alternative to nephrectomy in these resistant patients.[108-110]

Excessive hair growth on the face and chest has been reported to be caused by minoxidil, especially in patients with impaired renal function. It has been reported to induce pulmonary hypertension in some patients.

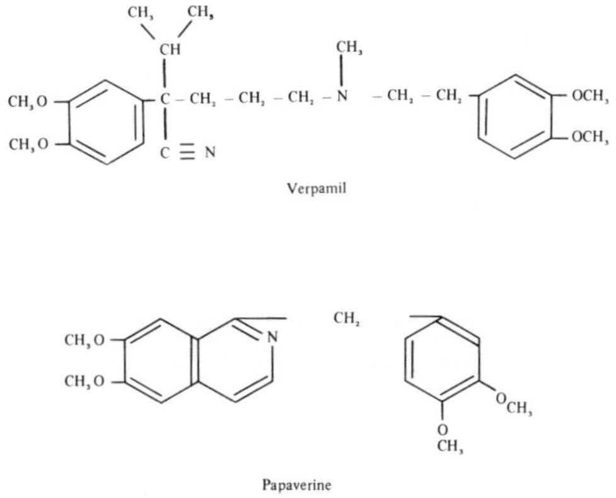

Verpamil

Papaverine

FIGURE 14. The standard formulas of verapamil
and papaverine.

Myocardial necrosis occurring mainly in the left ventricular papillary muscles has
been reported in dogs given oral minodixil in moderately large doses.[111] Tachycardia
and electrocardiographic ST segment depression also occurred. Pretreatment with digoxin and propranolol did not alter the incidence of these lesions.[111] Similar lesions
have not been seen in other species, nor have similar findings in man been reported.
It has been reported that hydralazine, diazoxide, and guancydine induce similar lesions.[112]

D. Guancydine

Guancydine is a vasodilator drug of moderate potency with properties similar to
those of hydralazine. Following oral administration of 250 to 270 mg, Freis and Hammer[113] found a fall in blood pressure and tachycardia. The peak effect occurred 3 hr
after administration, and the duration of effect was from 6 to 8 hr. Gupta and Goldberg[114] found guancydine in combination with propranolol and quinethazone (a benzothiadiazine diuretic) to be a more effect antihypertensive drug than hydralazine in
combination with the same drugs. However, the drug has been reported to cause gynecomastia, galactorrhea, and some central nervous system excitatory responses.[115]

E. Verapamil

This substance has a structure resembling that of papaverine, in that both have a
dimethoxybenzene grouping at each of the molecule (Figure 14). The drug was introduced in 1962[116] as a coronary arterial dilator and has recently been reported to have
antihypertensive properties. Verapamil has been reported to impede the passage of
calcium across the plasma membrane of cardiac and vascular smooth muscle.[117] In this
respect, it resembles papaverine, which also reduces the permeability of the cell membrane and/or the sarcoplasmic reticulum to calcium and has the effect of decreasing
the availability of activator calcium for the contractile mechanism of smooth muscle.[118]

Papaverine has also been reported to inhibit phosphodiesterase activity, which has
not been reported for verapamil.

Verapamil is well absorbed after oral administration, but undergoes extensive biotransformation on its first hepatic circulation, so that 70 to 80% of the drug is metabolized on its first pass through the liver. As with propranolol, continuing administration leads to stable plasma levels of the drug.[119] Acute administration usually leads to
a small fall in cardiac output, with a fall in total peripheral resistance.[120]

Although devoid of β-adrenoceptor-blocking properties, verapamil sems to induce

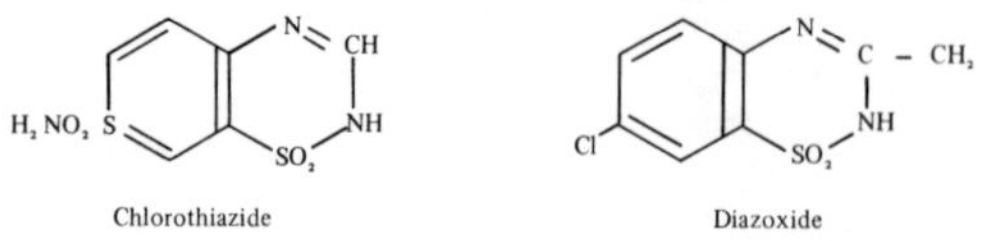

FIGURE 15.   The structure of chlorothiazide and diazoxide.

rather comparable clinical effects, presumably by its action in reducing contractility of the heart. Its place in the management of hypertension is not yet established, but initial reports are of promise.

F. Diazoxide

Diazoxide is a structurally similar drug to benzothiadiazine diuretics (Figure 15), but is, however, devoid of saluretic action. It relaxes arterial smooth muscle, and like papaverine and nitroglycerine, leads to an increase in cyclic AMP content in arterial smooth muscle.[125] It acts predominantly in arteries.

Diazoxide has the capacity to block vasoconstriction in the rat aorta induced by the barium ion. It also increases the concentration of calcium required to restore responsiveness to norepinephrine in a calcium-free medium and appears to block a calcium receptor with smooth muscle.[126] Thus, its primary vasodilator effect appears to be linked with calcium-activated contraction.

It is rapidly bound to serum albumin, which inactivates the drug,[127] and for this reason, its antihypertensive effect is mainly evident following rapid i.v. injection.[128] Slow infusion i.v. or oral administration is usually ineffective. After a rapid i.v. injection, the maximal fall in blood pressure occurs within a few minutes and persists for up to 12 hr. Like most potent peripheral vasodilating drugs, diazoxide induces tachycardia, an increase in cardiac output, stimulates a rise in plasma renin activity, and induces marked sodium retention .

Its major use has been in situations in which a rapid fall in blood pressure is required, such as hypertensive encephalopathy, severe malignant hypertension, subarachnoid hemorrhage, or hemorrhagic stroke.[128] Repeated doses may be given as necessary. Abrupt falls of blood pressure to dangerously hypotensive levels may occur. Transient hyperglycemia may occur. This is usually of little significance, but can be prevented by pretreatment with tolbutamide.

G. Sodium Nitroprusside

Although the antihypertensive effects of sodium nitroprusside were described almost 50 years ago,[129] major interest in the clinical use of this interesting compound has been most marked in the last 3 to 4 years.

Page et al.[130] reported that sodium nitroprusside reacted with sulfydryl-containing amino acids located within erythrocytes and suggested that its action on smooth muscle followed intracellular penetration of the drug. The drug depresses the contraction of saphenous vein strips caused by electrical stimulation, tyramine, potassium, barium, norepinephrine, and acetylcholine.[88] Preincubation with the phosphodiesterase inhibitor, 3-isobutyl-1-methylxanthine, did not affect the depressant action of sodium nitroprusside, suggesting that the action of the drug is independent of the accumulation of cyclic AMP.

Verghaeghe and Shepherd[88] further suggested that the drug may prevent or reverse mobilization of calcium from intracellular stores. The depression also occurred in a calcium-free medium and after calcium influx had been prevented by verapamil. Such a mechanism of action would be consistent with the depressant action of barium-induced contraction, since barium is thought either to mobilize intracellular calcium or act directly on the contractile protein. The effects on vascular smooth muscle seem specific in that uterine and duodenal smooth muscle is 100 times less sensitive than vascular tissue.

Whole animal studies reveal a fall in arterial pressure and total peripheral resistance with minimal effects on heart rate.[130] Cardiac output may increase, but the effect on output is variable and inconsistent. The effect probably depends on the relative magnitude of effects in arterial and venous smooth muscle in different individuals and may vary with the initial state of contraction of these vessels. The effects on renal blood flow are also variable,[130] with a fall in renal vascular resistance and arterial blood pressure, leading sometimes to an increase and sometimes to a fall in renal blood blow.

Intravenous administration causes a prompt fall in blood pressure, which is transitory, so that for a sustained antihypertensive effect, i.v. infusions need to be used. The dose required is variable. As little as 1 $\mu g/kg/min$ often induces a satisfactory response in man, but larger doses can be used.[131]

Nitroprusside is probably converted to cyanide by combination with sulfydryl groups in erythrocytes, and the cyanide is converted in the liver to thiocyanate, which is subsequently excreted in the urine, with a half-life of about 5 to 7 days.[130] Toxic manifestations are probably mainly due to accumulation of thiocyanate and occur with plasma levels of 5 to 10 gm/$c\ell$. Toxic symptoms include fatigue, nausea, disorientation, and, rarely, features of hypothyroidism.

The main use of sodium nitroprusside is in the emergency control of blood pressure in hypertensive encephalopathy (Figure 16), hemorrhagic stroke,[131] and dissecting aneurysm.[132] More recently, Franciosa et al.[133] have described the use of sodium nitroprusside in patients with acute myocardial infarction in whom a fall in ventricular end diastolic pressure was consistently associated with improvement in the manifestations of left ventricular failure. Chatterjee et al.[134] claim that mortality from cardiogenic shock following myocardial infarction is significantly reduced by controlled hypotension induced by sodium nitroprusside and external counterpulsation.

For the acute emergency situation, sodium nitroprusside appears to have considerable advantages over diazoxide in that its effects are rapidly reversed by discontinuing the infusion, so that the desired degree of antihypertensive effect is more readily controlled. Longer term administration may lead to undesirable toxicity.

H. Benzothiadiazines

These diuretic drugs inhibit phosphodiesterase activity,[122] which may be significant in their antihypertensive actions. It has not been finally resolved whether in addition to their effect in reducing extracellular fluid volume and exchangeable sodium, these drugs also affect vascular smooth muscle or its reactivity to pressor agents. Zoster, Heart and Radde[135] reported that after treatment with hydrochlorothiazide for 6 to 10 weeks, norepinephrine produced significantly smaller responses in the mesenteric artery and vein of rabbits than in untreated controls. The effects of acetylcholine, barium, angiotensin, papaverine, and ATP were not altered. The same authors found that in dogs pretreatment with hydrochlorothiazide depressed contractile responses to both norepinephrine and sympathetic nerve stimulation. On the other hand, Jandhayala et al.[136] found that treatment with hydrochlorothiazide of dogs for 12 months did not alter either the response to intra-arterial norepinephrine or sympathetic nerve stimulation, although resting sympathetic tone was found to be reduced.

It is quite uncertain whether the antihypertensive action of the benzothiadiazines has a significant component resulting from an action on vascular smooth muscle. It is clear that a major (sole, in the view of many investigators) action is related to the

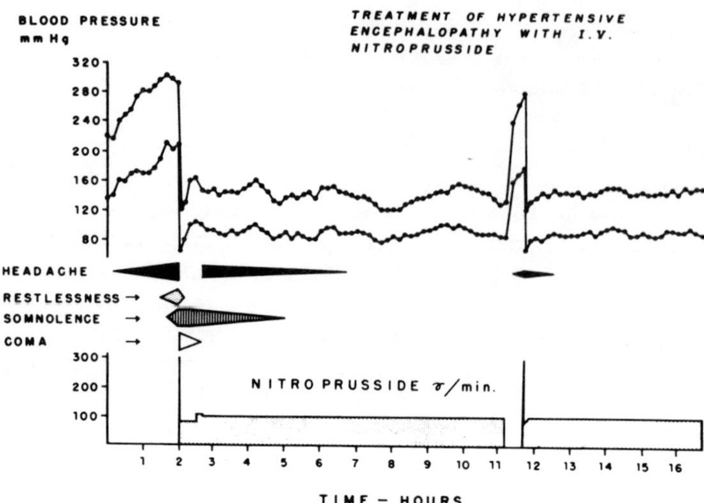

FIGURE 16.   Treatment of hypertensive encephalopathy with i.v. infusion of sodium nitroprusside. The patient was first somnolent, then comatose. The upper third shows the effect on arterial pressure; the middle, signs and symptoms; and lower third, the amount of nitroprusside in μg/min. (From Page, I. H., Corcoran, A. C., Dustan, H. O., and Koppanyi, T., *Circulation*, 11, 188, 1955. With permission.)

volume-depleting action of these drugs. If there is an action on vascular smooth muscle, it may be mediated via phosphodiesterase inhibitory action, or may be related to alterations in the ionic composition of the smooth muscle cell or its extracellular surroundings. The diuretic action of these drugs is discussed in Volume 1, Chapter 1.

REFERENCES

1. Zweifach, W., Local regulation of capillary pressure, *Circ. Res.*, 28 (Suppl. 1), 1, 1971.
2. Huxley, A. F. and Nidergerke, R., Structural changes in muscle during contraction: interference microscopy of living muscle fibres, *Nature (London)*, 173, 971, 1954.
3. Huxley, H. E. and Hansson, J., Changes in the cross striations of muscles during contraction and stretch and their structural interpretation, *Nature (London)*, 173, 973, 1954.
4. Somlyo, A. P., Devine, C. E., Somlyo, A. V., and Rice, R. V., Filament organization in vertebrate smooth muscle, *Philos. Trans. R. Soc. Lond. Ser. B.*, 265, 223, 1973.
5. Murphy, R. A., Structural proteins in the myofilaments and regulation of contraction in vertebrate smooth muscle, *Fed. Proc. Fed. Am. Soc. Exp. Biol.*, 35, 1302, 1976.
6. Bohr, D. F., Vascular smooth muscle updated, *Circ. Res.*, 32, 665, 1973.
7. Somlyo, A.V. and Somlyo, A. P., Strontium accumulation by sarcoplasmic reticulum and mitochondria in vascular smooth muscle, *Science*, 174, 955, 1971.
8. Devine, C. E., Somlyo, A. V., and Somlyo, A. P., Sarcoplasmic reticulum and excitation-contraction coupling in mammalian smooth muscle, *J. Cell. Biol.*, 52, 690, 1972.
9. Baudouin, M., Meyer, P., Fermandjian, S., and Morgat, J., Calcium release induced by interaction of angiotensin with its receptors in smooth muscle cell microsomes, *Nature (London)*, 235, 336, 1972.
10. Somlyo, A. P. and Somlyo, A.V., Vascular smooth muscle. II. Pharmacology of normal and hypertensive vessels, *Pharmacol. Rev.*, 22, 249, 1970.
11. Haeusler, G., Differential effect of verapamil on excitation-contraction coupling in smooth muscle and on excitation-secretion coupling in adrenergic nerve terminals, *J. Pharmacol. Exp. Ther.*, 180, 672, 1972.

12. **Somlyo, A. P. and Somlyo, A. V.,** Pharmacology of excitation-contraction coupling in vascular smooth muscle and in avian slow muscle, *Fed. Proc. Fed. Am. Soc. Exp. Biol.,* 28, 1634, 1969.
13. **Andersson, R. and Nilsson, I.,** Relaxation in intestinal smooth muscle: role of cyclic AMP and calcium, *Nature (London),* 238, 119, 1972.
14. **Andersson, R.,** Role of cyclic AMP and Ca^{++} mechanical and metabolic events in isometrically contracting vascular smooth muscle, *Acta Physiol. Scand.,* 87, 84, 1973.
15. **Volicer, L. and Hyme, S.,** Effect of catecholamines and angiotensin on cyclic AMP in rat aorta and tail artery, *Eur. J. Pharmacol.,* 15, 214, 1971.
16. **Nesheim, B.-I., Osnes, J.-B., and Øye, I.,** Role of cyclic adenosine 3′,5′-monophosphate in the isoprenaline-induced relaxation of the oestrogen dominated rabbit uterus, *Br. J. Pharmacol.,* 53, 403, 1974.
17. **Moncada, S., Grylewski, R., Bunting, S., and Vane, J. R.,** An enzyme isolated from arteries transforms prostaglandin endoperoxides to an unstable substance that inhibits platelet aggregation, *Nature (London),* 263, 663, 1976.
18. **Dusting, G.J., Moncada, S., and Vane, J. R.,** Prostacyclin (PGX) is the endogenous metabolite responsible for relaxation of the coronary arteries induced by arachidonic acid, *Prostaglandins,* 13, 3, 1977.
19. **Gorman, R. R., Bunting, S., and Miller, O. V.,** Modulation of human platelet adenyl cyclase by prostacyclin (PGX), *Prostaglandins,* 13, 377, 1977.
20. **Malik, K. U. and McGiff, J. C.,** Modulation by prostaglandins of adrenergic transmission in the isolated perfused rabbit and rat kidney, *Circ. Res.,* 35, 599, 1975.
21. **Armstrong, J. M., Blackwell, G. J., Flower, R. J., McGiff, J. C., Mullane, K. M., and Vane, J. R.,** Genetic hypertension in rats is accompanied by a defect in renal prostaglandin catabolism, *Nature (London),* 260, 582, 1976.
22. **Armstrong, J. M., Bell, C., Lattimer, N., McGiff, J. C., and Mullane, K. M.,** Contribution of prostaglandins to the renal vascular supersensitivity to vasoconstrictor agents exhibited by New Zealand genetic hypertensive rats, *Clin. Sci. Mol. Med.,* 51, 275s, 1976.
23. **Sitrin, M. D. and Bohr, D. F.,** Ca and Na interaction in vascular smooth muscle contraction, *Am. J. Physiol.,* 220, 1124, 1971.
24. **Hering, H. E.,** *Die Karotissinus Reflexe auf Herz und Gefasse,* Steinkopff, Leipzig, 1927.
25. **Doyle, A.E. and Black, H.,** Reactivity to pressor agents in hypertension, *Circulation,* 12, 974, 1955.
26. **McCubbin, J. W., Green, J. H., and Page, I. H.,** Baroreceptor function in chronic renal hypertension, *Circ. Res.,* 4, 205, 1956.
27. **Barnett, A. J. and Fraser, J. R. E.,** The mechanism of arterial hypertension: a comparison of the effects of hexamethonium bromide in hypertensive and normotensive persons, *Aust. Ann. Med.,* 3, 152, 1954.
29. **Duff, R. A.,** Adrenaline sensitivity of peripheral blood vessels in hypertension, *Br. Heart J.,* 19, 45, 1957.
30. **Doyle, A.E., Fraser, J. R. E., and Marshall, R. J.,** Reactivity of forearm vessels to vasoconstrictor substances in hypertensive and normotensive subjects, *Clin. Sci.* 18, 441, 1959.
31. **Fatheree, T. J. and Brown, G. E.,** Digital arterioles of normal and hypertensive individuals: their response to intravenous administration of epinephrine as measured by cutaneous temperature, *Am. Heart J.,* 13, 1, 1937.
32. **Greisman, S. E.,** The reaction of the capillary bed of the nail fold to the continuous intravenous infusion of levo-norepinephrine in patients with normal blood pressure and with essential hypertension, *J. Clin. Invest.,* 33, 975, 1954.
33. **Mendlowitz, M., Naftchi, N., Wolf, R. L., and Gitlow, S. E.,** Reactivity of the digital blood vessels to angiotensin II in normotensive and hypertensive subjects, *Am. Heart J.,* 62, 221, 1961.
34. **Mendlowitz, M., Gitlow, S. E., Wolf, R. L., and Naftchi, N. E.,** Mechanisms in essential hypertension, *Am. J. Cardiol.,* 9, 100, 1962.
35. **Mendlowitz, M., Naftchi, N. E., Bobrow, E. B., Wolf, R. L., and Gitlow, S. E.,** The effect of aldosterone on electrolytes and on digital vascular reactivity to L-norepinephrine in normotensive, hypertensive and hypotensive subjects, *Am. Heart J.,* 65, 93, 1963.
36. **Moulon, R., Spencer, A. G., and Willoughby, D. A.,** Noradrenaline sensitivity to hypertension measured with a radioactive sodium technique, *Br. Heart J.,* 20, 224, 1958.
37. **Lee, R. E. and Holze, E. A.,** Peripheral vascular hemodynamics in the bulbar conjuctiva of subjects with hypertensive vascular disease, *J. Clin. Invest.,* 30, 539, 1951.
38. **Jackson, W. B.,** The functional activity of the human conjunctival capillary bed in hypertensive and normotensive subjects, *Am. Heart J.,* 56, 222, 1958.
39. **Barany, F. R. and James, P.,** The sensitivity to L-noradrenaline of patients with high blood pressure, *Clin. Sci.,* 18, 543, 1959.

40. **Sivertsson, R.,** Haemodynamic importance of structural vascular changes in essential hypertension, *Acta Physiol. Scand. Suppl.,* 343, 6, 1970.
41. **Folkow, B.,** Haemodynamic consequences of adaptive structural changes of resistance vessels in hypertension, *Clin. Sci.,* 41, 1, 1971.
42. **Doyle, A. E. and Fraser, J. R. E.,** Essential hypertension and inheritance of vascular reactivity, *Lancet,* 2, 509, 1961.
43. **McQueen, E. G.,** Vascular reactivity in experimental renal and renoprival hypertension, *Clin. Sci.,* 15, 523, 1956.
44. **Hinke, J. A. M.,** In vitro demonstration of vascular hyper-responsiveness in experimental hypertension, *Circ. Res.,* 17, 359, 1965.
45. **Hinke, J. A. M.,** Effect of Ca^{++} upon contractility of small arteries from DCA-hypertensive rats, *Circ. Res.,* 18, (Suppl. 1), 23, 1966.
46. **McGregor, D. D.and Smirk, F. H.,** Vascular responses in mesenteric arteries from genetic and renal hypertensive rats, *Am. J. Physiol.,* 214, 1429, 1968.
47. **McGregor, D. D.and Smirk, F. H.,** Vascular responses to 5-hydroxytryptamine in genetic and renal hypertensive rats, *Am. J. Physiol.,* 219, 687, 1970.
48. **Haeusler, G. and Finch, L.,** Vascular resistance and reactivity to various vasoconstrictor agents in hypertensive rats, in *Spontaneous Hypertension,* Okamoto, K., Ed., Igaku Shoin, Tokyo, 1972, 97.
49. **Folkow, B., Hallback, M., Lundgren, Y., and Weiss, L.,** Background of increased flow resistance and vascular reactivity in spontaneously hypertensive rats, *Acta Physiol. Scand.,* 80, 93, 1970.
50. **Collis, M. G. and Alps, B. J.,** Vascular reactivity to noradrenaline, potassium chloride, and angiotensin II in the rat perfused mesenteric vascular preparation during the development of renal hypertension, *Cardiovasc. Res.,* 9, 118 1975.
51. **Berecek, K. H. and Bohr, D. F.,** Structural and functional changes in vascular resistance and reactivity in the deoxycorticosterone acetate (DOCA)-hypertensive pig, *Circ. Res.,* 40 (Suppl. 1), 1, 1977.
52. **Friedman, S. M. and Friedman, C. L.,** The ionic matrix of vasoconstriction, *Circ. Res.,* 20 (Suppl 2), 147, 1967.
53. **Redleaf, P. D. and Tobian, L.,** The question of vascular hyperresponsiveness in hypertension, *Circ. Res.,* 6, 185, 1958.
54. **Mallov, S.,** Comparative reactivities of aortic strips from hypertensive and normotensive rats to epinephrine and levarterenol, *Circ. Res.,* 7, 196, 1959.
55. **Spector, S., Fleisch, J. H., Maling, H. M., and Brodie, B. B.,** Vascular smooth muscle reactivity in normotensive and hypertensive rats, *Science,* 166, 1300, 1969.
56. **Bohr, D. F. and Sitrin, M.,** Regulation of vascular smooth muscle contraction, *Circ. Res.,* 26 and 27 (Suppl. 2), 83, 1970.
57. **Holloway, E. T. and Bohr, D. F.,** Reactivity of smooth muscle in hypertensive rats, *Circ. Res.,* 33, 678, 1973.
58. **Shibata, S. and Kurahashi, K.,** Possible mechanisms of vascular reactivity differences in spontaneously hypertensive and normotensive rat aortae, in *Spontaneous Hypertension,* Okamoto, K., Ed., Igaku Shoin, Tokyo, 1972, 115.
59. **Bevan, J. A., Bevan, R. D., Chang, P. C., Pegram, B. L., Purdy, R. E., and Su, C.,** Analysis of changes in reactivity of rabbit arteries and veins two weeks after induction of hypertension by coarctation of the abdominal aorta, *Circ. Res.,* 37, 183, 1975.
60. **Bevan, R. D., Van Marthens, E., and Bevan, J. A.,** Hyperplasia of vascular smooth muscle in experimental hypertension in the rabbit, *Circ. Res.,* 38 (Suppl. 2), 2, 58, 1976.
61. **Busse, R., Bauerm, R. D., and Summa, Y.,** Comparison of the visco-elastic properties of the tail artery in spontaneously hypertensive, and normotensive rats, *Pflugers Arch.,* 364, 175, 1976.
62. **Friedman, S. M., Nakashima, M., and Mar, M.,** Morphological assessment of vasoconstriction and vascular hypertrophy in sustained hypertension in the rat, *Microvasc. Res.,* 3, 416, 1971.
63. **Short, D.,** Morphology of the intestinal arterioles in chronic human hypertension, *Br. Heart J.,* 28, 184, 1966.
64. **Tobian, L. and Binion, J. T.,** Tissue cations and water in arterial hypertension, *Circulation,* 5, 754, 1952.
65. **Tobian, L. and Binion, J. T.,** Arterial wall electrolytes in renal and DCA hypertension, *J. Clin. Invest.,* 33, 1407, 1954.
66. **Raab, W., Humphreys, R. J., and Lepeschkin, E.,** Potentiation of pressor effects of norepinephrine and epinephrine in man by desoxycorticosterone acetate, *J. Clin. Invest.,* 29, 1397, 1950.
67. **Raab, W.,** The integrated role of catecholamines, mineralocorticoids and sodium in hyper- and hypotension, *J. Mt. Sinai Hosp., New York,* 19, 233, 1952.
68. **Bunting, C. H. and Bunting, H.,** Acid mucopolysaccharides of the aorta, *Arch. Path.,* 55, 257, 1953.

69. **Manley, G. and Hawsworth, J.,** Distribution of mucopolysaccharides in the human vascular tree, *Nature (London),* 206, 1152, 1965.

70. **Farber, S.J. and Schubert, M.,** Binding of cations to chondroitin sulphate, *J. Clin. Invest.,* 36, 1715, 1957.

71. **Crane, W. A. J.,** Sulphate utilization and mucopolysaccharide synthesis by the mesenteric arteries of rats with experimental hypertension, *J. Pathol. Bacteriol.,* 84, 113, 1962.

72. **Hollander, W., Madoff, I. M., Kramsch, D., and Yagi, S.,** Arterial wall metabolism in experimental hypertension of coarctation of the aorta, in *Hypertension,* American Heart Association, New York, 1965, 61.

73. **Constantopoulos, G., Kusumoto, M., Boucher, R., and Genest, J.,** Étude des methodes de détermination de la teneur en eau et en electrolytes dan les tissus, *Union Med. Can.,* 102, 918, 1973.

74. **Headings, V. E., Rondell, P. A., and Bohr, D. F.,** Bound sodium in artery wall, *Am. J. Physiol.,* 199, 783, 1960.

75. **Friedman, S. M., Mar, M., and Nakashima, M.,** Lithium substitution analysis of Na and K phases in a small artery, *Blood Vessels,* 11, 55, 1974.

76. **Jones, A.W. and Swain, M. L.,** Chemical and kinetic analyses of sodium distribution in canine lingual artery, *Am. J. Physiol.,* 223, 1110, 1972.

77. **Constantopoulos, G., Kusumoto, M., Rojo-Ortega, J. M., Granger, P., Bouchier, R., and Genest, J.,** Arterial water, cations and norepinephrine in early and late hypertension, *Am. J. Physiol.,* 228, 1415, 1975.

78. **Halpern, B., Meyer, P., Milliez, P., and Lagrue, G.,** Increase in sodium content in the arterial walls during experimental hypertension, *Nature (London),* 201, 505, 1964.

79. **Nagoaka, A., Kikuchi, K., and Aramaki, Y.,** Participation of tissue electrolytes and water to the spontaneous hypertension in rats, *Jpn. Circ. J.,* 34, 489, 1970.

80. **Mallov, S.,** Effects of sodium ion and solution toxicities on reactiveness of rat aortic strip, *Am. J. Physiol.,* 198, 1019, 1960.

81. **Bohr, D. F., Brodie, D. C., and Chen, D. H.,** Effects of electrolytes in arterial muscle contraction, *Circulation,* 17, 746, 1958.

82. **Harris, G. S. and Palmer, W. A.,** The effect of enzymatic depolymerization of arterial mucoploysaccharides on sodium ion content and vessel reactivity, *Clin. Sci.,* 40, 293, 1971.

83. **Harris, G. S. and Palmer, W. A.,** Effect of increased sodium ion on arterial sodium and reactivity, *Clin. Sci.,* 42, 301, 1972.

84. **Friedman, S. M. and Friedman, C. L.,** Cell permeability, sodium transport, and the hypertensive process in the rat, *Circ. Res.,* 39, 433, 1976.

85. **Jones, A. W. and Hart, R. G.,** Altered ion transport in aortic smooth muscle during deoxycorticosterone acetate hypertension in the rat, *Circ. Res.,* 37, 333, 1975.

86. **Fries, E. D.,** The collapse produced by venous congestion of the extremities or by venesection following certain hypotensive agents, *J. Clin. Invest.,* 30, 435, 1951.

87. **Dustan, H. P., Tarazi, R. C., and Bravo, E. L.,** Dependence of arterial pressure on intravascular volume in treated hypertensive patients, *N. Engl. J. Med.,* 286, 861, 1972.

88. **Verghaege, R. H. and Shepherd, J. T.,** Effect of nitroprusside on smooth muscle and adrenergic nerve terminals in isolated blood vessels, *J. Pharmacol. Exp. Ther.,* 199, 269, 1976.

89. **Gross, F., Druey, J., and Meier, R.,** Eine neue gruppe blutdrucksenkender substanzen von besonderum wirkungscharakter, *Experientia,* 6, 19, 1950.

90. **Åblad, B., Johnsson, G., and Henning, M.,** The effect of intra-arterially administered hydrallazine on blood flow in the forearm and hand, *Acta Pharmacol. Toxicol.,* 18, 165, 1961.

91. **Åblad, B.,** Site of action of hydrallazine and dihydrallazine in man, *Acta Pharmacol. Toxicol.,* 16, 113, 1959.

92. **Åblad, B. and Johnsson, G.,** Comparative effects of intra-arterially administered hydrallazine and sodium nitrite on blood flow and volume of the forearm, *Acta Pharmacol. Toxicol.,* 20 (Suppl. 1), 1, 1963.

93. **Moore-Jones, D. and Perry, H. M.,** Radioautographic localization of Hydralazine-1-C^{14} in arterial walls, *Proc. Soc. Exp. Biol. Med.,* 122, 576, 1966.

94. **Freis, E. D., Rose, J C., Higgins, T. F., Finnerty, F. A., Kelley, R. T., and Partenope, E. A.,** The hemodynamic effects of hypotensive drugs in man. IV. 1-Hydrazinophthalazine, *Circulation,* 8, 199, 1953.

95. **Zacest, R. and Koch-Weser, J.,** Relation of hydralazine plasma concentration to dosage and hypotensive action, *Clin. Pharmacol. Ther.,* 13, 420, 1972.

96. **Perry, H. M.,** Late toxicity to hydrallazine resembling systemic lupus erythematosus or rheumatoid arthritis, *Am. J. Mcd.,* 54, 58, 1973.

97. **Hess, H. J.,** Biochemistry and structure-activity studies with prazosin, in *Prazosin — Evaluation of a New Antihypertensive Agent,* Cotton, D. W. K., Ed., Excerpta Medica, Geneva, 1974, 3.

98. **Constantine, J. W., McShane, W. K., Scriabine, A., and Hess, H.-J.,** Analysis of the hypotensive action of prazosin, in *Hypertension: Mechanisms and Management,* Onesti, G., Kim, K. E., and Moyer, J. H., Eds., Grune & Stratton, New York, 1973, 429.

99. **Rand, M. J.,** personal communication.

100. **Fernandes, M. and Onesti, G.,** Clinical pharmacology of prazosin, in *New Antihypertensive Drugs,* Scriabine, A. and Sweet, C. S., Eds., Spectrum Publications, New York, 1976, 481.

101. **Lund-Johansen, O.,** Hemodynamic changes at rest and during exercise in long term prazosin therapy of essential hypertension, in *Prazosin — Evaluation of a New Antihypertensive Agent,* Cotton, D. W. K., Ed., Excerpta Medica, Geneva, 1974, 103.

102. **Graham, R. M., Muir, M. R., and Hayes, J. M.,** Effects of prazosin on blood pressure and plasma renin activity in the anaesthetized dog, *Aust. N. Z. J. Med.,* 4, 424, 1974.

103. **Hayes, J. M., Graham, R. M., O'Connell, B. P., Muir, M. R., Speers, E., and Humphrey, T. J.,** Experience with prazosin in the treatment of patients with severe hypertension, *Med. J. Aust.,* 1, 562, 1976.

104. **Massingham, R. and Hayden, M. L.,** A comparison of the effects of prazosin and hydrallazine on blood pressure, heart rate and plasma renin activity in conscious renal hypertensive dogs, *Eur. J. Pharmacol.,* 30, 121, 1974.

105. **DuCharme, D. W., Freyburger, W. A., Graham, B. E., and Carlson, R. G.,** Pharmacologic properties of minoxidil; a new antihypertensive agent, *J. Pharmacol. Exp. Ther.,* 184, 662, 1973.

106. **Gilmore, E., Weil, J., and Chidsey, C.,** Treatment of essential hypertension with a new vasodilator in combination with beta-adrenergic blockade, *N. Engl. J. Med.,* 282, 521, 1970.

107. **Gottlieb, T. B., Katz, F. H., and Chidsey, C. A.,** Combined therapy with vasodilator drugs and beta-adrenergic drugs in hypertension. A comparative study of minoxidil and hydrallazine, *Circulation,* 45, 571, 1972.

108. **Pettinger, W. A. and Mitchell, H. C.,** Minoxidil: an alternative to nephrectomy for refractory hypertension, *N. Engl. J. Med.,* 289, 167, 1973.

109. **Limas, C. J. and Freis, E. D.,** Minoxidil in severe hypertension with renal failure: effects of its addition to conventional antihypertensive drugs, *Am. J. Cardiol.,* 31, 355, 1973.

110. **Dormois, J. C., Young, J. L., and Nies, A. S.,** Minoxidil in severe hypertension. Value when conventional drugs have failed, *Am. Heart J.,* 90, 360, 1975.

111. **Balags, T., Herman, E., Earl, F. L., and Wolff, F.,** Cardiotoxicity studies with diaoxide, reserpine, guanethidine and combinations of diazoxide and propranolol in dogs, *Toxicol. Appl. Pharmacol.,* 20, 442, 1975.

112. **Balags, T., Herman, E., and Earl, F. L.,** Myocardial necroses induced by diazoxide and minoxidil in dogs, and the effects of propranolol and digoxin on the minoxidil-induced lesions, in *New Antihypertensive Drugs,* Scriabine, A. and Sweet, C. S., Eds., Spectrum Publications, New York, 1976, 535.

113. **Freis, E. D. and Hammer, J.,** Guancydine, a new type of antihypertensive agent, *Med. Ann. D. C.,* 38, 69, 1969.

114. **Gupta, N. and Goldberg, L. I.,** Guancydine, a new vasodilator: comparison with hydralazine in a regime including propranolol and guimethazone, in *Hypertension, Mechanisms and Management,* Onesti, G., Kim, K. E. and Moyer, J. H., Eds., Grune & Stratton, New York, 1973, 351.

115. **Clark, D. W. and Goldberg, L. T.,** Guancydine: a new antihypertensive agent. Use with guinethiazone and guanethidine or propranolol, *Am. Intern. Med.,* 76, 1972, 579.

116. **Haas, H. and Hartfelder, F.,** α-Isopropyl-α[(N-methyl-N-)-α-aminopropyl]-3-4 dimethoxyphenylacetonitril, eine substanz nut coronargefasserweiternden eigenschaften, *Arzneim. Forsch.,* 12, 549, 1962.

117. **Nayler, W. G. and Szeto, J.,** Effect of verapamil on concontractility, oxygen utilization, and calcium exchangeability in mammalian heart muscle, *Cardiovasc. Res.,* 6, 120, 1972.

118. **Carpenedo, F., Toson, G. C., Furlannt, M., and Ferrari, M.,** Effects of papeverine and eupaverin on calcium uptake by isolated sarcoplasmic vesicles, *J. Pharm. Pharmacol.,* 23, 502, 1971.

119. **Schomerus, M., Spiegelhalcher, B., Stieren, B., and Eichelbaum, M.,** Physiological disposition of verapamil in man, *Cardiovasc. Res.,* 10, 605, 1975.

120. **Livesley, B., Catley, P. F., Campbell, R. C., and Oram, S.,** Double blind evaluation of verapamil, propranolol and isorbide-dinitrate against placebo in the treatment of angina pectoris, *Br. Med. J.,* 1, 375, 1973.

121. **Grant, R. H. E., McDevitt, D. G., and Shanless, R. C.,** Is verapamil a β-blocker?, *Lancet,* 1, 362, 1968.

122. **Vohra, J., Hunt, D., and Sloman, J. G.,** Clinical experience with verapamil, *Med. J. Aust.,* 2, 417, 1975.

123. Andreasan, F., Boye, E., Christoffersen, E., Dalsgaard, P., Henneberg, E., Kallenbach, A., Lade-
foged, S., Lithquist, K., Mikkelsen, E., Norderø, E., Olsen, J., Pedersen, J. K., Pedersen, V., Bruun
Petersen, G., Schroll, J., Schultz, H., and Seidelin, J., Assessment of verapamil in the treatment of
angina pectoris, *Eur. J. Cardiol.*, 2, 443, 1975.

124. Lewis, G. R. J., Morley, K., Lewis, B. M., and Bones, P., The treatment of hypertension with verapamil, *N. Z. Med. J.*, 1978, in press.

125. Moore, P. F., The effect of diazodie and benzothiadiazine diuretics upon phosphodiesterase, *Ann.
N. Y. Acad. Sci.*, 150, 26, 1968.

126. Wohl, A. J., Hausler, L. M., and Roth, F. E., The role of calcium in the mechanism of the antihypertensive action of diazoxide, *Life Sci.*, 7, 381, 1965.

127. Sellers, E. M., and Koch-Weser, J., Protein binding and vascular activity of diazoxide, *N. Engl. J.
Med.*, 281, 1141, 1969.

128. Mroczek, W. J., Leibel, B. A., Davidov, M., and Finnerty, F. A. Jr., The importance of the rapid
administration of diazoxide in accelerated hypertension, *N. Engl. J. Med.*, 285, 603, 1971.

129. Johnson, C. C., The actions and toxicity of sodium nitroprusside, *Arch. Int. Pharmacodyn. Ther.*,
35, 480, 1929.

130. Page, I. H., Corcoran, A. C., Dustan, H. O., and Koppanyi, T., Cardiovascular actions of sodium
nitroprusside in animals and hypertensive patients, *Circulation*, 11, 188, 1955.

131. Palmer, R. F. and Lasseter, K., Drug Therapy. Sodium nitroprusside, *N. Engl. J. Med.*, 292, 294,
1975.

132. Palmer, R. F., Seelman, R. C., and Wheat, M. W., Pharmacological approach to the therapy of
acute dissecting aneurysm of the aorta, *Clin. Res.*, 13, 27, 1965.

133. Franciosa, J. A., Guiha, N. H., Limas, C. F., Rodriguera, E., and Cohn, J. N., Improved left
ventricular function during nitroprusside infusion in acute myocardial infarction, *Lancet*, 1, 650,
1972.

134. Chatterjee, K., Parmley, W.W., Ganz, W., Forrester, J., Walinsky, P., Crexells, C., and Swan, H.
J. C., Hemodynamic and metabolic responses to vasodilator therapy in acute myocardial infarction,
Circulation, 48, 1183, 1973.

135. Zoster, T. T., Hart, F., and Radde, I. C., Mechanism of antihypertensive action of prolonged administration of hydrochlorothiazide in rabbit and dog, *Circ. Res.*, 27, 717, 1970.

136. Jandhayala, B. S., Cavero, I., and Buckley, J. P., Effects of prolonged hydrochlorothiazide administration on neurogenic tone in the hind limb vasculature, *Eur. J. Pharmacol.*, 17, 357, 1972.

Chapter 3

THERAPEUTICS OF HYPERTENSION

I. INTRODUCTION

In the last quarter of a century, there has been a revolution in the therapeutics of high blood pressure due to the introduction of pharmacological agents capable of producing large falls of blood pressure in hypertensive patients and to the demonstration that such treatment improves prognosis and alters the pattern of mortality and morbidity in patients with severe hypertension. The earlier drugs, notably the ganglion-blocking drugs, had grave disadvantages. They needed to be given by injection, produced large and often unpredictable falls in blood pressure, often of a magnitude to promote cerebral or cardiac ischemia, and additionally had a high incidence of severe side effects which caused numerous symptoms. It is therefore not surprising that in the early phase of the use of antihypertensive drugs, treatment was generally offered only to those in whom the short term prognosis was clearly very poor. Since that time, numerous new antihypertensive drugs have led to easier control of blood pressure and have mostly had side effects of a less dramatic nature than did the earlier ganglion-blocking drugs. Nevertheless, all drugs at present available for the treatment of hypertension have some disadvantages, and most patients still require comparatively skilled medical supervision, although for many patients this can be of a lower order than was formerly the case.

The administration of any form of treatment for any disease always involves a cost-benefit analysis being carried out. In the case of the patient with hypertension, the most important questions to be resolved are, firstly, what are the risks of not treating the patient; secondly, what diminution of these risks is to be expected from treatment; and thirdly, what, if any, are the disadvantages and disabilities which may result from the treatment? There are also a number of logistical questions which have to be answered in relation to the patient with hypertension. These relate to methods of detecting symptomless hypertensives within the community and to the very high costs, both of drugs and of medical supervision, involved in managing all cases of hypertension. Clearly, these questions only become of importance if the benefits of treatment can be shown to be worthwhile and to outweigh the disadvantages of prolonged treatment with drugs. Finally, perhaps the most important question to be considered is the possibility that patients with hypertension may be divisible into subsets, each carrying a different prognosis unrelated to the levels of blood pressure. Linked with this question is the important aspect of pathogenesis of hypertension and the possibility of defining several distinct etiological types of hypertension, each carrying a different prognosis and each amenable to a specific form of therapy. Finally, there exists the important question of the presence of definable risk factors other than the level of blood pressure; this matter, although linked with pathogenesis, may exist independently of the causes of hypertension and may relate to genetic or environmental factors.

This section deals with the practical aspects of patient management, with chapters in clinical aspects of hypertension, selection of patients for treatment, the selection of the appropriate drug, the results of treatment, and a few specific types of hypertension in which investigation or management raises special problems.

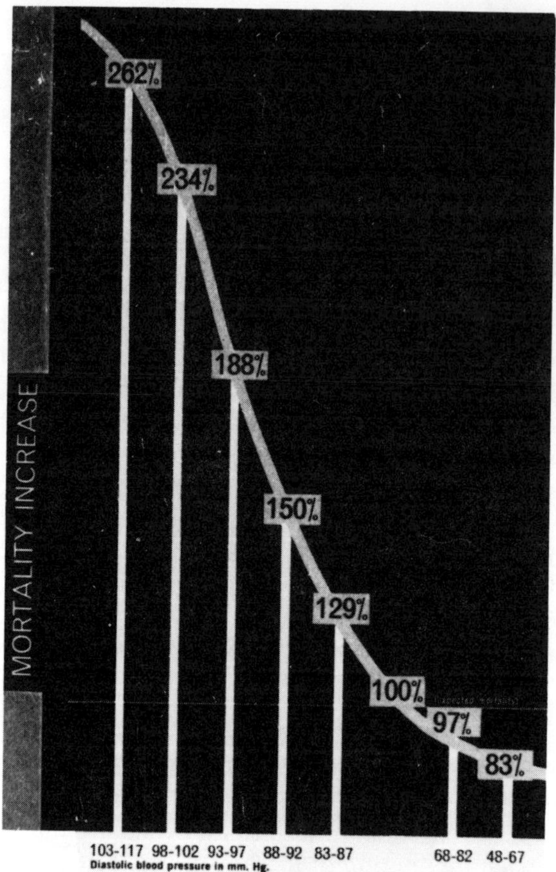

FIGURE 1.   The relationship between diastolic blood pressure during examination for life assurance and mortality. (From Society of Actuaries, *Build and Blood Pressure Study*, Vol. 1, Society of Actuaries, Chicago, 1959. With permission.)

II. ESSENTIAL HYPERTENSION

A. Clinical Aspects

1. Casual Blood Pressure

There is very strong evidence, which mostly derives from life insurance statistics, that any elevation of blood pressure leads on the average to earlier death from cardiovascular disorders. Thus, figures published by the life insurance companies[1] based on casual estimates of blood pressure in several million people examined for life insurance purposes showed a very close relationship between the level of diastolic blood pressure and excess mortality (Figure 1). In this study, individuals with diastolic blood pressures of about 75 mmHg were shown to exhibit the expected mortality for their age and sex, but individuals whose diastolic blood pressure was 88 to 92 mmHg had an increased mortality of 150%, and those with diastolic pressures between 103 to 117 mmHg had a mortality rate two- and one half times the average. Significantly, also, individuals with diastolic blood pressures lower than 75 mmHg showed decreased mortality and prolonged life expectancy. There is thus clear evidence that the level of blood pressure

TABLE 1

Life Expectancies in Slight and Moderate Hypertension

Age	Blood Pressure	Life expectancy (years)	
		Men	Women
35	Normal	41.5	—
	130/90	37.5 (reduction of 4 years	—
	140/95	32.5 (reduction of 9 years)	—
	150/100	25 (reduction of 16½ years)	—
45	Normal	32	37
	130/90	29 (reduction of 3 years)	35.5 (reduction of 1½ years)
	140/95	26 (reduction of 6 years)	32 (reduction of 5 years)
	150/100	20.5 (reduction of 11½ years)	28.5 (reduction of 8½ years)
55	Normal	23.5	27.5
	130/90	22.5 (reduction of 1 year)	27 (reduction of ½ year)
	140/95	19.5 (reduction of 4 years)	24.5 (reduction of 3 years)
	150/100	17.5 (reduction of 6 years)	23.5 (reduction of 4 years)

From Lew, A., *An Actuarial View of Hypertension,* Monographs on Hypertension, Merck & Co., 1973.

has an important effect in inducing early death and also that quite modest elevations of diastolic pressure are associated with early death.

Other evidence is available to show the effects of such marginal elevations on life expectancy and on the effect of blood pressure rises in the two sexes and at various ages. Thus, the figures of the Society of Actuaries[2] show that for American men aged 35 years with blood pressures of 120/80 or below presenting for life insurance, the average life expectancy was 42 years, and for men in the same age group, the life expectancy with a presenting blood pressure of 150/100 was reduced by 17 years to 25 years (Table 1). For men aged 45, the average life expectancy was 32 years; with blood pressures of 150/100, it was reduced to about 20 years. For women of 45 years, average life expectancy was reduced by 8.5 years.

Figures published by the Society of Actuaries, Chicago, provide further evidence on the relationship between casual insurance blood pressure readings and mortality at various ages of presentation.[2] These indicate that at the age of 30 to 39 years, there is a steady increase in mortality as the initial systolic pressure rises, so that, whereas deaths in individuals of this age are only about 1 per 1000 per annum when the systolic pressure is 125 mmHg, deaths in persons with initial systolic pressures of 165 mmHg are about 10 per 1000 per annum. At 50 to 59 years the deaths rise from 20 per 1000 per annum for normotensives to 50 per 1000 per annum in mild hypertensives. Such figures indicate that when very large numbers of persons are involved, quite modest elevations of blood pressures in people of 50 to 59 years lead to an excess mortality of 30,000 per million per annum. Moreover, these mortality figures, impressive though they are, take no account of morbidity. The studies of the Society of Actuaries[2] indi-

TABLE 2

Major Causes of Death Among Hypertensives

	Mortality ratio (standard risk = 100%)	
Cause of Death	Men (%)	Women (%)
Heart disease	258	340
Cerebral hemorrhage	546	525
Nephritis	424	—
Influenza and pneumonia	136	—
Digestive disease	153	—

From Lew, A., *An Actuarial View of Hypertension,* Monographs on Hypertension, Merck & Co., 1973.

cate that the mortality increase is accounted for mainly by stroke and cardiovascular disease and that the increased mortality from stroke in persons with blood pressures in the range 148/93 to 177/102 is six times that of individuals with diastolic pressures below 83 mmHg (Table 2).

The Framingham study[3] has underlined the significant role of hypertension in the causation of stroke and vascular disease. In men aged 30 to 62 at entry, both hemorrhagic stroke and non hemorrhagic stroke were more than three times as common in those with systolic blood pressure on entry of 160 mmHg or more and diastolic blood pressure of 95 mmHg or more, as they were in those with lower blood pressures. In the same study,[4] the incidence of congestive heart failure was almost six times greater in the hypertensive group than in the normotensive. Mortality from coronary heart disease is also substantially greater in persons with hypertension than those without,[5] and there seems good evidence that all the clinical manifestations of coronary heart disease, such as angina, myocardial infarction, congestive heart failure, and sudden death, are significantly related to the antecedent level of both systolic and diastolic blood pressure.

There is therefore little doubt about the adverse effect of even modest rises of blood pressure on mortality and morbidity in American individuals, and most evidence suggests that these figures are applicable to other westernized communities. The magnitude of the problem has already been mentioned. Prevalence studies carried out in a number of areas of the world have demonstrated that as many as 15% of the population aged 50 or more years have casual diastolic pressures of 95 mmHg or more. Thus, Prineas, Stephens, and Lovell,[6] in a study in an Australian country town, found a percentage of this order in a population sample aged 50 to 59 years. Similarly, in a survey in Atlanta, Georgia, hypertension was found in 23% of a mainly black population.[7] Studies in Europe have shown a similar prevalence.[8,9] It is evident, therefore, that many communities contain large numbers of patients with mild hypertension, and that in these patients, morbidity and mortality from cardiovascular diseases and stroke can be expected to be substantially greater than in the population at large.

Given the clear relationships between the incidence of cardiovascular complications and the preceding level of blood pressure, it might be supposed that the only useful indication for treatment would be an elevated blood pressure, yet the value of a single casual blood pressure reading as a sole indication for treatment may have only a limited value. From a clinical standpoint, a single elevated reading is seldom an indication for

TABLE 3

Changes in Blood Pressure Over a 2-Year Period in Male Employees of the Metropolitan Life Insurance Company

Systolic Pressure

	Initial pressure of 128 to 147 mmHg			Initial pressure of 148 mmHg or higher		
2 years later	Ages 38—45 years (%)	Ages 46—55 years (%)	Ages 56—68 years (%)	Ages 38—45 years (%)	Ages 46—55 years (%)	Ages 56—68 years (%)
Lower blood pressure	28.0	21.1	19.0	47.5	30.0	22.8
Same blood pressure	34.0	27.4	28.6	21.3	31.4	26.3
Higher blood prssure	38.0	51.4	52.4	31.1	38.6	50.9
Very much higher blood pressure	12.2	20.6	19.0	14.8	22.9	21.1

Diastolic Pressure

	Initial pressure of 83—92 mmHg			Initial pressure of 93 mmHg or higher		
2 years later	Ages 38—45 years (%)	Ages 46—55 years (%)	Ages 56—68 years (%)	Ages 38—45 years (%)	Ages 46—55 years (%)	Ages 56—58 years (%)
Lower blood pressure	28.3	30.2	14.0	27.8	28.2	31.0
Same blood pressure	49.7	44.4	56.1	43.1	42.3	47.6
Higher blood pressure	21.9	25.4	29.8	29.2	29.9	21.4
Very much higher blood pressure	2.1	0.8	7.0	4.2	5.6	2.4

From Lew, A., *An Actuarial View of Hypertension,* Monographs on Hypertension, Merck & Co., 1973.

the immediate initiation of treatment, unless it is associated with other evidence of hypertensive disease. The finding of a diastolic blood pressure of 90 mmHg or higher justifies repeated measurement within a few days. Casual diastolic blood pressures which remain persistently 100 mmHg or higher are a firm indication for the institution of treatment irrespective of other findings, particularly when measured over a period of 1 to 2 weeks with multiple measurements of blood pressure.[10]

Pressures below 100 mmHg and above 90 mmHg constitute borderline hypertension, when based on multiple blood pressure measurements under standard conditions and on separate days. [10]

Patients with these blood pressure levels should be reexamined at yearly intervals as a minimum, and treatment should be considered in those showing additional risk factors.

It has to be emphasized that many individuals whose blood pressure is marginally elevated may be found on rescreening to be normotensive. The study in Göteborg[11] identified 531 men with borderline hypertension. Two years later 3% of these had developed symptoms of hypertension and were being treated, and in 7.5% the blood pressure had risen to between 95 to 115 mmHg. However, in 46% the blood pressure remained borderline, and in 38% the blood pressure had fallen to normal levels. Thus, only about 10% of this borderline group became definitely hypertensive in 2 years, while 38% had become normotensive. Similar data were recorded in the Framingham study[12] and by the Metropolitan Insurance Company[1] (Table 3).

The level of the casual blood pressure may vary considerably with the circumstances of measurement. Pain or discomfort, anxiety, or anger may lead to transient rises of pressure, which although often exaggerated in hypertensive individuals, may also occur in people whose blood pressures are usually normal. Inaccuracies in technique of recording blood pressure, particularly in fat people with obese arms, may lead to spuriously high pressures being recorded. It is necessary to stress the value of repeated measurements of casual blood pressure rather than single observations as a means of deciding whether treatment should be instituted. Unless repeated measurement reveals diastolic blood pressures consistently 100 mmHg or higher, there is usually little to be lost by withholding active antihypertensive therapy.

2. Basal Blood Pressure

Some of the difficulties inherent in the evaluation of the significance of casual blood pressures can be avoided by the use of basal blood pressures. The term basal blood pressure was first used by Addis[13] and later by Alam and Smirk (1939),[14] and the prognostic value of the basal blood pressure has been extensively studied by Smirk and colleagues over some years. According to Smirk, the casual blood pressure reading is composed of two components: the basal, which is comparatively stable for any given individual, and the supplemental, which is the labile component. The basal blood pressure is measured after an overnight rest with a barbiturate by repeated measurement until a stable level is attained. Using this technique, it is claimed that the basal blood pressure remains approximately constant from one occasion to the next. Smirk has adduced strong evidence that a high basal blood pressure carries a very poor prognosis[15] and has suggested that this technique allows identification of those hypertensive patients most at risk and hence most in need of antihypertensive therapy. More recently, Smirk (1976)[16] has shown that first degree relatives of patients with hypertension have higher basal blood pressures than do control populations with no hypertension in close relatives. The basal blood pressures in the hypertensive's relatives increased with age to a greater degree than did those of the normal propositi (Figure 2). The technique, although simple, is time consuming and has not been widely

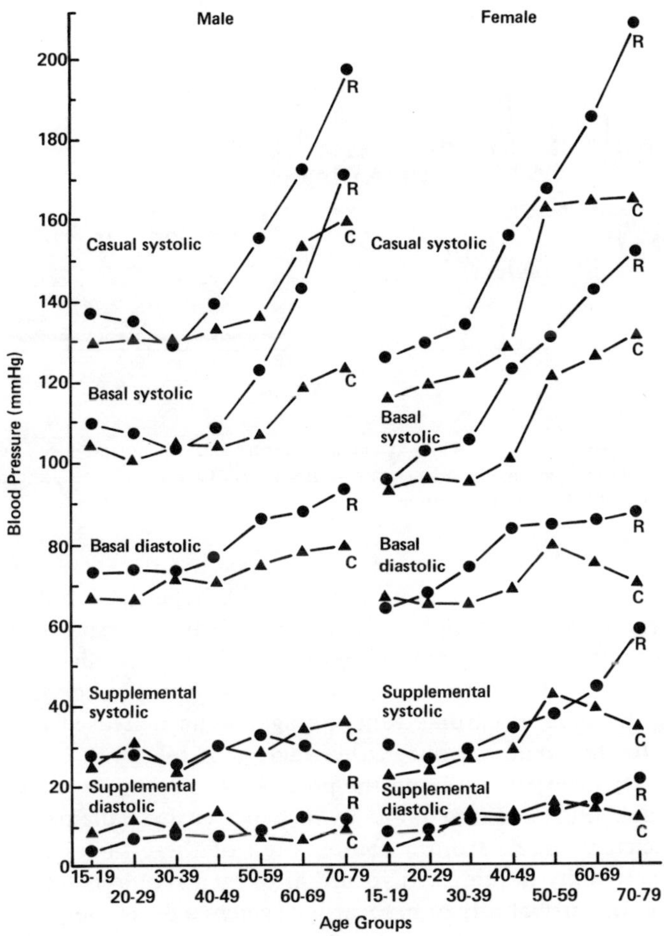

FIGURE 2. Comparison of blood pressures of relatives (•, R) of patients with essential hypertension and pressures of population control subjects (▲, C). (From Smirk, F. H., *Clin. Sci. Mol. Med.*, 51, 135, 1956. With permission.)

adopted. It is of value in emphasizing that persistent elevation of blood pressure is considerably more sinister than transient elevation. The data of Smirk and colleagues have been to some degree confirmed by the use of continuous recordings of blood pressure[17] which have emphasized the great variability which may occur between readings recorded under different circumstances and in particular the very low blood pressures which can be recorded during sleep, both in normotensive and hypertensive patients[18] (Figure 3). From a clinical point of view, the patient whose blood pressure falls rapidly on rest is likely to have a better prognosis than the one whose blood pressure remains elevated after hospitalization or a period of bed rest. Nevertheless, it has to be emphasized that patients with labile hypertension cannot in any way be regarded as having a normal expectation of life. Increased risk of cardiovascular disease is present even with labile hypertension, although certainly to a lesser degree than in people with fixed elevation of basal blood pressure.[19]

3. The Heart

a. Cardiac Failure

Although cardiac decompensation and death from heart failure are common seque-

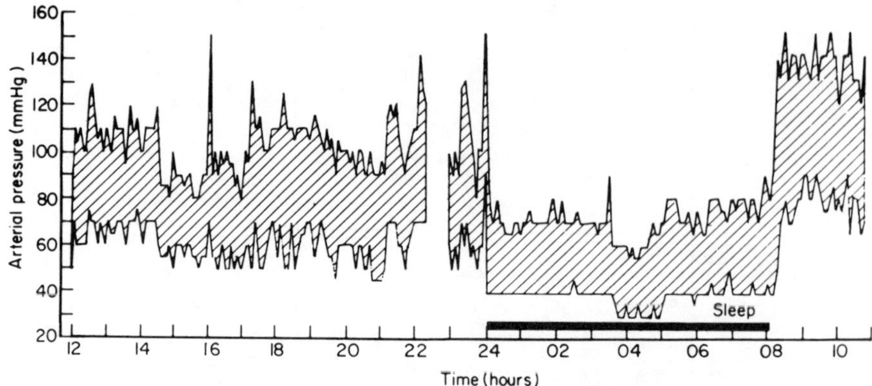

FIGURE 3.   Arterial pressure while awake and during sleep in normotensive (upper panel) and hypertensive (lower panel) subjects. (From Bevan, A. T., Honor, A. J., and Scott, F. H., *Clin. Sci.*, 36, 329, 1969. With permission.)

lae of untreated hypertension,[4] not all patients with hypertension develop evidence of cardiac enlargement or hypertrophy, and some patients may survive hypertension for many years without developing any symptoms or signs of cardiac involvement.[20] It is clear that the elevated blood pressure is only one important factor among many others in determining the state of cardiac function against an increased pressure load; even though it may be the dominant one. Other factors of relevance obviously include the extent of coronary artery disease and the presence or absence of ischemia or ischemic necrosis of cardiac muscle. In the majority of hypertensive patients, it is probable that cardiac insufficiency results from a combination of these factors. Moreover, as left ventricular hypertrophy develops, myocardial oxygen requirements increase,[21] which further increases the probability of myocardial ischemia developing.[22]

The early stages of labile or borderline hypertension are commonly associated with a cardiac output which is higher than the normal average, particularly in young patients. These changes have been well documented.[23,24] The elevated cardiac output was associated with only slightly elevated or in some instances, a normal peripheral resistance. In patients with moderate to severe hypertension, cardiac output was either normal or even lower than normal, the latter particularly in patients with evidence of heart failure. The same authors noted that an increased heart rate was observed in all stages of hypertension, which may be related to the observation of Lund-Johansen that hypertensive patients are less able than normotensives to increase stroke output.[25]

Frohlich et al.[26] have also described the clinical and physiological correlates of cardiac involvement in hypertension. The patients with essential hypertension were devided into three groups according to the severity of cardiac involvement (Figure 4). They were those exhibiting no cardiac involvement, those having electrocardiographic evidence of left atrial abnormalities,[27] and those having evidence of left ventricular enlargement, either radiological, electrocardiographic, or clinical. These authors demonstrated that these indexes of cardiac involvement correlated well with hemodynamic measurements. Arterial pressure and peripheral resistance were highest in those having left ventricular enlargement, lowest in those with no cardiac involvement, and intermediate in the group with left atrial abnormalities. The cardiac index likewise fell progressively in the three groups, whereas the pressure time per beat (which is an index of left ventricular tension) rose progressively, as cardiac involvement became more severe.

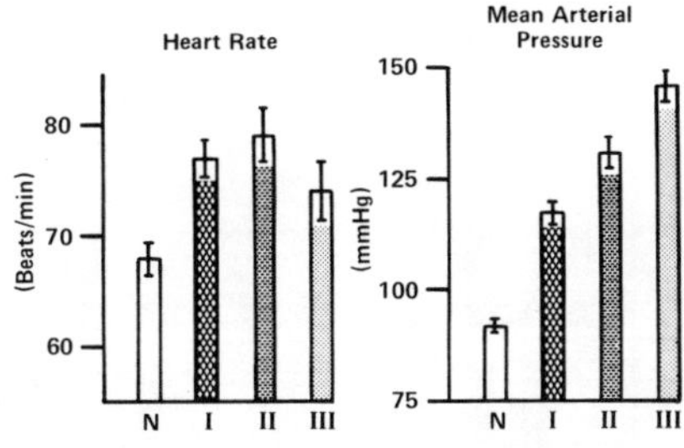

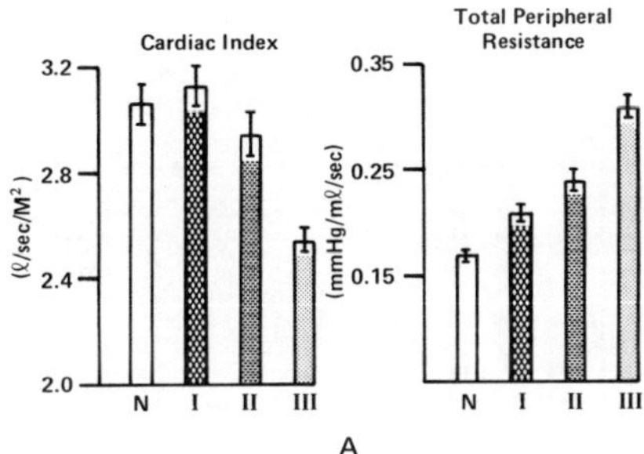

A

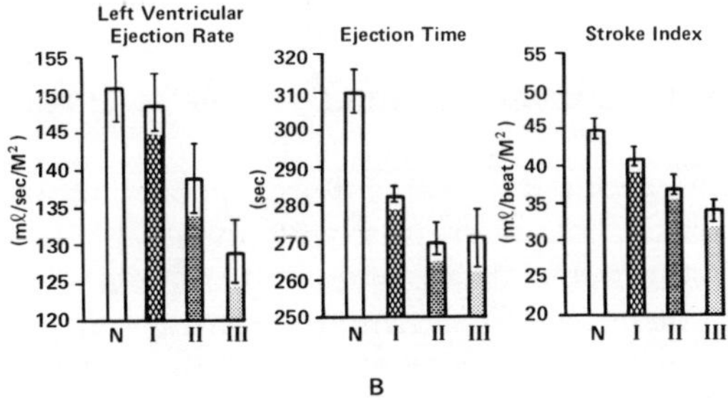

B

FIGURE 4. Hemodynamic indexes in 25 normotensive volunteer subjects (N) and three groups of patients with essential hypertension: group I, 54 patients having normal-sized hearts; Group II, 20 patients having left atrial abnormality; and group III, 23 patients having left ventricular hypertrophy. (A) Heart rate, mean arterial pressure, cardiac index, and total peripheral resistance. (B) Left ventricular ejection rate (index), ejection time, and stroke index. (C) Four derived left ventricular functions. All bars represent the mean for the group (± 1 standard error of the mean). (From Frohlich, E. D., Tarazi, R. C., and Dustan, H. P., *Circulation*, 44, 446, 1971. With permission.)

The genesis of hypertensive heart disease appears to develop over a substantial time and to be related to the severity of the hypertension. The probable sequence of events is a rise in peripheral resistance, leading to a rise in aortic pressure, with a consequent increase in left ventricular wall tension, with an increase in left ventricular and diastolic pressure. This leads to left atrial and to left ventricular hypertrophy and increased wall thickness which would restore wall tension to normal with a consequent reduction in myocardial oxygen requirement (per 1 gm of tissue).[21] The extent to which a balance in these factors occurs probably depends in part on the extent to which the pressure

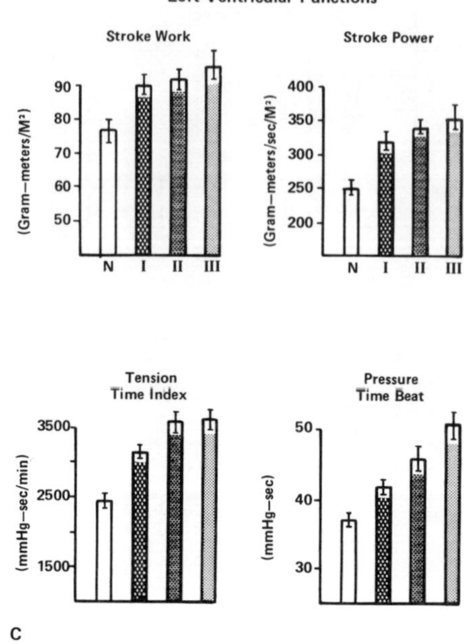

Figure 4C

continues to rise and partly on the rate at which it does so. It must also depend on the extent to which the hypertrophied muscle can be supported by the coronary circulation. The development of frank congestive heart failure has been shown to be accompanied by an increased left ventricular filling pressure with no increase in end diastolic volume, suggesting a fall in left ventricular compliance.[28] These authors have suggested that sudden rises in pressure in the nonhypertrophied ventricle or sudden rises in arterial pressure might induce myocardial hypoxia by producing sudden dilatation with a consequent increase in myocardial oxygen consumption. The same authors rightly point out that myocardial hypoxia because of coronary artery disease might also lead to a similar decrease in diastolic ventricular compliance, such as has been observed in acute myocardial infarction and angina pectoris.

From a clinical viewpoint, any evidence of cardiac enlargement whether clinical, radiological, or electrocardiographic indicates a poor prognosis and can be regarded as an unequivocal indication for drug treatment. Sokolow and Perloff,[29] in a study of prognosis in untreated hypertensives, reported a dramatic reduction in survival in relation both to electrocardiographic evidence of left ventricular enlargement and to radiological evidence of cardiac enlargement (Figure 5).

Evidence from the Framingham study[4] indicates that persons with hypertension have an incidence of congestive heart failure between four to six times that in normotensive people. These risks rise very steeply when there is evidence of cardiac involvement, whether electrocardiographic or radiological.

Symptoms of cardiac involvement usually occur late in the course of hypertension. Most patients with severe hypertension, even when there is objective evidence of cardiac involvement, deny any significant exertional dyspnea. The development of breathlessness on exertion in untreated hypertension is usually followed by evidence of congestive heart failure within a few months. In many patients, the initial symptom may be an attack of paroxysmal nocturnal dyspnea due to left ventricular failure.

Clinical evidence of left ventricular enlargement with a heaving displaced apex beat

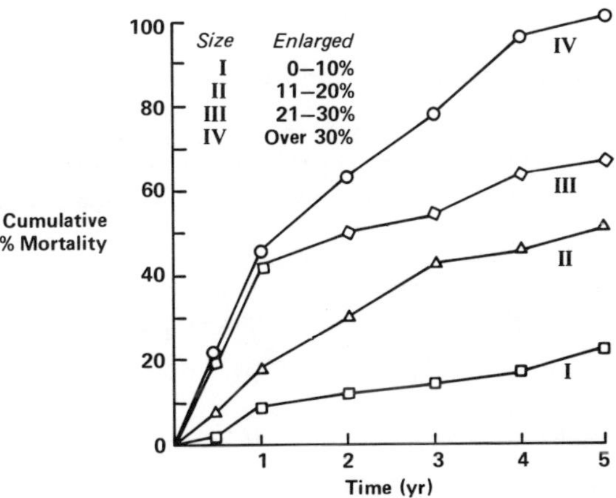

FIGURE 5. Relationship between cumulative mortality and radiological estimate of heart size in untreated hypertensive patients. (From Sokolow, M. and Perloff, D., *Circulation*, 34, 697, 1961. With permission.)

may precede the development of heart failure by months or years, as may the occurrence of an atrial sound (presystolic gallop rhythm).

By contrast, acute rises of blood pressure, such as occur in acute glomerulonephritis, phaeochromocytoma, or some cases of malignant hypertension, may lead to paroxysmal nocturnal dyspnea, pulmonary edema, or congestive heart failure with little clinical or electrocardiographic evidence of left ventricular hypertrophy, although cardiac enlargement, presumably due to dilation of the heart, is usually evident radiologically.

To summarize, raised blood pressure is a potent cause of heart failure. Evidence of left ventricular hypertrophy, whether clinical, radiological, or electrocardiographic, carries an unfavorable outlook and must be regarded as an unequivocal indication for antihypertensive therapy.

b. Coronary Artery Disease

Hypertension is a major, perhaps the main, risk factor in the pathogenesis of ischemic heart disease. The higher the pressure, the greater the risk of clinical manifestations of coronary artery disease including angina, myocardial infarction, and sudden death. Hypertension appears to be independent of, but additive to, other risk factors, such as elevated serum cholesterol, cigarette smoking, diabetes, obesity, and the male sex[19] (Table 4).

There is no doubt that the development of either frank myocardial infarction or ischemia significantly adds to the chances of a hypertensive patient developing congestive heart failure, often at lower levels of blood pressure than in patients without coronary artery disease.

There is no clear evidence that antihypertensive drug treatment significantly alters the incidence of myocardial infarction or sudden death. However, as will be discussed later, recent studies have suggested that β-adrenergic blocking drugs may reduce the incidence of a further episode after an initial infarction. It remains possible that antihypertensive treatment with these drugs may lead to a reduction in the incidence of myocardial infarction as a complication of hypertension.

i. Angina Pectoris

Angina pectoris may occur in up to 20% of hypertensive patients[29] and follows the

TABLE 4

Mortality Ratios Among Male Hypertensives with Other Impairments

	Mortality ratio (standard risks = 100%)			
Nature of hypertension	Without any known minor impairments (%)	With mild overweight as minor impairment (%)	With albuminuria as minor impairment (%)	With early cardiovascular-renal family history (%)
Normal systolic and normal diastolic (98—137/48—82	85	100	105	125
Moderately elevated systolic with normal diastolic (138—147/48—82)	135	165	165	165
Normal systolic with moderately elevated diastolic (98—137/83—92)	120	135	150	180
Moderately elevated systolic and moderately elevated diastolic (138—147/83—92)	155	180	175	180
High systolic with normal to moderately elevated diastolic (148—177/48—92)	180	225	270	—
Normal to moderately elevated systolic with high diastolic (98—147/93—102)	175	210	—	—
High systolic and high diastolic (148—177/93—102)	250	250	—	—

From Lew, A., *An Actuarial View of Hypertension,* Monographs on Hypertension, Merck & Co., 1973.

classical pattern of gripping retrosternal chest pain, induced by effort or by emotion and relieved by rest or glyceryl trinitrate.

Angina pectoris in hypertension is usually caused by inadequate blood supply to the myocardium as a result of coronary artery disease. However, because the high pressure load leads to left ventricular hypertrophy with a consequently increased myocardial oxygen demand, angina may occur more readily in the hypertensive patient than in people with normal levels of blood pressure. There are thus two components, one related to the increased cardiac work, and the other related to the severity of coronary artery disease. In general, it may be said that the higher the blood pressure in a hypertensive patient with angina, the greater the possibility that antihypertensive drug treatment will relieve the angina. In very severe hypertension with diastolic blood pressures of 140 to 150 mmHg, reduction of blood pressure by any form of therapy commonly relieves angina. Presumably in such patients, the angina is almost wholly due to the increased work load. The situation is analogous to that prevailing in patients with aortic valve disease, where angina may be found in patients with markedly dilatated and undiseased coronary arteries.[30] Harrison and Wood[31] concluded from an autopsy study of hypertensive patients with angina that in many cases, angina occurred with dilated rather than narrowed coronary arteries, and Doyle and Kilpatrick[32] described similar findings in some, but not all, patients with hypertension and angina. On the other hand, coronary artery disease is common in hypertensive patients, and reduction of aortic blood pressure may reduce coronary blood flow considerably, so that drug treatment of hypertension may sometimes exacerbate rather than relieve angina.[32]

Angina of effort need not be regarded in most patients as a contraindication for antihypertensive drug treatment. In patients with severe hypertension, it may be regarded as an additional indication. In patients with modest hypertension, angina is usually related to disease of coronary arteries and relief of this symptom is less certain. Coronary angiography and bypass surgery may need to be considered in some patients.

ii. Myocardial Infarction

Myocardial infarction is several times commoner in hypertensive than in normotensive patients and is probably the commonest cause of death in the treated hypertensive patient. Goldning and Chasis[33] found that 13% of 1264 untreated patients reviewed at autopsy died of myocardial infarction.

Immediately following myocardial infarction in a hypertensive patient, the blood pressure may fall to normotensive levels, but in some it remains elevated. In either event, the blood pressure usually rises again to previous levels within 10 to 21 days of the episode unless heart failure develops.

Antihypertensive drug treatment is usually discontinued following a myocardial infarction, but should be reinstituted as soon as the blood pressure rises again. β-Adrenergic blocking drugs may be used to diminish the risks of arrhythmias during the acute phase.

4. The Brain

The major effects of hypertension on the brain are exerted through the effect on the cerebral vasculature, leading to cerebrovascular accidents or to other manifestations. Even small elevations of blood pressure increase the risk of stroke from four to six times.[3]

An adequate cerebral blood flow is essential to the function of the brain, and in normal people, the cerebral blood flow is maintained at a very constant level.[34] This is achieved in part by baroreceptor mechanisms, particularly the aortic and carotid baroreceptors, which regulate blood pressure in the arterial supply to the brain and in part by the capacity of the cerebral circulation to autoregulate flow by dilatation in response to falls and constriction in response to rises of blood pressure.[35,36] In normal persons, cerebral blood flow can be maintained at normal levels with a mean blood pressure as low as 70 mmHg. Below this level, cerebral blood flow falls rapidly as the blood pressure falls, leading to faintness and loss of consciousness.

In hypertension, the cerebral vessels constrict with an increase in brain vascular resistance, which approximately matches the rise in blood pressure with the result that cerebral blood flow is usually in the normal range.[17]

Hypertensive patients may exhibit a variety of symptoms or disorders of the brain.

a. Headache

Headache is a common symptom in hypertensive patients, although its relationship to the elevated pressure itself is controversial. The classical hypertensive headache is described as occipital, usually present when the patient awakens and wearing off an hour or two later. Occasionally, typical migraine may occur, often developing as a recurrence of the symptom in patients who had previously experienced migraine.

Not all headaches appear to be due to the hypertension, and the development of headaches not infrequently follows rather than precedes the discovery of the elevated blood pressure, suggesting that they may be aggravated by concomitant anxiety. Nevertheless, severe and persistent headache and particularly migraine in hypertensive patients are usually dramatically relieved when the blood pressure is lowered, and for this reason, this symptom can be regarded as an indication for therapy.

b. Transient Ischemic Attacks (TIA)

Episodes of temporary focal cerebral ischemia are not uncommon in hypertensive patients. The manifestations of the episodes depend on the site of the ischemia and may present as transient aphasia, weakness of an arm or leg, or occasionally transient blindness. These episodes usually develop rapidly, and the neurological deficit may last from a few minutes to several hours. Characteristically, the pattern of each episode is very uniform, both in the pattern of neurological deficit and in duration. The pattern of neurological symptoms differs depending upon whether focal ischemia is in the carotid or basilar territory. Vertebro basilar episodes cause dysarthria, vertigo, dysphagia, visual loss, and sensory symptoms, sometimes with weakness on one or both sides. Carotid ischemic episodes usually lead to hemiparesis, dysphasia, hemianopia, or sensory disturbances on one side of the body.

These episodes often result from carotid or vertebrobasilar stenosis, and when this can be demonstrated angiographically, surgical relief of the stenosis, if feasible, is indicated. On occasions, however, particularly when associated with severe hypertension or with sudden elevations of blood pressure, no major arterial lesion is demonstrable. Such episodes are best regarded as being symptoms of focal ischemia induced by hypertension, presumably having a mechanism similar to that demonstrated by Byrom[38] in the rat and can be regarded as an indication for antihypertensive therapy.

c. Hypertensive Encephalopathy

This syndrome is usually considered to consist of very high blood pressure, epileptiform fits, and altered consciousness and is usually, but not always, associated with the retinal manifestations of malignant hypertension. The syndrome is uncommon and has to be distinguished from intracerebral hemorrhage. It usually occurs in patients with renal failure and hypertension and is probably a manifestation of cerebral edema; it is particularly likely to occur in situations in which there is fluid overload such as acute oliguric glomerulonephritis, eclampsia, or uremia. However, the syndrome may occur in malignant hypertension, usually with some renal failure, during a hypertensive crisis in phaeochromocytoma or after ingestion of tyramine in patients taking monoamine oxidase inhibitors.

In these patients urgent reduction of blood pressure and often hemodialysis is essential.

d. Cerebral Hemorrhage

Intracerebral hemorrhage is the classical variety of hypertensive stroke. Cole and Yates[39] found that intracerebral hemorrhages occurred almost exclusively in hypertensive patients. The condition has a very high mortality.

Cerebral hemorrhage may develop as a result of a sudden rise in blood pressure induced by coitus, straining at stool, or cessation of antihypertensive drug treatment, but may occur in the absence of any of these. The underlying pathological lesion may be an atherosclerotic lesion of a major- or medium-sized cerebral artery, but these are probably not often responsible for intracerebral hemorrhage.[40] The frequency with which cerebral hemorrhage occurs in malignant hypertension suggests that fibrinoid necrosis of smaller arteries may be the underlying pathological cause in some patients.[41]

The presence of small aneurysms in the brain of hypertensive patients was described by Charcot and Bouchard in 1868.[42] They are distributed in the basal ganglia, pons, cerebellum, and subcortex. They were redescribed by Ross Russell in 1963.[43] Fisher[44] discussed the relationship between these lesions and the presence of recurrent small strokes or massive brain hemorrhage.

About 80% of intracerebral hemorrhages occur in the cerebral cortex, and not infrequently the hemorrhage may involve the intracerebral ventricles. The remaining hemorrhages occur in the brain stem or cerebellum.[45]

The onset of symptoms is usually not abrupt, but there is usually rapid progression of neurological signs with progressive clouding of consciousness, usually proceeding to stupor. There is usually profound hemiplegia and often conjugate deviation of the eyes towards the affected hemisphere. Periodic respiration, hyperpyrexia, and a secondary rise of blood pressure to very high levels commonly occur.

The mortality rate of major cerebral hemorrhage is extremely high.[46] Although early investigation with computerized axial tomography will usually reveal the site and progress of the lesion, surgical exploration seldom, except in the case of intracerebellar hemorrhage, improves the prognosis.

Patients who recover usually have profound disability. Antihypertensive drug therapy is of value in preventing this type of stroke, but has little to offer in the established case.

e. Lacunar Infarction

Multiple small cystic infarctions are commonly found in the brains of hypertensive patients at autopsy. They probably result from Charcot Bouchard aneurysms which have become thrombosed and occluded.[44] They may produce no symptoms, but may be associated with a type of organic dementia associated with bilateral pyramidal tract signs and some features of Parkinson's disease, when they occur in the region of the basal ganglia. This syndrome occurs usually in middle-aged men with severe hypertension. In fully established cases, antihypertensive drug treatment is not indicated, but progression may be halted in early cases due presumably to the arrest of the pathological vascular process.

f. Cerebral Infarction

Major cerebral infarction usually results from atherosclerotic disease of the larger intracerebral arteries.[40] While there is no doubt that atherosclerotic cerebral vascular disease occurs more intensively and at a younger age in patients with hypertension, it also occurs in normotensive people, particularly diabetics, and in many elderly people. Cerebral infarction leads to hemiplegia with a varying degree of residual recovery.

It seems to be generally agreed that in patients with hypertension with no previous history of stroke, antihypertensive drug treatment reduces the risk.[46] In patients with a previous history of stroke, the value of antihypertensive drug treatment is less certain, presumably because of the presence of preexisting cerebral atherosclerosis.[47] However, there is no evidence that stroke recurrence is made more frequent by drug treatment, and hence in view of the possible benefits in terms of stroke recurrence and the prevention of cardiac failure, a completed stroke should not be regarded as a contraindication for drug treatment. However, benefit is likely to be most obvious in younger patients and in those with the highest levels of blood pressure.[48]

5. The Retina

The retinal vessels are easily seen with an ophthalmoscope, and changes occuring in the optic fundus have been known to be a useful guide to prognosis since the classification of fundoscopic changes by Keith et al. in 1939.[49] More recently, studies of the retinal circulation using fluorescein angiography and retinal photography have given more precise insights into the mechanism of retinal circulatory disturbances.[50]

Changes in the retinal arteries may occur as a result of hypertension or as a result of aging or both. Hypertension leads to hypertrophy of vascular smooth muscle. In long-standing hypertension, some muscle fibers may be replaced by fibrous tissues. Similar thickening commonly occurs in aging. Both processes lead to an increased reflection of light from the arterial wall, giving rise to the silver wire appearance and many also lead to an appearance of obstruction of veins at arterio venous crossings. In severe hypertension, there is often either generalized narrowing of the lumen, focal narrowings of the lumen, or focal narrowings of the arteries.[51]

The pathological processes which develop in the retina result mainly from ischemia of the retina, sometimes as a result of thrombotic occlusions, but more commonly because of fibrinoid necrosis and associated occlusion of arterioles.[52] These latter changes in the retinal vessels usually reflect similar changes elsewhere in the vascular system, notably the kidney, and indicate the onset of accelerated or malignant hypertension. However, none of the changes in the retina are unique to hypertensive vascular disease and may result from other pathological processes, such as severe anemia, hypoxia, diabetic vascular disease, or other causes of vasculitis, such as scleroderma, systemic lupus erythematosis, or polyarteritis nodosa.

Complete or partial occlusion of the arterioles leads to capillary ischemia, retinal edema, or retinal underperfusion. Ischemic damage to capillary walls results in hemorrhages. These characteristically occur in the nerve fiber layer of the retina, usually close to the disc, and are very rarely lateral to the macula. The hemorrhages are usually bright red in color, lie superficial to the retinal arteries, and are irregular in shape. By contrast, hemorrhages due to arteriosclerosis or venous occlusion usually occur in the more peripheral areas of the fundus and are darker in color and occur in the deeper layers of the retina.

Superficial hemorrhages occurring in the nerve fiber layer due to severe hypertension disappear rapidly with successful reduction of blood pressure. Effective antihypertensive treatment almost immediately stops the occurrence of new hemorrhages and existing hemorrhages usually disappear within 2 to 3 weeks.

Hard exudates appear as white or yellowish shiny particles, usually in the region of the macula or between the macula and the optic disc. They are composed of fat, fibrin, and cellular debris and are believed to result from edema which has leaked from damaged capillaries. Although they most commonly are present in accelerated hypertension, they occasionally occur without other manifestations, such as hemorrhage and soft exudate, and under these circumstances do not carry the same poor prognosis.

Soft exudates, or cotton wool spots, are the result of ischemic infarction of nerve fibers, and the appearances are due to intracellular edema of the nerve fibers.[54] In hypertensive patients, they indicate the onset of malignant hypertension. They may, however, result from other pathological causes of arteriolar obstruction, such as systemic lupus erythematosis, dermatomyositis, retinal artery occlusion, diabetes, or emboli. As the name cotton wool spots implies, they look fluffy and soft; they are usually congregated in the region of the disc and macula where the nerve fibres are most concentrated. They usually enlarge rapidly and may continue to grow in size for a few days after the institution of drug treatment. New patches rarely develop, however, and the existing ones usually disappear within 3 to 4 weeks of effective treatment.

Papilledema occurs in the most advanced form of malignant hypertension. It begins as a pinkness of the optic disc, usually with a loss of distinction of the nasal margin. As it develops, the disc becomes swollen, and both edges become obscured, and the veins, which often appear engorged, can be seen to be deformed by the swollen disc. Papilledema is almost always associated with hemorrhages and cotton wool spots. Visual loss may occur, particularly when there is associated retinal edema. Papilledema usually responds dramatically to drug treatment, and visual loss is usually restored within days of commencing treatment. Occasionally, prolonged untreated malignant hypertension with papilledema may be followed by secondary optic atrophy and persistent visual loss.

The development of flame-shaped hemorrhage, cotton wool spots, and papilledema constitute the syndrome of malignant hypertension. Without treatment, prognosis is extremely poor with a mean survival time of about 4 to 5 months from diagnosis. The changes in the retinal vessels are usually similar to those in the kidney, where they lead to progressive renal ischemia and renal failure. The whole process may develop very rapidly. It is more common in hypertension due to preexisting renal disease, such as glomerulonephritis, but may complicate almost any variety of hypertensive disease process. While the syndrome usually develops in patients known previously to have had high blood pressure, in a few, it may apparently develop *de novo.*

The appearance on ophthalmoscopic examination of flame-shaped hemorrhages, cotton wool spots, or papilledema in hypertensive patients is an unequivocal indication for antihypertensive drug treatment as a matter of urgency, since delay in treatment may lead to a cerebral hemorrhage or to rapidly developing renal failure.

6. The Kidney

The association between kidney disease and hypertension was first postulated by Richard Bright before the development of clinical methods for measuring blood pressure.

Almost any type of kidney disease appears to be able to initiate hypertension, although as has been discussed earlier, the mechanisms involved have so far remained obscure. Clinically, the situation is further complicated by the fact that vascular disease, secondary to the high blood pressure itself, may lead to disturbances of renal function both in patients with and without preexisting disease of the kidneys.

a. Parenchymal Renal Disease

Most types of diffuse renal disease appear to cause hypertension. Thus, hypertension is an almost invariable complication of mesangiocapillary glomerulonephritis, the diabetic kidney, membranous glomerulonephritis, renal amyloidosis, and polycystic kidney and is commonly associated with chronic pyelonephritis and analgesic nephropathy.

i. Glomerulonephritis

In acute poststreptococcal glomerulonephritis, some rise in blood pressure occurs very frequently. This elevation in blood pressure is usually not of severe degree, and the blood pressure usually subsides within 7 to 21 days. Occasionally, very severe hypertension may develop and persist, usually with evidence of malignant hypertension in the fundus occuli, but this course is extremely unusual.

In the great majority of patients with acute poststreptococcal glomerulonephritis, the prognosis is good; the disease process apparently resolving completely with no sequelae. There seems to be no doubt, however, that in a proportion of patients, the acute episode may be followed by progression to chronic nephritis. The frequency with which this has been recognized varies between different studies, some, notably in children, reporting an incidence of about 1%,[55,56] whereas other series[57-59] suggest a considerably higher incidence, particularly in adults. Since episodes of acute glomerulonephritis may escape detection clinically,[60] the possibility that apparent essential hypertension may be due to chronic glomerulonephritis needs to be borne in mind. The diagnosis is not easy to make, since renal biopsy may reveal no specific features other than hyalinisation of some glomeruli and arterial changes. However, in the absence of any specific therapy for chronic glomerulonephritis, the distinction is mainly of academic interest.

ii. Pyelonephritis

Acute infection of the renal pelvis with parenchymatous involvement is not commonly associated with hypertension. Moreover, recurrent or persistent urinary tract infections do not appear to be associated with hypertension either.[61] By contrast, patients with chronic atrophic pyelonephritis, defined by radiological means[62] or by pathological appearances,[63] have a high incidence of hypertension. It appears from the studies of Kincaid-Smith[61,64] that hypertension in patients with pyelonephritis is associated significantly with the presence of parenchymal scars in the kidney. Kincaid-Smith[61] drew attention to the frequency with which lesions of the arcuate arteries and arterioles occurred in atrophic pyelonephritis, and she suggested that these vascular lesions might be due to the infection leading to vascular injury. However, the relative absence of hypertension in patients with recurrent or persistent infections and the frequency with which hypertension occurs in patients with atrophic pyelonephritis cast some doubt as to whether the radiological and pathological features of what is described as atrophic pyelonephritis can be necessarily ascribed to previous infection. It remains possible that these changes may result from rather than cause hypertension, or that they may be due to some other noninfective disease process, such as infarction.

Clinically there is little to distinguish the patient with chronic pyelonephritis from those with essential hypertension. Proteinuria is not common, overt urinary infection is unusual, and the hypertension may be of any grade of severity.

iii. Analgesic Nephropathy

The relationship between a high intake of analgesics containing aspirin and phenacetin has been recognized since 1957,[65] initially in Europe and subsequently, very extensively in Australia.[66-68] While chronic interstitial nephritis appears to be the common underlying pathological process in Europe, most patients with analgesic nephropathy in Australia have papillary necrosis.[66] The incidence of associated hypertension seems to be considerably higher in Australian patients[69] than in the European reports. These differences may reflect differences in the analgesics ingested or may be due to other environmental factors. Hypertension is usually associated with moderate to severe degrees of renal failure and is probably a comparatively late development in the course of the illness.

iv. The Diabetic Kidney

Patients with diabetes, usually of long standing, may develop the characteristic lesions of glomeruli and renal arterioles described by Kimmelstiel and Wilson in 1936.[70] High blood pressure commonly develops early in the course of the disease process and is almost invariably accompanied by proteinuria and by evidence of diabetic retinopathy. The nephrotic syndrome develops commonly with edema and hypoproteinemia. This is usually followed by renal failure. The course of the renal failure may be accelerated by the development of malignant hypertension with superadded appearances of hypertensive changes in the retina.

v. Polycystic Kidneys

Most patients with the adult form of polycystic kidneys develop hypertension which is usually present at the time of dignosis. Characteristically, the kidneys are enlarged and can be felt clinically. Excretion pyelography confirms the diagnosis. As with other forms of renal disease, the development of hypertension with secondary vascular changes in the renal arteries may hasten the development of renal failure, and treatment of hypertension may effectively slow the development of renal insufficiency.

b. Renal Vascular Disease (Renovascular Hypertension)

It is possible that in parenchymal renal disease, malignant hypertension, and in such illness as radiation nephritis or thrombotic microangiopathy, the hypertension develops as a result of renal ischemia due to occlusion of small arteries and arterioles with resultant renal ischemia. However, the term "renovascular hypertension" is usually reserved for hypertension resulting from occlusive lesions of the major renal arteries or their main branches. Such obstruction may be due to atherosclerotic disease with or without secondary thrombosis, fibromuscular dysplasia affecting predominantly the media of the arteries, or to a few less common causes. This condition is discussed in detail in a later section.

B. Results of Treatment

Effective antihypertensive drug treatment was introduced in the early 1950s. Before this time, severe hypertension had been treated by bilateral thoracolumbar sympathectomy,[71] bilateral removal of the adrenal glands,[72] or by severe sodium restriction.[73] The synthesis of the methonium compound series in 1949 and the study of their parmacological actions by Paton and Zaimis[74] in the same year led to clinical trials being undertaken in the use of C_5 and C_6 members of the series, namely hexamethonium and pentamethonium salts. Smirk and Alstedt in 1951[75] reported on the results of treatment of severe hypertension with these compounds, for which a complex regime had been devised, involving the s.c. administration of these drugs to patients with very severe hypertension. In this publication and in subsequent ones, Smirk[76,77] reported that in patients with malignant hypertension, papilledema and retinopathy disappeared and that survival time was prolonged. He also reported that in patients with intractable hypertensive heart failure, antihypertensive drug treatment resulted in a diuresis, a reduction in heart size, and a marked increase in exercise tolerance. These results in severe hypertension were soon widely confirmed by others.[78-80]

These spectacular results in severe or malignant hypertension were widely assumed to be transferable to less severe hypertension with the result that few control studies were performed. However, Hamilton et al.[81] reported a controlled trial of the effects of antihypertensive drugs in 61 symptomless hypertensives all of whom had diastolic blood pressures of 110 mmHg or more. The study was continued over 6 years, and all treated cases received a minimum of 2 and a maximum of 6 years treatment. There were 22 men in the series. Of these, 10 cases were treated, none of whom developed any complication, whereas of the 13 untreated cases, 4 suffered strokes, 1 suffered a myocardial infarction, and 3 developed a progressive increase in heart size necessitating treatment. These differences were highly significant. In the 20 women treated, there were 5 complications, namely 3 strokes, 1 myocardial infarction, and 1 increase in heart size. In the 19 female controls, there were 3 strokes, 2 myocardial infarctions, and 3 patients in whom treatment had to be given because of an increasing heart size. Although the difference in the incidence of complications between treated and untreated women was not statistically significant, four of the five complications in the treated patients occurred in women whose blood pressures were not well controlled. Of 16 women whose blood pressures were adequately controlled, there was only 1 complication, whereas in the 23 women whose blood pressure was either inadequately treated or untreated, there were 6 strokes and 12 complications in all. The Veteran's Administration Co-Operative Study gave similar results for severe hypertension in the groups with a diastolic pressure above 115 mmHg.[48] The incidence of major complications in the control group was so high that the trial was discontinued after 20 months. The incidence of stroke was four times greater in the control group, and there was also a substantial reduction in the incidence of heart failure and uncontrolled

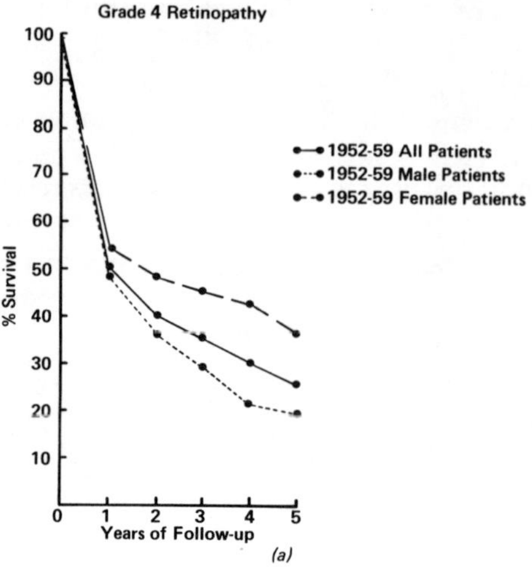

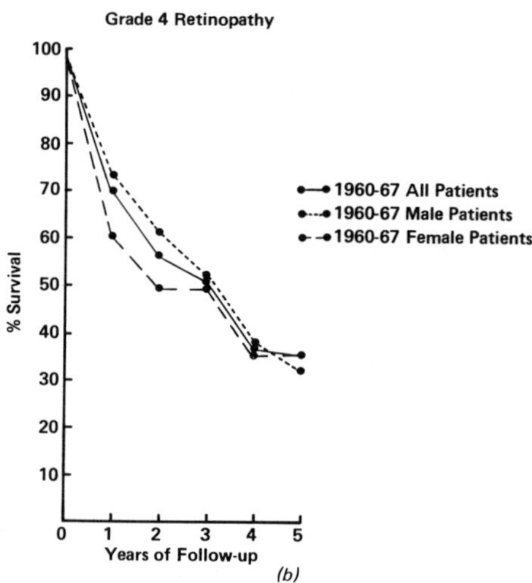

FIGURE 6.   Prognosis of patients with grade 4 retinopathy seen in (a) 1952 to 1969 and (b) 1960 to 1967. (From Breckenridge, A., Dollery, C. T., and Parry, E. O. H., *Q. J. Med.,* 39, 411, 1970. With permission.)

hypertension with diastolic pressures above 140 mmHg. In a later study,[82] the effects of antihypertensive drug treatment were assessed in patients whose diastolic pressures were between 90 and 115 mmHg. The results in this study, which had an average follow-up of 39 months, again showed a substantial reduction in the incidence of stroke and heart failure.

A major study on the prognosis of treated hypertension was reported by Breckenridge et al. in 1970.[83] These authors reported on the prognosis in 1294 patients treated between January 1952 and December 1967. This study found that in patients with malignant hypertension, there was a 25% 5-year survival rate in patients treated between 1952 and 1959 and a 34% survival rate in patients treated between 1960 and 1967 (Figure 6). Commenting on these results, these authors suggest that the most important single factor determining the outlook of patients with malignant hypertension was the presence or absence of renal failure before treatment commenced. Using

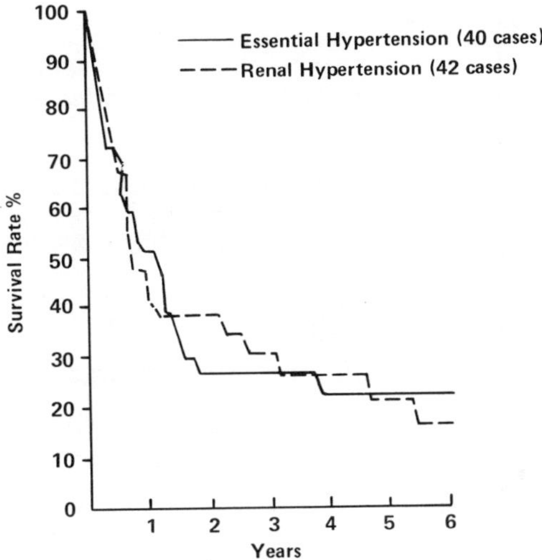

FIGURE 7. The survival of patients with treated malignant hypertension divided into those with a renal lesion and essential hypertension. The survival curves are similar. (From Harrington, M., Kincaid-Smith, P., and McMichael, J., *Br. Med. J.*, 2, 969, 1959. With permission.)

these criteria, patients with an initial blood urea of below 40 mg% had a survival rate of 83% in 1952 to 1959 and 84% in 1966 to 1967, whereas those with blood ureas higher than 40 mg% had a 5-year survival rate of 17% in 1952 to 1959 and 23% in 1960 to 1967. Harrington et al.[84] reported a 5-year survival rate in treated malignant hypertension of about 30% (Figure 7). Dustan et al.[85] reported a similar 5-year survival rate in 84 patients with malignant hypertension.

The outlook for patients with fundal hemorrhages of exudates, but no papilledema (grade III hypertensive retinopathy), was substantially better in Breckenridge's series, with approximately a 70% survival rate in both periods of observation. Again, the prognosis was better in those without initial evidence of renal failure; the 5-year survival rates for those with normal renal function was 82 and 84% in the two periods, whereas those with blood urea levels above 40 mg% had survival rates of between 50 and 55% over 5 years (Figure 8).

The 5-year survival rate in patients with nonexudative retinopathy was substantially better (Figure 9). The 5-year survival rates of 85% were recorded in the years 1952 to 1959 and 88% in 1960 to 1967. The influence of preexisting renal failure seemed much less in such patients.

Breckenridge et al.[83] also noted that the prognosis of female patients was better than male patients in each 8-year period. Examining the prognosis of patients according to the initial diastolic blood pressure, Breckenridge et al. found that initial blood pressures between 90 and 140 mmHg had little influence on overall survival, whereas there was a sharp fall in survival in patients presenting initially with diastolic blood pressures above 140 mmHg (Figure 10). In this series, the commonest cause of death, both between 1952 and 1959 and 1960 and 1967, was uremia (Table 5). Death from stroke accounted for 28% of the deaths between 1952 and 1959 and 21% of the deaths be-

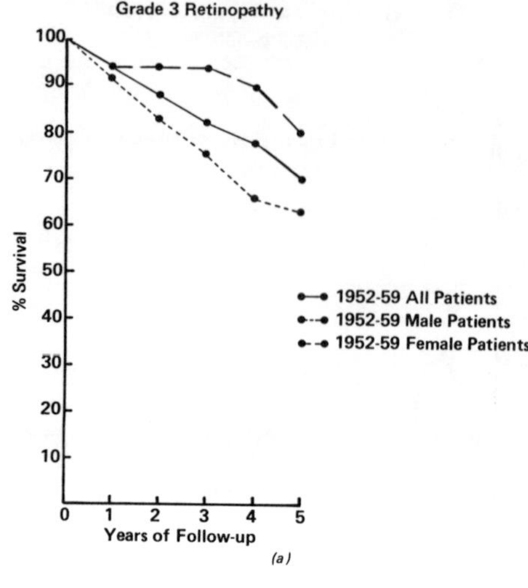

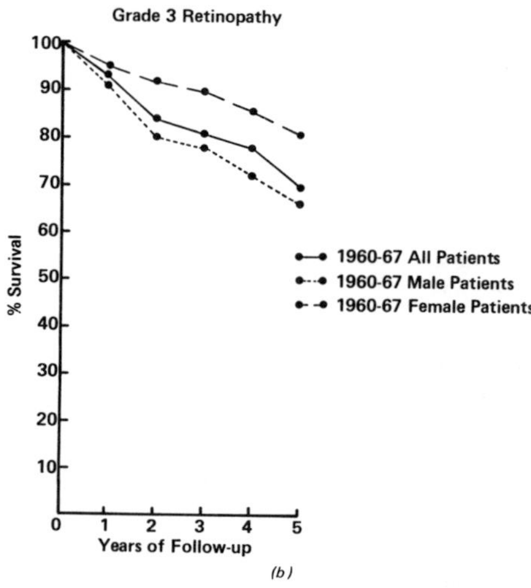

FIGURE 8.   Prognosis of patients with grade 3 retinopathy seen in (a) 1952 to 1959 and (b) 1960 to 1967. (From Breckenridge, A., Dollery, C. T., and Parry, E. H. O., *Q. J. Med.,* 39, 411, 1970. With permission.)

tween 1960 and 1967. Myocardial infarction accounted for only 7% of the deaths between 1952 and 1959, but 27% of the deaths between 1960 and 1967. Of the 97 patients dying from chronic renal failure, 81% had a blood urea above 40 mg/100 mℓ when first seen. Of the 66 patients who died from stroke, 44% had evidence on physical examination of previous cerebral vascular disease when first seen. Of the 60 patients who died of myocardial infarction, 38% had evidence of ischemic heart disease, either angina pectoris or a previous myocardial infarction before treatment commenced. These authors were unable to comment in detail as to whether the blood pressures of those who had died were significantly less well controlled than those who had survived. They found no difference in the degree of blood pressure control in patients dying of uremia, stroke, or myocardial infarction.

The other major point of interest in this study was the time at which deaths occurred

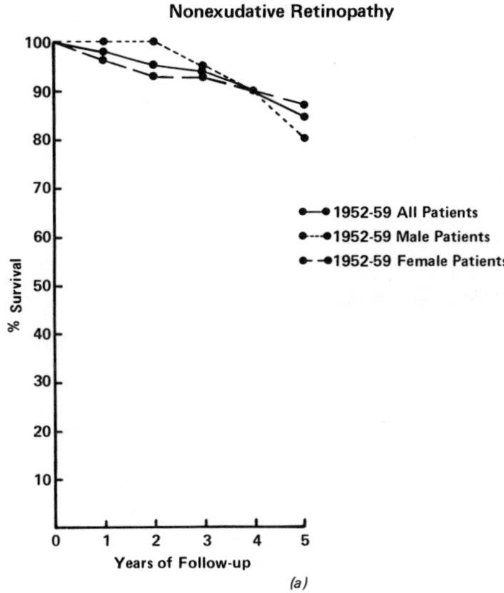

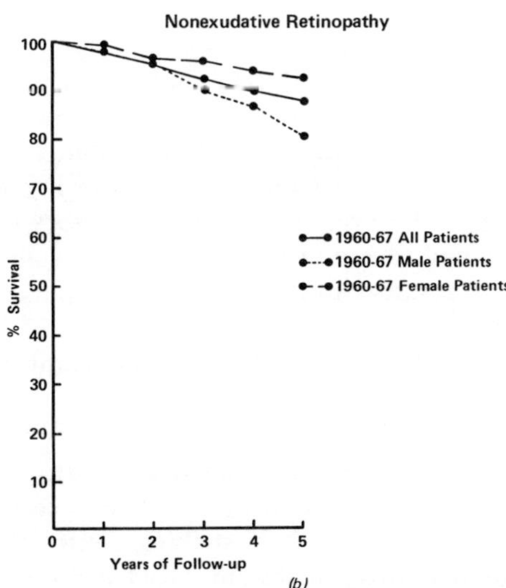

FIGURE 9.   Prognosis of patients with nonexudative retinopathy seen in (a) 1952 to 1959 and
(b) 1960 to 1967. (From Breckenridge, A., Dollery, C. T., and Parry, E. H. O., *Q. J. Med.,* 39,
411, 1970. With permission.)

in relation to the onset of treatment. The early deaths, within the first year of treatment, were predominantly due to renal failure, the incidence of which fell progressively
with the length of treatment. Death from cerebrovascular disease was also highest in
the first year and also diminished progressively with increasing duration of treatment.
By contrast, deaths from myocardial infarction showed no early peak, and from the
fifth year of treatment onwards, myocardial infarction emerged as the commonest
single cause of death (Figure 11).

It has to be emphasized that all the studies cited above have dealt with patients with
severe hypertension. The one possible exception is the Veteran's Co-Operative Study[82]
in which patients with diastolic blood pressures between 90 and 115 mmHg were ad-

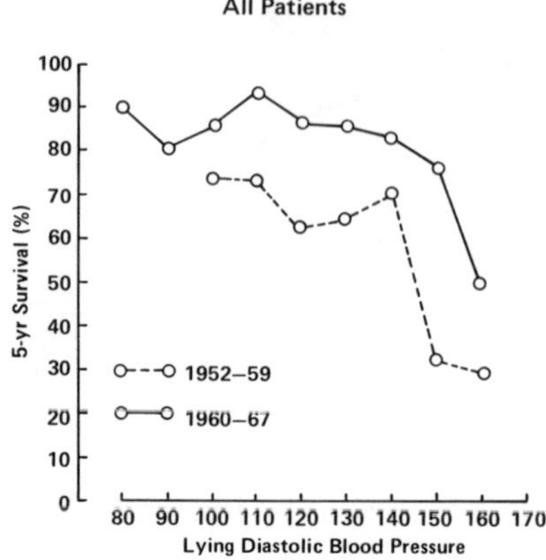

FIGURE 10.   Prognosis of all patients according to initial diastolic pressure seen in 1952 to 1959 and 1960 to 1967. (From Breckenridge, A., Dollery, C. T., and Parry, E. H. O., *Q. J. Med.*, 39, 411, 1970. With permission.)

mitted. However, in these patients the diastolic blood pressure was recorded after some days in hospital, and 58% of the patients in the study had had cardiac, central nervous system, or renal abnormalities at the time of randomization; 25% had enlarged hearts, 15% had abnormal renal function, 7% had had a previous myocardial infarction, 8% had a previous history of heart failure, and 5% had a history of stroke, so that these patients seem likely to have had severe hypertension and certainly had associated vascular disease. Whether these results can be transferred to patients with milder hypertension is not as yet certain.

Some aspects of the results of treatment deserve closer examination.

1. Results in Heart Disease

As had already been stated, effective antihypertensive drug treatment virtually prevents death from congestive heart failure in hypertension except where this is a complication of myocardial infarction. This is in striking contrast to the situation which obtained before antihypertensive drug treatment. Goldring and Chassis[33] in their large series claimed that heart failure caused death in 42% of patients, whereas the study of Breckenridge et al.[83] with a rather similar number of patients revealed that only 16 out of 1294 patients died of congestive heart failure. This difference is almost certainly due to a reduction on the cardiac work load. There is evidence[86] that the electrocardiogram may revert towards normal in successfully treated hypertensive patients. Reduction in heart size on radiological examination also occurs.[77]

a. Myocardial Infarction

Most reported studies suggest that myocardial infarction is now the major cause of death in treated hypertensive patients. Thus, in a group of severely hypertensive patients reported by Doyle,[87] death from myocardial infarction occurred over a 5-year period in 16 of 140 men and 4 of 140 women. A further 26 men and a further 15 women suffered nonfatal myocardial infarctions in this period. Thus, in the whole series, almost one fourth of the men and approximately one fifth of the women had myocardial infarctions over a 5-year period. Myocardial infarction, either fatal or nonfatal, appeared to occur with equal frequency in patients whose blood pressures had

TABLE 5

The Causes of Death in Patients Attending the Hammersmith Hospital Hypertensive Clinic Between 1952 and 1967

Causes of Death	1952—1959	1960—1967	Total
Deaths due to hypertension			
Uremia	38 (44%)	59 (29%)	97
Cerebrovascular disease	24 (28%)	42 (21%)	66
Myocardial infarction	6 (7%)	54 (27%)	60
Sudden cardiac death	—	3	3
Congestive heart failure	5	11	16
Aneurysm of aorta	5	10	15
Dissection	5	7	—
Ruptured abdominal aneurysm	—	3	—
Death due to drugs	4	3	7
P. ileus	4	1	—
Overdose of hypotensive drugs	—	1	—
Suicide	—	1	—
Deaths due to other causes	2	16	18
Carcinoma	—	12	—
Chronic bronchitis	—	2	—
Post operative	1	2	—
Disseminated lupus erythematosus	1	—	—
Unknown	3	5	8
Total	87	203	290

From Breckenridge, A., Dollery, C. T., and Parry, E. H. O., *Q. J. Med.*, 39, 41, 1970.

been well controlled as in those in whom it had not. This contrasted with the fact that the incidence of stroke was reduced and that strokes occurred predominantly in those patients whose blood pressure had not been well controlled. Smirk and Hodge[88] reported that coronary artery disease accounted for 42% of all deaths in their treated series and was the commonest single cause of death in treated hypertensive patients, and in the series reported by Breckenridge et al.,[83] deaths from myocardial infarction did not decline with time of follow-up and after the first 4 years of treatment had become the leading cause of death.

Myocardial infarction is due presumably to factors related to coronary artery disease, and as has been stated, hypertension appears to be additive to other risk factors, such as elevated cholesterol, cigarette smoking, obesity, and the male sex. It may not be surprising under these circumstances that deaths and morbidity from myocardial infarction remain common in treated hypertensive patients. Dollery and Bulpitt[89] have pointed out that when the incidence of myocardial infarction in the various control trials is compared to those of control groups, the incidence of myocardial infarction has fallen by 49% and suggest therefore that these pooled estimates may suggest that a possible benefit has occurred.

There is certainly no evidence that antihypertensive drug treatment prevents myocardial infarction absolutely, and it may not even reduce its incidence. This statement applies, however, to the results of therapeutic intervention before the introduction of β-adrenergic blocking drugs, and a possible new dimension has been introduced by the use of these agents. Wilhelmsen and colleagues[90] reported in 1974 that treatment with alprenolol appeared to reduce the incidence of sudden death in patients who had previously suffered myocardial infarction. In this important study, patients who had suffered a myocardial infarction were randomized and treated on a double-blind basis with alprenolol over a period of two years. These data were confirmed by Ahlmark et

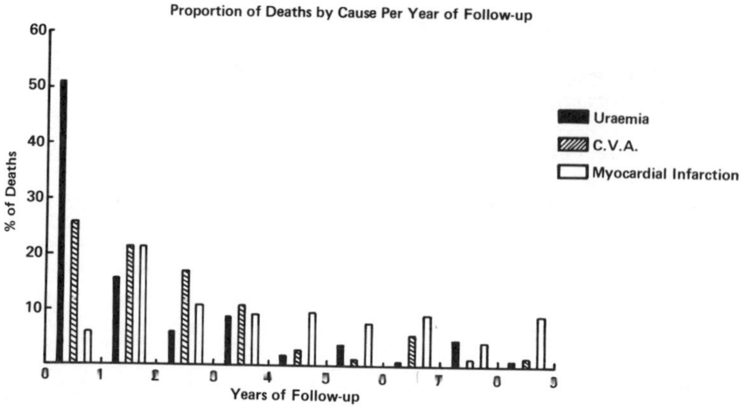

FIGURE 11.   Causes of death at various years of follow up. (From Brecken-ridge, A., Dollery, C. T., and Parry, E. H. O., *Q. J. Med.*, 39, 411, 1970. With permission.)

al.,[91] who agreed that alprenolol reduced the incidence of sudden death and suggested that it might also have reduced the incidence of reinfarction. Fox and colleagues[92] compared the incidence of myocardial infarction in a group of patients who had been previously treated with β-blocking drugs for angina with the incidence in an age-matched group also admitted to a coronary care unit and found a significantly lower incidence of infarction in the treated group. These results have been confirmed by a multicenter controlled trial using practolol.[93] Stewart[94] compared the incidence of a first myocardial infarction in hypertensive patients being treated with propranolol or being treated with a regime excluding a β-receptor blocker. A total of 169 patients with severe uncomplicated hypertension was divided into two groups. Of these, 121 were given long-term treatment containing propranolol, and 48 were treated with antihypertensive agents which excluded any β-blocking drug. There were no significant differences in other risk factors for myocardial infarction between the two groups. After a mean follow-up of 5¼ years, 9 of the 121 subjects (7.5%) in the propranolol-treated group had suffered first infarctions, and 15 of the 48 patients in the non- β-blocking group (31%) had suffered first infarctions. These differences were statistically highly significant. It is thus possible that antihypertensive drug treatment containing β-receptor blocking drugs will prove to be more effective than other forms of antihypertensive therapy in the primary prevention of myocardial infarction.

Recently, Berglund et al.[95] have reported on the effects of long-term antihypertensive drug treatment in a group of men with comparatively mild hypertension. The study was an open one with no placebo-treated control group. The treatment group and the control group were chosen according to blood pressure levels at a second screening examination. Those whose blood pressures were greater than 175/115 mmHg at both examinations were treated, while the control group consisted of those whose blood pressures at the second examination had fallen to a lower level. The total incidence of death from coronary heart disease and nonfatal myocardial infarction was 23 out of 635 treated cases in 5 years, which is 3.6%, whereas in the control group of 391, 27 (6.9%) had a fatal or nonfatal myocardial infarction (Figure 12). In 3696 men with blood pressures below 160/95 mmHg, 56 (1.5%) suffered a fatal or nonfatal myocardial infarction. Life table analysis for nonfatal myocardial infarction and death from ischemic heart disease showed that the benefit of treatment occurred early and continued throughout the period of follow-up (Figure 13). Other risk factors, such as cholesterol, age, and cigarette smoking seemed comparable in the various groups.

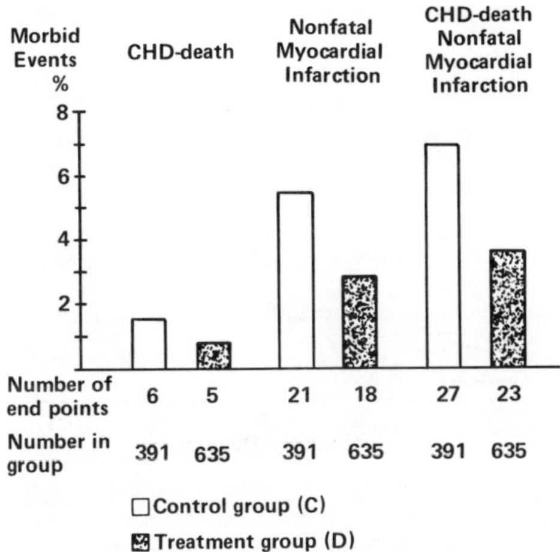

FIGURE 12.   Incidence of fatal and nonfatal coronary heart disease. (From Berglund, G., Wilhelmsen, L., Sannerstedt, R., Hansson, L., Andersson, O., Sivertsson, R., Wedel, H., and Wikstrand, J., *Lancet*, 1, 485, 1970. With permission.)

This study seems to suggest that long-term antihypertensive drug treatment in a mildly hypertensive group of men may reduce or delay the incidence of myocardial infarction, suggesting that early treatment given before the development of clinical evidence of coronary heart disease may be effective in reducing the incidence of myocardial infarction.

An alternative explanation which needs to be considered is the fact that in most patients, the antihypertensive regime included a β-adrenoceptor blocking drug and that this factor, rather than early treatment, might be a component. The available evidence does not allow a conclusion to be drawn as to which of these factors is responsible.

It needs to be noted that in this study, although the incidence of nonfatal myocardial infarction and death from coronary heart disease apparently fell from 6.9% in the untreated hypertensive group to 3.6% in the treated group, that the incidence in the nonhypertensive group was lower still at 1.5%, so that treatment does not totally reduce the added risk of hypertension. Furthermore, as the authors point out, in this milder group of patients, death from diseases apparently related to hypertension account for only 40% of all deaths.

b. Angina of Effort

Conventional antihypertensive drug therapy (excluding β-blocking drugs) may be effective in the prevention of angina, particularly when this is related to very severe hypertension.[32] These authors thought that in the patients with hypertension who obtained relief from angina after reduction in blood pressure, the reduction in cardiac work was probably greater than the reduction in coronary blood flow. They found some patients in whom angina was aggravated and concluded that in these the fall in coronary blood flow was probably more pronounced than the reduction in cardiac work. In the majority of patients, no very striking change in the severity or frequency of angina occurred. This situation has been changed by the introduction of β-adrenergic blocking drugs which are often very effective in the treatment of angina without hypertension.

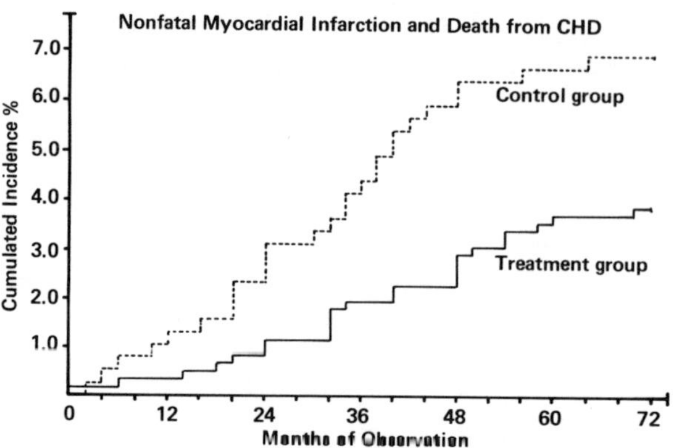

FIGURE 13.   Cumulative incidence of nonfatal myocardial infarction and death from chronic heart disease by life-table analysis. (From Berglund, G., Wilhelmsen, L., Sannerstedt, R., Hansson, L., Andersson, O., Sivertsson, R., Wedel, H., and Wikstrand, J., *Lancet*, 1, 485, 1970. With permission.)

2. Cerebrovascular Disease

In all series so far reported, it has been found that a major contribution to the reduction in mortality and morbidity has been due to the reduced incidence of stroke. Thus, in their controlled trial conducted by Hamilton and colleagues referred to earlier,[81] the differences between the treated and control group was largely due to the differences in incidence of stroke. In the Veteran's Administration Co-Operative study,[48] hemorrhagic stroke occurred in 19 control patients and in 6 treated patients. The effectiveness of treatment was greater in patients under the age of 60 years, although it was demonstrable at all ages. It also appeared to be more effective in preventing strokes in patients whose diastolic blood pressures exceeded 105 mmHg than those with levels below that value.

The effects of antihypertensive drug treatment on the recurrence of stroke in hypertensive patients is in dispute. Carter[96] conducted a randomized prospective study in 97 stroke survivors who had hypertension. After 2-5-years follow-up, the mortality from all causes was 46% in the control group and 26% in the treated group. Nonfatal recurrence of strokes occurred in 23% of the control group, but in only 14% of the treated group. There was little or no reduction in incidence among the patients who were 65 years of age or over at the onset of the study. In a larger and more recent study by the Hypertension Stroke Co-Operation Study Group,[47,97] a fixed drug combination of diserpidine and methylclothiazide was given in a randomized double-blind study to lower the blood pressure in half of a group of 452 patients, who had had a cerebrovascular episode in the preceding year. The control group received placebos. The mean age of the patients was 59 years and 80% were black. In the treated group, 37 strokes occurred, and 42 occurred in the placebo group. The type of the initial cerebrovascular episode did not affect the outcome, neither patients with completed stroke or those with transient ischemic attacks having a significant difference in the incidence of stroke between the treated and the control group. There was some suggestion in this study that the whites, who comprised only 20% of the whole group, might have had a greater reduction in stroke recurrence than the blacks. From these conflicting data certain conclusions may be drawn. Firstly, in severe hypertension, antihypertensive drug treatment clearly diminishes the risk of hemorrhagic stroke. Secondly, cerebral infarction due to thrombosis is not always prevented by antihypertensive drug treatment; the probability of protection being effective seems to depend on the age of the patient and on the severity of the hypertension.

The incidence of cerebral infarction seems to be significantly reduced in patients with severe hypertension below the age of 60 years. Its incidence seems unrelated to treatment in older patients. Presumably, in the more severe hypertensive patients, cerebral infarction results from the Charcot Bouchard aneurysm or fibrinoid necrosis, whereas in the less severely hypertensive or older patient, it results from cerebral atheroma. Importantly, there seems to be no evidence that antihypertensive drug treatment increases the risk of stroke.

3. Renal Failure

Severe hypertension is a potent cause of renal failure. Renal failure from other causes may also be complicated by the development of severe hypertension. The findings from the Hammersmith Hospital, London,[83] suggested that the commonest cause of death was uremia, particularly in patients with malignant hypertension. The great majority of patients who died of uremia had evidence of impaired renal function when first seen.

The treatment of hypertensive patients with renal failure is difficult. The patients are commonly anemic, fluid overloaded, and often have congestive heart failure. Because most drugs are excreted by the kidney and are hence retained in renal failure, antihypertensive drug therapy is difficult, and responses to drugs may be prolonged and unpredictable. Before treatment of end-stage renal disease with hemodialysis was used, attempts to lower the blood pressure often precipitated further deterioration in renal function, and it is probably not surprising that most of the earlier literature reported a very poor prognosis in patients with severe hypertension and end-stage renal failure.

The introduction of hemodialysis has greatly improved the prognosis of this group of patients. The majority of patients treated with hemodialysis and sodium restriction improve considerably, and the institution of this regime may reduce the blood pressure substantially, even in those in whom the blood pressure did not fall to satisfactory limits using antihypertensive drugs. Control of the blood pressure once dialysis is commenced can be achieved in most patients. There are, however, a small group of patients in whom the hypertension appears to be resistant to removal of sodium and water by dialysis accompanied by dietary sodium restriction. These patients remain hypertensive during dialysis and are often resistant to antihypertensive therapy. In most it is necessary to produce hypovolemia in order to obtain control over blood pressure levels, and this is usually accompanied by postural hypotension, weakness, and thirst; in most of these patients, plasma renin levels are markedly elevated. These findings have led to the suggestion that in these patients, the hypertension is renin dependent, and certainly bilateral nephrectomy often leads to a fall in both blood pressure and plasma renin activity without any change in either total body sodium or body fluids. This situation seems to have been improved by the introduction of β-blocking drugs. Whether the beneficial effects of these drugs are due in these patients to an effect on renin is not certain, but it seems probable, and the great majority of patients of end-stage renal disease can now have their blood pressure satisfactorily managed without bilateral nephrectomy. The introduction of hemodialysis has substantially improved the outlook of patients who present with end-stage renal disease. Five-year survivals of about 70% are claimed for patients on chronic dialysis. While patients with preexisting severe hypertension almost certainly have an increased incidence of myocardial infarction, it is likely that their prognosis is very much better than it was before the introduction of supportive treatment for renal failure.

4. The Retina

Effective reduction of blood pressure by pharmacological or other means has a striking effect on the lesions in the fundus. Patients with impaired vision usually report improvement within 48 to 72 hr, and vision usually returns to normal within 1 week or 10 days of commencing treatment. Papilledema commonly resolves rapidly and usually disappears within 2 weeks of control of the blood pressure being obtained. Flame-shaped hemorrhages likewise resolve rapidly,and it is unusual to see new hemorrhages develop once effective antihypertensive drug treatment has been commenced. Cotton wool spots may continue to appear for a few days after the institution of antihypertensive treatment and may take 3 to 4 weeks to disappear altogether. Hard exudate is more resistant to antihypertensive therapy; with continued effective control, it usually diminishes gradually in size and may disappear completely within 1 to 2 years of control of blood pressure. There are no convincing effects of antihypertensive drug treatment on the retinal arteries or veins.

5. Borderline Hypertension

While there is clear evidence concerning the effects of antihypertensive drug treatment on severe hypertension or on the complicating effects of it, there is as yet no firm evidence as to the effects of drug treatment on borderline or mild hypertension. This situation is complicated by the fact that many patients with borderline hypertension become normotensive without treatment and is further complicated by the placebo effects which have been demonstrated in the U.K. in the Medical Research Council trial of mild hypertension,[98] the Australian National Blood Pressure Study,[99] and in the US Public Health Service Study.[100] In the Australian study, the blood pressure fell by about 8 mmHg in both systolic and diastolic between the first and second screening examination, and the blood pressure in the placebo treated group has continued to fall over the first 4 yr of treatment. Evidence that the pharmacological treatment of mild hypertension reduces either the morbidity or mortality from the disease is not unequivocally available. The results of a 10-year feasibility trial in the treatment of mild hypertension,[100] however, are suggestive, although the numbers are small. The incidence of cerebrovascular accident was six in the placebo group to one in the treated group; nine patients developed retinopathy in the placebo group and one in the treated group. There was no difference between the groups in the incidence of myocardial infarction or coronary heart disease. The average admission blood pressures for this study were about 150/100 mmHg. Although no claims were made, it appears to the author that these results are highly suggestive that hypertensive complications occurred sufficiently often in the placebo group compared to those in the treatment group to suggest that people with these levels of blood pressure need treatment.

In this study, the incidence of coronary events was not altered by the treatment regimen which consisted of a benzothiadiazine diuretic and rauwolfia, in contrast to the study of Berglund et al.[95] in which most treated patients received β-receptor-blocking drugs. This suggests that prevention of the clinical manifestation of coronary artery disease may well be additionally assisted by the latter drugs.

6. Summary of Results of Treatment

There is clear evidence that sustained reduction of blood pressure by pharmacological or other means effectively prevents these manifestations of hypertension which are directly due to the high arterial pressure, such as heart failure, hemorrhagic stroke, and fibrinoid arteriolar necrosis. The effects of hypertension related to acceleration or aggravation of atherosclerotic vascular disease, such as myocardial infarction, cerebral infarction, or other secondary manifestations of vascular disease, are less obviously ameliorated. The widespread use of antihypertensive drug treatment has altered the pattern of morbidity in hypertension so that atherosclerotic phenomena, such as myocardial infarction, have now emerged as the major complication in treated hypertensive patients.

The fundamental and as yet unsolved question, is whether treatment instituted early in the course of the disease will delay or prevent the development of vascular disease. If the answer to this question is affirmative, then early treatment of all grades of severity, including the mildest forms of hypertension, would be plainly justifiable. If, however, the answer is negative, it would be a logical consequence that treatment could be reserved for those most likely to suffer direct consequences of the raised intravascular pressure, namely those with the highest pressures or with evidence of end organ involvement. Resolution of this problem will depend on large-scale intervention trials, prolonged over a sufficient period to allow observation of the effects of control of blood pressure on the development of vascular complications in patients with mild hypertension.

A second very important question which has been only partly answered is whether differing antihypertensive drugs exert different effects on the various complications of hypertension. Evidence does appear to be emerging that β-adrenoceptor blocking drugs reduce or delay the incidence of myocardial infarction and sudden death, both in nonhypertensive patients and in hypertensive. If further studies confirm these early impressions, the field of antihypertensive drug therapy will widen considerably and will involve the prophylactic use of these drugs in even mild hypertension to reduce the risk of myocardial infarction. Final evidence on this matter awaits the outcome of a number of large multicenter studies.

III. THE APPROACH TO THE INDIVIDUAL PATIENT

The decision as to whether and how to treat an individual patient can be clear-cut or can be a complex and difficult matter. The aim of management in hypertension, as in any other chronic disease, is to relieve symptoms and to improve prognosis. In hypertension, it is important to achieve these ends without imposing new and unnecessary restrictions on the patient's life and without inducing new symptoms or disabilites as a result of treatment or investigations.

A number of questions need to be answered before the management of any individual patient can be aproached rationally. In the section which follows, the questions will be posed, the methods of obtaining the answers outlined, and the consequence of the information evaluated.

A. Does This Patient Have High Blood Pressure?

Patients may consult physicians because they suspect they have or have been told they have high blood pressure. Such a presentation may follow a life insurance examination, participation in a blood pressure screening program, advice from another physician, seeing a television program, reading about hypertension in a magazine, anxiety because a relative has hypertension, or as part of a routine health check.

The answer to this question depends on careful measurement of blood pressure without any specific precautions to allay anxiety or to promote optimal conditions of comfort.

Blood pressure needs to be measured with a mercury sphygmomanometer, using a carefully applied cuff of appropriate size to the upper arm, by the auscultatory method. Three estimations are usually made. The diastolic pressure should be taken at the point of sudden muffling of the Korotkoff Sounds (Phase IV). The point of disappearance of these sounds (Phase V) should also be noted.

1.   If the patient's diastolic blood pressure is persistently below 90 mmHg (Phase IV), it can be assumed that the patient is not hypertensive, providing that he is not taking antihypertensive drugs and providing that there has been no recent episode to suggest that the blood pressure has been lowered, such as might occur following an infection, blood loss, or chest pain. The finding of a diastolic pressure persistently below 90 mmHg in an otherwise healthy adult allows the patient to be reassured that he is not hypertensive and that a repeat examination will not need to be made for 12 months.
2.   If the diastolic blood pressure is between 90 and 109 mmHg, the patient may or may not have hypertension. This leads to the need to continue the diagnostic process.
3.   If the diastolic blood pressure is above 110 mmHg, the patient is almost certainly hypertensive and will require full evaluation and probably treatment.

B. This Patient's Diastolic Blood Pressure is Above 90 mmHg. Are There Other Features Which Suggest the Need for Treatment?

The answer to this question depends on a careful history, a complete physical examination, and a few investigations.

1. History

Age — The significance of the finding of borderline hypertension is considerably influenced by the patient's age. In patients below the age of 45 years the presence of a blood pressure of this level is more likely than not to indicate that treatment will be needed, since blood pressures on the average rise considerably between the ages of 45 to 65, so that patients below this age with borderline hypertension more often will be found subsequently to have developed unequivocal hypertension. Patients over 65 are less likely to need treatment unless other indications are present.

Sex — For any given level of blood pressures, males have a worse prognosis than females. This is not to imply that women do not need to be treated, but that hypertension is a more severe illness in men than women.

How recently has this level of blood pressure developed? — Patients with hypertension may have information about previous levels of blood pressure. If the evidence suggests that the blood pressure has been marginally elevated for some years, it is less likely that treatment will be urgently required than if there is information that blood pressure was normal less than 1 year previously, since the latter fact raises the possibility either that some underlying cause has developed or that the patient is in a phase in which the blood pressure is rising rapidly.

Are there any symptoms suggesting end organ damage as a result of hypertension? — Specific inquiry needs to be made about the presence or absence of breathlessness, either on exertion or during recumbency, angina of effort, previous episodes suggesting transient cerebral ischemic attacks, visual disturbances, and nocturia. A few patients will have had breathlessness due to hypertensive heart disease, but dyspnea may be due to chronic obstructive airways disease or to bronchial asthma. Angina of effort or a past history of myocardial infarction may be present as may a history of transient ischemic attacks. Both these may be related more to associated atherosclerosis than to hypertensive vascular disease. Retinopathy leading to visual disturbances is uncommon but must be enquired about.

Are there any features in the history which suggest that the hypertension is due to

some underlying pathological cause? — Close enquiry should be made about possible renal causes. These include a past history of poststreptococcal glomerulonephritis, urinary tract infections, ureteric colic due to stone or papillary necrosis, loin pain, unexplained hematuria, and analgesic tablet intake. The importance of such a history is not that it is likely to influence a decision concerning treatment, but that it indicates the need for further investigation of a possibly remediable cause.

Symptoms related to less common pathological causes should also be sought. Muscular weakness or tetany, manifested as carpopedal spasm, may suggest primary aldosteronism. Episodes of paroxysmal headache, sweating, abnormal palpitations, particularly with bradycardia or unexplained sensations of anxiety, are features of pheochromocytoma, and although all these occur commonly in other patients, their presence suggests the need to exclude this disease.

Are there other risk factors for vascular disease present? — Hypertension is a major risk factor for the development of vascular disease. The presence of other risk factors needs to be evaluated, particularly obesity, cigarette smoking, a family history of arterial disease, diabetes, or gout. Alcohol intake needs to be evaluated. Evaluation of these factors are important in determining the probable risk of the development of vascular complications and will affect management and prognosis.

What kind of person is this patient? — This evaluation is often very difficult at a first consultation. It has considerable relevance to subsequent management because if antihypertensive drug treatment is required, the personality of the patient and his or her relationship to the physician may be an important factor in deciding whether or not the patient will cooperate in continuing drug treatment. Moreover, the blood pressure in overtly anxious patients is more likely to be spuriously high on a first visit so that in such patients, reassurance and repeated measurement may be helpful in the final assessment.

2. Physical Examination

Physical examination is directed to answering two main questions.

1. Is there evidence of end-organ damage attributable to hypertension which would alter management?

Evidence of end-organ damage needs to be sought in the heart, the blood vessels, the retinas, and in the central nervous system.

In the heart, evidence of left ventricular enlargement, a presystolic (atrial) triple rhythm, elevation of the jugular venous pressure, or manifestations of congestive cardiac failure are all indications for the need to institute antihypertensive treatment.

In the retina, the presence of retinal hemorrhages, cotton wool spots, hard exudate, or papilledema are also clearcut indications for the need for treatment. Changes in the blood vessels of the retina need to be noted, but have to be interpreted in the relation to the patient's age. They are probably of little value in diagnosis in patients over 50 years.

In the central nervous system, evidence of past hemiparesis should be sought. The presence or absence of carotid murmurs should be noted because of the high incidence of obstructive lesions of the extracranial arteries in hypertensive patients. The abdominal aorta, femoral arteries, and peripheral arteries should be palpated. The finding of evidence of occlusive vascular disease may indicate the need for angiography and corrective surgery.

2. Is there evidence of an underlying pathological cause for the hypertension which might alter management?

Some of the secondary causes of hypertension are detectable clinically. Most, however, need special investigation for their detection or confirmation.

Cushing's Syndrome can usually be suspected on clinical grounds. Although it is uncommon as a cause of hypertension, blood pressure is usually elevated in the disease. Clinically, Cushing's Syndrome should be suspected in patients with the florid moon face, truncal obesity, limb weakness, and striae. It may be difficult to distinguish from simple obesity, particularly in middle aged women who are often florid and not uncommonly have striae.

Hypertension secondary to renal vascular occlusive disease may be suspected in patients with hypertension, particularly of recent onset, who have a murmur audible in the epigastrium or towards the flanks. This sign is not confined to patients with renal artery stenosis. Polycystic kidneys are usually, but not always, palpable clinically; their presence should be routinely sought. Coarctation of the aorta, although rare, should aways be considered. The femoral arteries should be palpated routinely, and where there is difficulty in palpating them, the blood pressure should be measured in the popliteal fossa by using a large cuff applied around the thigh. Confirmatory evidence of collateral arteries around the scapulas and the presence of a bruit audible posteriorly and medial to the right scapula should be sought.

3. Investigations

At the initial consultation, only simple investigations are necessary to allow a decision as to whether treatment should be considered, unless features in the history or the physical examination have suggested the need for more complex studies.

Examination of the urine — Examination of the urine can be regarded as an extension of the physical examination. Proteinuria, particularly if accompanied by casts, red blood cells, or pus cells indicates the need for further evaluation of the renal tract. Some degree of proteinuria is common in hypertensive patients. Its presence is significantly associated with a considerably increased risk of death from cardiovascular causes in both men and women as shown by both the Framingham study and by life insurance statistics (Table 4), the risk being increased four to six times by the presence of proteinuria. The finding of proteinuria should be regarded as an indication for treatment.

The electrocardiogram (EKG) — The EKG gives information about cardiac rhythm, the presence of previous myocardial infarction, or the presence of left atrial or left ventricular hypertrophy. The presence of evidence of electrocardiographic abnormalities was a highly unfavorable indication for the development of cardiovascular morbid events in the Framingham study and can be regarded as an unequivocal indication for antihypertensive therapy.

Blood chemistry — Fasting values for serum sodium, potassium, creatinine, urea, uric acid, cholesterol, and triglycerides should be obtained.

C. This Patient Has a Diastolic Blood Pressure Above 90 mmHg. I Have Completed a History, Physical Examination, and Initial Investigation. Should He Be Treated for Hypertension at This Time?

Yes — This answer will include (1) all patients with diastolic pressures of 110 mmHg or greater; (2) all patients with proteinuria; (3) all patients with EKG evidence of left atrial or left ventricular hypertrophy; (4) all patients with retinal hemorrhages, exudate, or papilledema; (5) all patients with clinical evidence of cardiac enlargement; and (6) all patients with a familial history of hypertensive cardiovascular disease.

No — This answer will include all patients with diastolic blood pressures between 90 and 110 mmHg who have none of the additional criteria set out above.

D. How Should I Proceed With Those Specified in Section III. C Who Do Not Require Treatment at This Time?

These patients may or may not need antihypertensive drug treatment after further evaluation. This will need to be determined in the light of the subsequent progress of their blood pressure levels, which will need to be reevaluated at regular intervals of about 12 weeks to allow a decision to be made about antihypertensive drug treatment. Such patients should be told that while there is no clear indication for antihypertensive drug treatment on the basis of the observations so far made, subsequent progress will decide the need. As an immediate measure, patients who smoke or who are overweight or who have elevated cholesterol or triglyceride values should be advised of the known association between these factors and the incidence of vascular disease and advised about ways of solving these problems.

Opinions vary as to what level of blood pressure found on repeated measurement should be taken as an indication of treatment. In the absence of firm evidence, this is perhaps inevitable. In the author's opinion, patients who are found to have a diastolic pressure consistently between 100 mmHg and 109 mmHg should be offered treatment. Both patient and physician need to realize that treatment for mild hypertension in the absence of symptoms is designed to prevent or to minimize or to delay the risk of vascular disease developing later in life, that treatment needs to be continuing, perhaps for 30 or more years, and that the certainty of proof of benefit for any given individual can not be guaranteed in any way. The physician can be reasonably confident that treatment of 100 such patients will help some of them in the long term. What he cannot be sure of is whether any particular patient will be among those who will benefit. However, with the range of drugs available today, it is almost always possible to achieve a substantial fall of blood pressure without inducing uncomfortable or dangerous side effects, so that while the benefit of treatment is speculative in any given patient, the disadvantages are now so few that there is not much to be lost by offering treatment. Probably, the major disadvantage to the average patient is the need for regular medical supervision and for regular medication. Since, however, medical supervision is needed whether active treatment is given or not, this can probably be discounted.

To summarize, it is the opinion of the author that all patients who have diastolic blood pressures persistently above 100 mmHg should be given antihypertensive drug treatment. While it may not be generally agreed that patients in the lower levels should be treated, the other indications referred to above would be generally agreed with.

Once a decision has been made to treat a patient, a further series of decisions as to how to do so is needed. These are dealt with in the next section.

REFERENCES

1. **Lew, A.**, *An Actuarial View of Hypertension*, Monographs on Hypertension, Merck & Co. 1973.
2. Society of Actuaries, *Build and Blood Pressure Study*, Vol. 1, Society of Actuaries, Chicago, 1959.
3. **Kannell, W.B., Wolf, P. A., Verter, J., and McNamara, P. M.**, Epidemiological assessment of role of blood pressure in stroke: the Framingham study, *JAMA*, 214, 301, 1970.
4. **Kannel, W. B., Castelli, W. P., McNamara, P. M., McKee, P. A., and Feinleib, M.**, Role of blood pressure in the development of congestive heart failure: the Framingham study, *N. Engl. J. Med.*, 287, 781, 1972.
5. **Paul, O.**, Risks of mild hypertension: a ten year report, *Br. Heart J.*, 33, (Suppl.), 116, 1971.
6. **Prineas, R. J., Stephens, W. D., and Lovell, R. R. H.**, Early consequences of screening for hypertension in a community, *Clin. Sci. Mol. Med.*, 45, 47s, 1973.

7. **Wilber, J. A. and Barrow, J. G.,** Hypertension: community problem, *Am. J. Med.,* 52, 653, 1972.
8. **Bøe, J., Humerfelt, S., and Wedervang, F.,** The blood pressure in a population. Blood pressure readings and heights and weight determinations in the adult population of the city of Bergen, *Acta Med. Scand. Suppl.,* 321, 157, 1957.
9. **Lellouch, J. and Richard, J. L.,** La pression arterielle d'une population masculine active. Étude épidemiologique de 19, 714 sujets, *Presse Med.,* 79, 1749, 1971.
10. **Hatano, S., Shigematsu, I., and Strasser, T.,** *Hypertension and Stroke Control in the Community. Summary and Recommendations,* World Health Organization, Geneva, 1976.
11. **Werko, L.,** In discussion. in *Hypertension and Stroke Control in the Community,* Hatano, S., Shigematsu, T., and Strasser, T., Eds., World Health Organization, Geneva, 1976, 245.
12. **Kannel, W. B.,** in *Hypertension,* Genest, J., Koiw, E., and Kuchel, O., Eds., McGraw-Hill, New York, 1977, 889.
13. **Addis, T.,** Blood pressure and pulse rate levels, *Arch. Intern. Med.,* 29, 539, 1922.
14. **Alam, G. M. and Smirk, F. H.,** Casual and basal blood pressures. I. In British and Egyptian men. II. In essential hypertension, *Br. Heart J.,* 5, 152, 1943.
15. **Smirk, F. H., Veale, A. M. O., and Alstad, K. W.,** Basal and supplemental pressure in relationship to life expectancy and hypertension symptomatology, *N. Z. Med. J.,* 58, 711, 1959.
16. **Smirk, F. H.,** Casual, basal and supplemental blood pressures in 519 first-degree relatives of substantial hypertensive patients and in 350 population controls, *Clin. Sci. Mol. Med.,* 51, 13s, 1976.
17. **Bevan, A. T., Honor, A. J., and Stott, F. H.,** Direct arterial pressure recording in unrestricted man, *Clin. Sci.,* 36, 329, 1969.
18. **Littler, W. A., Honour, A. J., Carter, R. D., and Sleight, P.,** Sleep and blood pressure, *Br. Med. J.,* 3, 346, 1975.
19. **Shurtleff, D.,** Some characteristics related to the incidence of cardiovascular disease and death: the Framingham study, 18 year follow up, U.S. Department of Health, Education, and Welfare Publ. No. (NIH), 74-599, Sect. 30, 1974.
20. **Grant, R. P.,** Aspects of cardiac hypertrophy, *Am. Heart J.,* 46, 154, 1953.
21. **Sonnenblick, E. H., Ross, J., Jr., and Braunwald, E.,** Oxygen consumption of the heart. Newer concepts of its multifactorial determination, *Am. J. Cardiol.,* 22, 328, 1968.
22. **Lingbach, A. J.,** Heart failure from the point of view of quantitative anatomy, *Am. J. Cardiol.,* 5, 370, 1960.
23. **Dustan, H. P., Tarazi, R. C., and Bravo, E. L.,** Physiologic characteristics of hypertension, *Am. J. Med.,* 52, 610, 1972.
24. **Frohlich, E. D., Dustan, H. P., and Tarazi, R. C.,** Hyperdynamic beta-adrenergic circulatory state. An Overview, *Arch. Intern. Med.,* 126, 1068, 1970.
25. **Lund-Johansen, P.,** Hemodynamics in early essential hypertension, *Acta Med. Scand.,* 181 (Suppl. 482), 1, 1967.
26. **Frohlich, E. D., Tarazi, R. C., and Dustan, H. P.,** Clinical physiological correlations in the development of hypertensive heart disease, *Circulation,* 44, 446, 1971.
27. **Tarazi, R. C., Miller, A., Frohlich, E. D., and Dustan, H. P.,** Electrocardiographic changes reflecting left atrial abnormality in hypertension, *Circulation,* 34, 818, 1966.
28. **Cohn, J. N., Rodriguera, E., and Guiha, N.,** in *Hypertension. Mechanisms and Management,* Onesti, G., Kim, K. E., and Moyer, J. H., Eds., Grunne & Stratton, New York, 1973, 191.
29. **Sokolow, M. and Perloff, D.,** The prognosis of essential hypertension treated conservatively, *Circulation,* 34, 697, 1961.
30. **Davis, D. and Klainer, M. J.,** Studies in hypertensive heart disease. I. The incidence of coronary atherosclerosis in cases of essential hypertension, *Am. Heart J.,* 19, 185, 1940.
31. **Harrison, C. V. and Wood, P.,** Hypertensive and ischaemic heart disease. A comparative clinical and pathological study, *Br. Heart J.,* 11, 205, 1949.
32. **Doyle, A. E. and Kilpatrick, J. A.,** Methonium compounds in the angina of hypertension, *Lancet,* 1, 905, 1954.
33. **Goldring, W. and Chasis, H.,** in *Hypertension and Hypertensive Disease,* Commonwealth Fund, New York, 1944.
34. **Kety, S. S. and Schmidt, C. F.,** The nitrous oxide method for the quantitative determination of cerebral blood flow in man. Theory, procedure and normal values, *J. Clin. Invest.,* 27, 476, 1948.
35. **Fog, M.,** The cerebral circulation. The reaction of the pial arteries to a fall in blood pressure, *Arch. Neurol. Psychiatry,* 37, 351, 1937.
36. **Harper, A. M.,** Autoregulation of cerebral blood flow. Influence of the arterial pressure on blood flow through the cerebral cortex, *J. Neurol. Neurosurg. Psychiatry,* 29, 398, 1966.
37. **Standgaard, S., Olesen, J., Skinhøj, E., and Lassen, N. A.,** Autoregulation of brain circulation in severe arterial hypertension, *Br. Med. J.,* 1, 507, 1973.

38. **Byrom, F. B.,** The pathogenesis of hypertensive encephalopathy and its relation to the malignant phase of hypertension. Experimental evidence from the hypertensive rat, *Lancet,* 2, 201, 1954.
39. **Cole, F. M. and Yates, P. O.,** Comparative incidence of cerebrovascular lesions in normotensive and hypertensive patients, *Neurology,* 18, 255, 1968.
40. **Prineas, J. and Marshal, J.,** Hypertension and cerebral infarction, *Br. Med. J.,* 1, 14, 1966.
41. **Fisher, C. M.,** Cerebral miliary aneurysms in hypertension, *Am. J. Pathol.,* 66, 313, 1972.
42. **Charcot, J. M. and Bouchard, C.,** Nouvelles recherches sur la pathogénie de l'hémarhagie cérébrale, *Arch. Physiol. Norm. Pathol. (Paris),* 1, 110, 1868.
43. **Ross Russell, R. W.,** Observations on intracerebral aneurysms, *Brain,* 86, 425, 1963.
44. **Fisher, C. M.,** The arterial lesions underlying lacunes, *Acta Neuropathol.,* 12, 11, 1969.
45. **Sandok, B. A. and Whisnant, J. P.,** Hypertension and the brain, *Arch. Intern. Med.,* 133, 947, 1974.
46. **Matsumoto, N., Whisnant, J. P., Kurland, L. T., and Okazaki, H.,** Natural history of stroke in Rochester, Minnesota, 1955 through 1969, *Stroke,* 4, 20, 1973.
47. Hypertension-Stroke Cooperative Study Group, Effects of antihypertensive treatment on stroke recurrence, *JAMA,* 224, 329, 1973.
48. Veteran's Administration Cooperative Study Group on Antihypertensive Agents, Effects of treatment on morbidity in hypertension: results in patients with diastolic blood pressures averaging 115 through 129 mm. Hg., *JAMA,* 202, 1029, 1967.
49. **Keith, N. M., Wagener, H. P., and Barker, N. W.,** Some different types of hypertension: their cause and prognosis, *Am. J. Med. Sci.,* 197, 332, 1939.
50. **Dodge, J. V. and Dollery, C. T.,** Retinal soft exudates, *Q. J. Med.,* 33, 117, 1964.
51. **Kagan, A., Aurell, E., and Tibblin, G.,** Signs in the fundus oculi and arterial hypertension, *Bull. W.H.O.,* 36, 231, 1967.
52. **Garner, A., Ashton, N., Tripathi, R., Kohner, E. M., Bulpitt, C. J., and Dollery, C. T.,** Pathogenesis of hypertensive retinopathy and experimental study in the monkey, *Br. J. Ophthalmol.,* 59, 3, 1975.
53. **Kirkendale, W. M. and Armstrong, M. L.,** Vascular changes in the eye of the treated and untreated patient with essential hypertension, *Am. J. Cardiol.,* 9, 663, 1962.
54. **Shakib, M. and Ashton, N.,** Focal retinal ischaemia, *Br. J. Ophthalmol.,* 50, 325, 1966.
55. **Perlman, L. V., Herdman, R. C., Kleinman, H., and Vernier, R. L.,** Streptococcal glomerulonephritis. A ten-year follow up of an epidemic, *JAMA,* 194, 63, 1965.
56. **Earle, D. P.,** in *Cornell Seminars in Nephrology,* Becker, E.L., Ed., John Wiley & Sons, New York, 1973, 73.
57. **Kushner, D. S., Armstrong, S. H., Dublin, A., Szanto, P. B., Markowitz, A., Madernos, B. P., Levine, J. M., Rivver, G. L., Glyman, T. N., and Pendras, J. P.,** Acute glomerulonephritis in the adult. Longitudinal, clinical, functional and morphologic studies of rates of healing and progression to chronicity, *Medicine (Baltimore),* 40, 203, 1961.
58. **Baldwin, D. S.,** in *Proc. 5th Int. Congr. Nephrology, Mexico,* Vol. 3, S. Karger, Basel, 1974, 36.
59. **Rodriguez-Iturbe, B., Garcia, R., Anzola, E., Cuenca, L., Treser, G., and Lange, L.,** Incidence of chronicity after an epidemic of acute poststreptococcal glomerulonephritis, in *Proc. 6th Int. Congr. of Nephrol.,* Giovanetti, S., Bononini, V., and D'Amico, G., Eds., S. Karger, Basel, 1975.
60. **Albert, M. S., Leeming, J. M., and Scaglione, P. R.,** Acute glomerulonephritis without abnormality of the urine, *J. Pediatr.,* 68, 525, 1966.
61. **Kincaid-Smith, P., Fairley, K. F., and Heale, W. F.** in *Hypertension, Mechanisms and Management,* Onesti, G., Kim, K. E., and Moyer, J. H., Eds., Grune & Stratton, New York, 1973, 697.
62. **Hodson, C.J. and Edwards, D.,** Chronic pyelonephritis and vesicoureteric reflux, *Clin. Radiol.,* 11, 219, 1960.
63. **Heptinstall, R. H.,** *Pathology of the Kidney,* 2nd ed., Little, Brown, Boston, 1974, 881.
64. **Kincaid-Smith, P.,** Vascular obstrucion in chronic pyelonephritic kidneys and its relation to hypertension, *Lancet,* 2, 1263, 1955.
65. **Moeschlin, S.,** Phenacetin suht und — schaden. (Innen körperanamien und interstitialle Nephritis), *Schweiz. Med. Wochenschr.,* 87, 123, 1957.
66. **Kincaid-Smith, P.,** Pathogenesis of the renal lesion associated with the abuse of analgesics, *Lancet,* 1, 859, 1967.
67. **Burry, A. F.,** The evolution of analgesic nephropathy, *Nephron,* 3, 185, 1968.
68. **Kincaid-Smith, P.,** Analgesic nephropathy. A common form of renal disease in Australia, *Med. J. Aust.,* 2, 1131, 1969.
69. **Dawborn, J. K., Fairley, K. F., Kincaid-Smith, P., and King, W. E.,** The association of peptic ulceration, chronic renal disease and analgesic abuse, *Q. J. Med.,* 35, 69, 1966.
70. **Kimmelstiel, P. and Wilson, C.,** Intercapillary lesions in glomeruli of kidney, *Am. J. Pathol.,* 12, 83, 1936.
71. **Smithwick, R. H.,** in *Hypertension,* Bell, E. T., Ed., University of Minnesota Press, Minneapolis, 1951, 429.

72. **Thorn, G. W., Harrison, J. H., Merrils, J. P., Criscitiello, M. G., Frawley, T. F., and Finkenstaedt, J. T.**, Clinical studies on bilateral complete adrenalectomy in patients with severe hypertensive vascular disease, *Ann. Intern. Med.*, 37, 972, 1952.

73. **Kempner, W.**, Treatment of hypertensive vascular disease with rice diet, *Am. J. Med.*, 4, 545, 1948.

74. **Paton, W. D. M., and Zaimis, E. M.**, The pharmacological actions of polymethylene bismethylammonium salts, *Br. J. Pharmacol. Chemother.*, 4, 381, 1949.

75. **Smirk, F. H. and Alstad, K. S.**, Treatment of arterial hypertension by penta- and hexamethonium salts based on 150 tests on hypertensives of varied aetiology and 53 patients treated for periods of two to fourteen months, *Br. Med. J.*, 1, 1217, 1951.

76. **Smirk, F. H.**, Results of methonium treatment of hypertensive patients. Based on 250 cases treated for periods up to 3½ years including 28 with malignant hypertension, *Br. Med. J.*, 1, 717, 1954.

77. **Smirk, F.H., Hamilton, M., McQueen, E. G., and Doyle, A. E.**, The treatment of hypertensive heart failure and of hypertensive cardiac overload by blood pressure reduction, *Am. J. Cardiol.*, 1, 143, 1958.

78. **McMichael, J. and Murphy, E. A.**, Methonium treatment of severe and malignant hypertension, *J. Chronic Dis.*, 1, 527, 1955.

79. **Burnett, C. F., Jr. and Evans, J. A.**, Drug therapy in hypertension with hemorrhagic hypertensive retinitis, *N. Engl. J. Med.*, 253, 395, 1955.

80. **Smith, K. S. and Fowler, P. B. S.**, Prevention and treatment of hypertensive heart failure by ganglion blocking agents, *Lancet*, 1, 417, 1955.

81. **Hamilton, M., Thompson, E. N., and Wisniewski, T. K. M.**, The role of blood pressure control in preventing complications of hypertension, *Lancet*, 1, 235, 1964.

82. Veteran's Administration Co-Operative Study Group on Antihypertensive Agents, II. Effect of treatment on morbidity and mortality: results of treatment in patients with diastolic blood pressures averaging 90 through 114 mm.Hg, *JAMA*, 213, 1143, 1970.

83. **Breckenridge, A., Dollery, C. T., and Parry, E. H. O.**, Prognosis of treated hypertension, *Q. J. Med.*, 39, 411, 1970.

84. **Harrington, M., Kincaid-Smith, P., and McMichael, J.**, Results of treatment in malignant hypertension: a seven-year experience in 94 cases, *Br. Med. J.*, 2, 969, 1959.

85. **Dustan, H. P., Schneckloth, R. E., Corcoran, A. C., and Page, I. H.**, The effectiveness of long term treatment of malignant hypertension, *Circulation*, 18, 644, 1958.

86. **Doyle, A. E.**, Electrocardiographic changes in hypertension treated by methonium compounds, *Am. Heart J.*, 45, 363, 1953.

87. **Doyle, A. E.**, Treatment of hypertension, *N. Y. State J. Med.*, 68, 256, 1968.

88. **Smirk, F. H. and Hodge, J. V.**, Causes of death in treated hypertensive patients, *Br. Med. J.*, 2, 1221, 1963.

89. **Dollery, C. T. and Bulpitt, C. J.**, in *Hypertension*, Genest, J., Koiw, E., and Kuchel, O., Eds., McGraw-Hill, New York, 1977, 1038.

90. **Wilhelmsson, C., Vedin, J. A., Wilhelmsen, L., Tabbling, G., and Werko, L.**, Reduction of sudden deaths after myocardial infarction by treatment with alprenolol, *Lancet*, 2, 1157, 1974.

91. **Ahlmark, G., Saetre, H., and Korsgren, M.**, Reduction of sudden death after myocardial infarction, *Lancet*, 2, 1563, 1974.

92. **Fox, K. M., Chopra, M. P., Portal, R. W., and Aber, C. P.**, Long term beta blockade: possible protection from myocardial infarction, *Br. Med. J.*, 1, 117, 175.

93. **Anon.**, Improvement in prognosis of myocardial infarction by long-term beta adrenoceptor blockade using practolol. A multicenter study, *Br. Med. J.*, 3, 735, 1975.

94. **Stewart, I. McD. G.**, Compared incidence of first myocardial infarction in hypertensive patients under treatment containing propranolol or excluding β-receptor blockade, *Clin. Sci. Mol. Med.*, 51 (Suppl. 3), 509s, 1976.

95. **Berglund, G., Wilhelmsen, L, Sannerstedt, R., Hansson, L., Andersson, O., Sivertsson, R., Wedel, H., and Wikstrand, J.**, Coronary heart disease after treatment of hypertension, *Lancet*, 1, 1, 1978.

96. **Carter, O.**, Hypertensive therapy in stroke survivors, *Lancet*, 1, 485, 1970.

97. Hypertension-Stroke Study Group, Stroke recurrence after anti-hypertensive therapy, *Circulation*, Suppl. 4, 84, 1973.

98. **Miall, W. E., Brennan, P. G., and Mann, A. H.**, Medical Research Council's treatment trial for mild hypertension: an interim report, *Clin. Sci. Mol. Med.*, 51 (Suppl. 3), 563s, 1976.

99. **Abernethy, J. D., Baker, J. L., Bullen, M. U., Lamb, M. L., and Stewart, M. R.**, Report on progress in the Australian National Blood Pressure Study (NBPS), *Clin. Sci. Mol. Med.*, 51 (Suppl. 3), 645s, 1976.

100. **McFate Smith, W.**, Treatment of mild hypertension. Results of a ten year intervention trial, U.S. Public Health Service Hospitals Cooperative Study Group, *Circ. Res.*, 40 (Suppl. 1), 1, 1977.

Chapter 4

PRINCIPLES OF MANAGEMENT AND THE USE OF DRUGS

I. INTRODUCTION

The aim of treating hypertension of whatever etiology or severity is to normalize the blood pressure or to achieve levels as close to normal as possible. In a substantial number of patients, this aim can be achieved without difficulty. In some patients, however, either the blood pressure cannot be reduced to normal levels no matter what therapeutic agents are used, or more commonly, reduction of blood pressure to normal levels can only be achieved with doses of antihypertensive drugs which are sufficiently high to lead to unwanted side effects. For these reasons, it is not possible to define an ideal treatment for all patients with hypertension, and it cannot be emphasized too strongly that the response of the individual patient to various drugs is at least as important a component of the successful management of hypertension as is the appropriate selection of drugs.

Generally, once antihypertensive drug treatment has commenced, it is likely to be necessary for the patient to continue with medication indefinitely. This is more likely to be successfully achieved in patients who have symptoms or disability related to their hypertension than in the uncomplicated symptom-free hypertensive patient. It is also likely to be more readily achieved if a regime can be devised which produces little or no side effects of an uncomfortable or disabling nature and if the dosage schedule can be devised so as to avoid major disruption to the patient's social and other everyday activities. All existing antihypertensive drugs have some disadvantages, the degree of which varies from one patient to the next. Moreover, all antihypertensive drug regimes require patients to take drugs at least once daily and most commonly at more frequent intervals. Drug treatment also involves the patient in recurring medical supervision. For these reasons, the problem of patient compliance is a major one in the therapeutics of hypertension. Thus, Sackett et al.[1] in a study of 230 Canadian steel workers with hypertension found that only 50 to 55% of patients studied had complied with suggested treatment 6 months after it had been initiated. They found that patients assigned to receive an educational program designed to give them the facts about hypertension, its effects upon target organs, health and life expectancy, the benefits of antihypertensive therapy, the need for compliance with medication, and some simple reminders for pill taking were no more compliant with therapy than patients who received none of these. Moreover, in the same study, it appeared to make no difference whether clinic attendances were arranged for the convenience of patients or not (Table 1). This latter finding is at variance with observations of Finnerty et al.,[2] whose study suggested that augmenting the convenience of care did lead to improved compliance.

Various strategies have been devised for measuring the compliance of patients given antihypertensive drug treatment. The ones most usually used are tablet counts, the measurement of drugs and/or metabolites in urine, and the identification of such changes as falls in serum potassium and elevations of uric acid in patients taking thiazide drugs. Using such criteria, Dollery,[3] in studies at the Hammersmith Hospital Hypertensive Clinic, found between 85 and 92% of the patients studied had measurable levels of drug in the plasma on the day of the clinic attendance. Tablet counts are commonly used, but patients may discard tablets without taking them, so that this method is not infallible. In spite of these difficulties, it is important that physicians managing patients with high blood pressure are aware of the rather low rates of patient compliance that have been reported. In spite of the negative results in the randomized

TABLE 1

Effects of Strategies upon Compliance

Strategy	No. of men placed on antihypertensive drugs	% (and number) of dropouts	% (and number) designated compliant at 6 months	% (and number) designated compliant and at goal BP[a]
Augmented convenience	87	7% (6)	54% (47)	23% (20)
Normal convenience	57	7% (4)	51% (29)	19% (11)
Undergoing mastery learning	80	10% (8)	50% (40)	24% (19)
Not undergoing mastery learning	64	3% (2)	56% (36)	19% (12)

[a] Blood pressure.

From Sackett, D. L., Haynes, R. B., Gibson, E. S., Hackett, B., Taylor, D. W., Roberts, R. S., and Johnson, A. L., *Lancet,* 1, 1205, 1975.

control trial of Sackett, it still seems reasonable to hope that compliance can be improved by an understanding of the problem of hypertension and its treatment by both physician and patient. This involves a full explanation, together with frequent visits to reinforce the information given during the early stages of treatment. It also demands that when possible the regime be suited to the patient's convenience, both in times of administration and in terms of the avoidance of side effects. It is likely that even with the best management, a substantial number of patients will fail to comply with the therapeutic regime. Nevertheless, the physician should be aware of the problem and be alert for evidence of noncompliance.

administration and in terms of the avoidance of side effects. It is likely that even with the best management, a substantial number of patients will fail to comply with the therapeutic regime. Nevertheless, the physician should be aware of the problem and be alert for evidence of noncompliance.

In the great majority of hypertensive patients, there is no great urgency about obtaining control of blood pressure levels. This is certainly true in the mild or borderline hypertensive who is symptomless, but also applies to some of the more severely hypertensive patients in whom the risk of delay in obtaining good control of blood pressure is small. However, patients with diastolic blood pressures persistently above 120 mmHg should be regarded as requiring more urgent treatment, as should patients with evidence of congestive heart failure, hemorrhages, exudates or papilledema in the optic fundus, or patients with evidence of renal insufficiency. In a few patients, emergency treatment may be needed. In patients in whom there is no urgency about obtaining control of the blood pressure, it is desirable to begin either with dietary sodium restriction or diuretics and to add additional drugs progressively until the blood pressure appears to be well controlled. Alterations in dose should be made at intervals of about 7 days. The whole process of stabilization may take 2 to 3 months, although in most patients the control of blood pressure can be obtained much more rapidly than this.

II. INITIAL ANTIHYPERTENSIVE TREATMENT

A. Control of Sodium Intake

The observations of Kempner[4] on the treatment of malignant hypertension by the

TABLE 2

Percentage of Patients with Mean Diastolic Blood Pressure (BP) below 95
mmHg or 90 mmHg 2 Years after Entering Study

Group	Number of patients	BP < 95 mmHg	BP < 90 mmHg
Normoten-sive	62	80%	60%
Borderline 1[a]	31	26%	16%
Borderline 2[a]	31	55%	32%
Borderline 3	31	74%	52%
Borderline 4	31	62%	42%

[a] B.P. of patients placed on medication taken as B.P. at time therapy
started.

From Morgan, T. O., Adam, W., Gillies, A., Wilson, M., Morgan, G.,
and Carney, S., *Lancet*, 1, 227, 1978.

rice diet indicated plainly that even patients with very severe hypertension could improve if they were markedly depleted of sodium. The rice diet, which consisted of rice
and fruit juices with a sodium content less than 10 mM/day, was moderately high in
potassium content. Marked improvement could be obtained in the majority of patients
who were able to tolerate such a diet.

The question as to whether dietary sodium should be restricted in less severe hypertensives is a controversial matter. Thus, an editorial in *Lancet*[5] suggested that "current
practice allows no place for a salt restriction in the management of hypertension" and
claimed that "the doctor who tells his hypertensive patient with normal renal function
to avoid salt is wrong on two grounds. First, the reduction in salt intake with such
advice falls far short of that required to produce a significant effect on blood pressure,
and second, existing drugs are potent enough to render the misery of an effective life-
long salt restriction unnecessary." On the other hand, there is evidence[6,7] that moderate reduction of sodium intake to less than 75 mM/day may produce a substantial
reduction in blood pressure in a number of moderately severely hypertensive patients.
Thus, Hunt[6] claimed that in mild hypertension with diastolic pressures between 90 and
104, 84% of patients responded with a fall of blood pressure to normotensive levels if
the 24-hr urine sodium could be kept below 75 mM/day, whereas with urinary sodium
excretion above 150 mM/day, only 11% responded. In patients with diastolic pressures
between 105 and 114, 64% responded if 24-hr urine sodium excretion was kept below
75 mM/day, and only 3% wi th urine sodium excretion above 150 mM/day. In more
severe hypertensives, the corresponding figures were 49 and 0%. Thus, Hunt's data
suggest that almost all the mild patients who cooperated had a substantial fall in diastolic blood pressure. Hunt further claims that there was a weight loss of almost 20 lb
and an average reduction of diastolic pressure of almost 30 mmHg. Morgan et al.[7]
have recently compared the effects of limiting sodim intake with the effects of no
treatment, treatment with thiazide diuretics, and treatment with propranolol. Patients
studied were men with borderline hypertension (diastolic blood pressures 94 to 109
mmHg). In 2 years after entering the study, 16% of the untreated patients had diastolic
blood pressures below 90 mmHg, whereas 32% of those given advice to reduce salt
intake, 52% of those given thiazides, and 42% of those given propranolol had blood
pressures below 90 mmHg (Table 2). The average changes in systolic and diastolic
blood pressure for the four groups are shown in Figure 1. Studies of urinary sodium

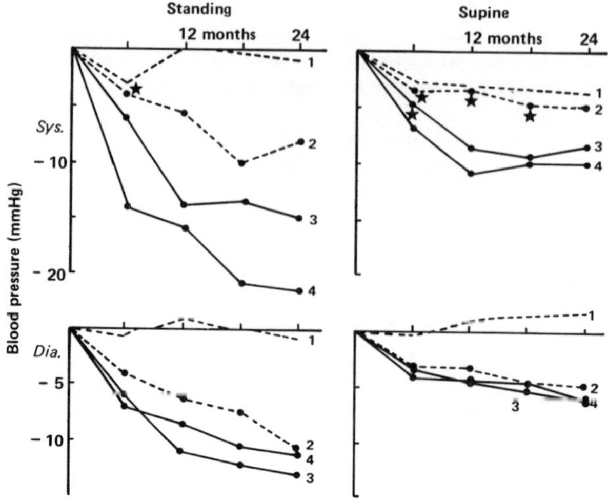

FIGURE 1.   Change in blood pressure, standing and supine, in the different groups, at 6 monthly intervals. The changes in systolic and diastolic blood pressure standing and supine are indicated. Changes in group 1 were not significantly different. All other changes except those marked with a star were significant (p < 0.05); S.E.M. was between 1 and 2 for diastolic blood pressure changes and between 2.5 and 4 for systolic blood pressure changes. The groups are as defined in Table 2. (From Morgan, T. O., Adam, W., Gillies, A., Wilson, M., Morgan, G., and Carney, S., *Lancet*, 1, 227, 1978. With permission.)

excretion revealed (Table 3 and Figure 2) that although the urinary sodium excretion was significantly reduced, the mean sodium excretion was still 157 mM/day in the group given dietary advice. This study suggests that modest restriction of sodium intake can reduce blood pressures, but also confirms that Australian veterans, at least, find difficulty in altering sodium intake. Kirkendall and Overturf[8] have presented evidence that the falls of systolic blood pressure induced by thiazides could be abolished by the ingestion of 12 gm of sodium chloride a day (Figure 3). To summarize this evidence, there is reasonably well-documented evidence that dietary sodium restriction of the order of 70 to 80 mM/day produces a substantial reduction of blood pressure in many hypertensive patients, particularly of mild degree, and where this can be achieved, such a regime would appear to have advantages over many forms of antihypertensive drug treatment. The major difficulty arises with such a regime that patients may find compliance difficult. This applies particularly to those whose occupations compel them to eat away from home frequently, but there is no firm evidence that compliance with a sodium-restricted diet is appreciably worse than compliance with antihypertensive drugs.

B. Diuretic Therapy

Regardless of whether dietary sodium intake is restricted or not, most agree that the first line of drug treatment for the majority of hypertensive patients is the use of a diuretic drug. A few authorities now prefer the initial use of a β-adrenoceptor-blocking drug. While not entirely free of side effects, the diuretics are usually well tolerated by hypertensive patients. The dose requirements are usually similar in various patients, particularly with the thiazide diuretics which have rather a flat dose-response curve.

TABLE 3

Urinary Excretion of Sodium

| | | Urinary Na | |
Urine sample	No. of samples	Mean (mmol/day)	SEM (mmol/day)
Initial sample (all patients)	107	191	6
Normotensive — subsequent sample	69	191	8
Group 1 — subsequent sample	58	180	9
Group 2 — subsequent sample	109	157	7[a]
Group 3 — subsequent sample	75	191	8
Group 4 — subsequent sample	55	189	10

Note: All patients had at least one urine collection and estimation after the initial visit. There were 126 patients in the trial; only two thirds (107) had an estimation of urinary Na at the start of the trial.

[a] Significantly less than all other values.

From Morgan, T. O., Adam, W., Gillies, A., Wilson, M., Morgan, G., and Carney, S., *Lancet*, 1, 227, 1978.

Aside from any intrinsic antihypertensive properties which they possess, they enhance the antihypertensive effects of almost all other antihypertensive drugs.

The mode of action of diuretics in lowering blood pressure is controversial. Following acute administration of thiazide diuretics, all investigators are agreed that a fall in extracellular fluid volume occurs, together with a fall of plasma volume and a loss of weight, usually of the order of 2 to 3 kg. Wilson and Freis[9] estimated that most patients lost about 2 ℓ of extracellular fluid, included in which were 300 to 400 mℓ of plasma volume. This comprised of about 10% of the extracellular fluid and about 15% of plasma volume. It has been reported[10] that the hypotensive action of diuretic agents could be reversed by reexpanding the plasma volume with salt-free dextran, and that by administering salt loads of between 15 and 30 gm per day by mouth, the loss in body weight can be reversed and the antihypertensive effect diminished or abolished.[8,11,12] The question as to whether the long-term effects of diuretics can be attributed exclusively to their dehydrating effect or whether there are additional effects on blood vessels is by no means clear. The balance of evidence suggests that although the plasma volume and extracellular fluid volume fall rapidly during the acute administration of thiazides, these parameters become stable after 2 to 3 weeks treatment. The persistent antihypertensive effect is thought by many to be due to the persisting hypovolemia. An alternative possible mechanism is a direct effect on the smooth muscle or vessels as has been discussed in an earlier chapter. The evidence for this rests largely on the similarities between thiazide diuretics and diazoxide which is a nondiuretic benzothiadiazine, and which acts directly on vascular smooth muscle to produce a prompt fall in arterial pressure. Both frusemide and ethacrynic acid seem to induce demonstrable effects on blood pressure even in anephric animals as has also been discussed previously. There is also some evidence that diuretics may lower blood pressure by decreasing vascular responses to pressor stimuli of various sorts, particularly catecholamines. The extent to which direct vascular effects or interference with pressor responsiveness contribute to the antihypertensive action of diuretics is not clear. What is generally agreed is that the hypovolemia which they induce is an important and predictable component of the antihypertensive mechanism.

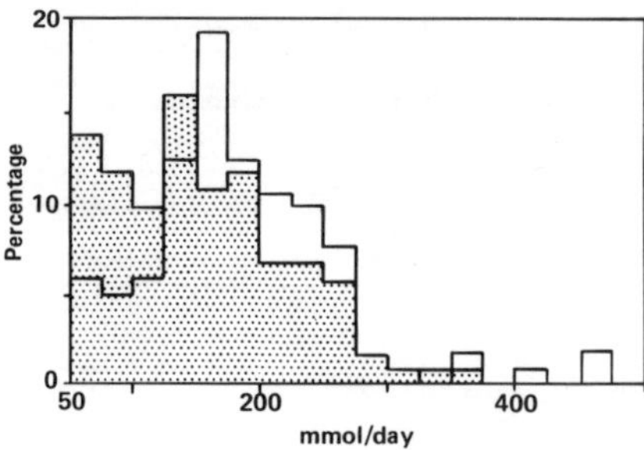

FIGURE 2.   Percentage distribution of urinary Na in 25 mmol/day increments. Solid line is the distribution for all patients before entering the study and is based on 107 urines from 107 patients. Hatched area is distribution of urinary sodium in the patients given dietary advice (based on 109 urines collected from 31 patients). (From Morgan, T. O., Adam, W., Gillies, A., Wilson, M., Morgan, G., and Carney, S., *Lancet,* 1, 227, 1978. With permission.)

The magnitude of the diuretic action and the fall in extracellular fluid volume and plasma volume depends in part on the dose of diuretic given and in part on the dietary sodium intake. The combination of dietary sodium restriction and thiazides produces additive effects on extracellular fluid volume and plasma volume, while as has already been mentioned, increases in dietary sodium intake lead to partial or complete reversal of the effects of diuretics. The fall in extracellular volume stimulates renin secretion which in turn leads to a secondary increase in aldosterone output in the adrenals. With continuing administration of large doses of diuretics, sodium excretion gradually returns to normal, and potassium excretion, promoted by an exchange of potassium for sodium in the distal and collecting tubules under the influence of aldosterone, increases sharply. If diuretic doses are too large, or dietary sodium restriction too severe in combination with these drugs, hypovolemia may proceed to the point where a fall in glomerular filtration rate occurs with consequent rises in blood urea, nitrogen, and creatinine. These changes occur most often with more powerful loop diuretics such as frusemide or ethacrynic acid.

Most classes of diuretics inhibit the tubular secretion of uric acid and may induce hyperuricemia and sometimes gout. Since about 25% of untreated hypertensive patients are reported to have hyperuricemia, additional uric acid retention due to diuretic therapy is a significant clinical problem. Although gout occurs in not more than 10% of patients receiving diuretics, serum uric acid levels may rise as high as 10 mg% in many more. Diuretic therapy commonly produces minor degrees of impaired carbohydrate tolerance. In a prospective study of hypertensives with normal glucose tolerance, however, fewer than 3 developed overt diabetes or marked impaired glucose tolerance over a 1 year period.[13] Nevertheless, in hypertensive patients, glucose tolerance may be occasionally substantially impaired following diuretic therapy.

1. The Benzothiadiazines

These diuretics, which are structurally related to sulfonamides and the carbonic anhydrase inhibitors, are the most commonly used diuretic agents in the treatment of hypertension. Individual drugs vary considerably in their potency and their duration

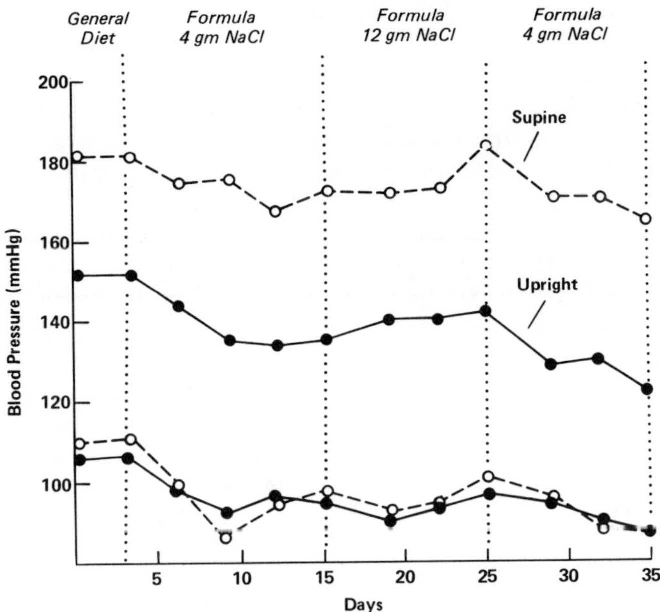

FIGURE 3.   Data from representative patient showing blood pressure responses to varying amounts of sodium chloride in diet. (From Kirkendahl, W. M., and Overturf, M. L., *Systemic Effects of Antihypertensive Agents,* Sambhi, M., Ed., Stratton Intercontinental, New York, 1976, 119. With permission.)

of action. The drugs are rapidly and almost completely absorbed from the GI tract so that oral administration produces satisfactory results.

In mild or borderline hypertension, these diuretics may be the only antihypertensive drug treatment required. In the Australian National Blood Pressure Study, well over half of the patients with borderline hypertension developed falls of blood pressure to below 90 mmHg with doses of chlorothiazide of 500 mg twice daily. In patients in whom there is no urgency about obtaining control over blood pressure, administration of a benzothiadiazine diuretic as the sole antihypertensive treatment should be tried for at least 14 days. If normalization of blood pressure occurs after this period, no additional therapy need be added. After approximately 3 months treatment with these diuretic agents, an estimation of serum potassium should be performed and compared with the pretreament levels. Serum potassium levels above 3.5 mM/l do not commonly require potassium supplements or the use of potassium-sparing diuretics unless the patient is concomitantly taking digitalis. With ordinary doses of benzothiadiazines in ambulant patients on normal dietary sodium intakes, hypokalemia below 3.5 mM/l occurs in less than 10% of patients. Hypokalemia occurs more commonly when maximal doses are used, when dietary sodium restriction is practiced in association with the diuretics, and is also more commonly seen with certain long-acting diuretics, notably chlorthalidone, a drug whose prolonged action seems to favour potassium depletion, particularly in doses of 50 mg daily or more. For routine use, the dose of chlorthalidone should not exceed 25 mg daily, and even this may induce hypokalemia in some patients.[13] The best method of management of hypokalemia induced by diuretics is not generally agreed. Some recommend the use of slow-release potassium tablets routinely as potassium supplements when diuretics are administered to prevent hypokalemia from developing, but others recommend measures to correct hypokalemia only when the serum potassium falls to 3.0 mM/ℓ.[14] Prichard[15] believes that potassium supplements are preferable to the use of potassium-sparing diuretics on the grounds that the latter are more expensive and have a higher incidence of side effects than oral potassium. On the other hand, potassium supplements may cause small bowel ulceration and stenosis[16,17] and are not always effective in overcoming hypokalemia.[18] As will be discussed later, potassium-sparing diuretics are generally well tolerated and effective, and in the author's opinion are preferable to the use of oral supplements of potassium. As has been mentioned above, these diuretics commonly induce hyperuricemia and frank episodes of gout may occur. These drugs, however, are so valuable in the treatment of hypertension that they should not be discontinued because of hyperuricemia or gout, and these manifestations may be treated by the additional use of a uricosuric agent such as probenecid or by the use of allopurinol. Interference with carbohydrate metabolism is rarely a problem of sufficient severity to justify the discontinuation of benzothiadiazine diuretics.[19] The major indication for discontinuing these drugs is the not uncommon development of skin rashes which may be photosensitive in nature. Other less common side effects include thrombocytopenia, nausea, and vomiting. In elderly patients, particularly in hot climates, marked hypovolemia may occur leading to symptoms of postural hypotension. Elderly patients usually require smaller doses of diuretics than younger patients.

2. Loop Diuretics

Ethacrynic acid and frusemide are rapidly acting and extremely powerful diuretics whose principal site of diuretic action is on the ascending limb of the loop of Henle. Both these diuretics have a rapid action of short duration and produce a large and often inconvenient diuresis shortly after the dose. Whether because of their brief action, or perhaps because they have no other action on vascular smooth muscle, the loop diuretics appear to be less effective antihypertensive agents than the benzothiadiazines. Their major disadvantage relates to their extreme potency and brevity of effect. In contrast to the benzothiadiazines, which have a flat dose-response curve, the loop diuretics have a steep dose-response curve so that excessive effects on sodium and water excretion are induced comparatively readily. Their use is best reserved for hypertensive patients with congestive heart failure and edema, in patients with renal hypertension, and the nephrotic syndrome. In some patients with renal disease, they may be used in combination with a high salt intake to increase urinary output. Ethacrynic acid induces a high incidence of GI disturbances, including nausea, dysphagia, vomiting, and diarrhea. It also has the major disadvantage of producing deafness, which may occasionally be permanent. The side effects of frusemide are much less common. Both drugs seem more likely to produce deafness when large doses are given to patients with renal failure.

3. The Potassium-Sparing Diuretics

There are two major types of potassium-sparing diuretics, both of which act on the distal and collecting tubules to prevent potassium exchange for sodium. These are the aldosterone antagonists, such as spironolactone, which are effective only as competitive inhibitors of aldosterone. The other class of potassium-sparing diuretics is represented by amiloride and triamterene, both of which block potassium exchange for sodium in the distal tubule, irrespective of the presence of aldosterone. They are weak diuretics and have their main use in combination with benzothiadiazines to promote sodium excretion and to reduce potassium loss.

As has been mentioned previously, marked hypokalemia is uncommonly encountered with conventional doses of benzothiadiazines, at least in patients with essential hypertension. Patients with primary aldosteronism, secondary aldosteronism secondary to renovascular hypertension or malignant hypertension, or patients who have become severely sodium depleted, may develop severe potassium depletion. In a small proportion of patients, the plasma potassium falls without any of these other conditions being present. Potassium-sparing diuretics may be combined with benzothiadiazines either routinely or to correct a deficiency in plasma potassium. The fixed combination of amiloride and hydrochlorothiazide (Moduretic®) has been widely accepted in the United Kingdom and Europe. The combination has the advantage that falls in plasma and total body potassium are usually prevented, and there is an enhanced antihypertensive and diuretic effect. The combination tablet seems well tolerated by the majority of patients, although occasional patients complain of nausea. Similarly, a fixed combination tablet of hydrochlorothiazide and spironolactone (Aldactazide®) is available and likewise has similar advantages. Spironolactone tends to be less well tolerated than amiloride, since it induces gynecomastia, breast tenderness, irregularities of menstruation, and impotence, particularly with large doses. It also not infrequently causes GI disturbances.

The major disadvantages of the potassium-sparing diuretics lie in the risk of inducing hyperkalemia. This is particularly likely to occur in patients with impaired renal functon, but may also occur if excessively large doses are used. The risks of hyperkalemia are greater with amiloride and triamterene than with spironolactone, since the latter is a competitive inhibitor of aldosterone. All three drugs cause sharp elevations of plasma renin. Whether this has any clinical significance is uncertain.

4. New Diuretic Agents

a. Indanone

This substance, which is 6,7,dichloro-2-methyl-l-oxo-2-phenyl-5-l-indaminoxy acetic acid, is a recently synthesized diuretic which has been claimed to have uricosuric properties.[20] It produces a steeper dose-response curve for sodium and chloride excretion than hydrochlorothiazide, but less steep than that of frusemide. The effect on reducing mean arterial pressure in spontaneous hypertensive rats appeared to be greater for indanone than for hydrochlorothiazide or frusemide at the doses given, and similar results were obtained in the renal hypertensive African green monkey. In the chimpanzee, indanone produced rather larger increases in sodium excretion than did ethacrynic acid or frusemide, very much the same effect on potassium excretion, but a marked increase in uric acid excretion. As far as can be judged, clinical trials using this substance have not been reported. It is clear, however, that a potent diuretic which does not lead to uric acid retention on a long-term basis would be an advance in the therapeutics of hypertension.

b. Indapamide

Indapamide (n-3-sulfamoyl-4-chlorobenzamedo)2 methyl indamine is a weak acid which has been reported to have diuretic properties.[21] It is a molecule made up of two distinct parts: a polar chlorosulfamoylbenzamide and a lipid soluble methyl indoline substituent. The drug appears to be highly lipid soluble, and to concentrate substantially in red cells, and to be strongly protein bound.[22] It is very slowly eliminated, taking up to 4 days before elimination is complete in some human subjects. On a daily dosage of 2.5 mg, mean plasma levels in six subjects reached a stable level within 24

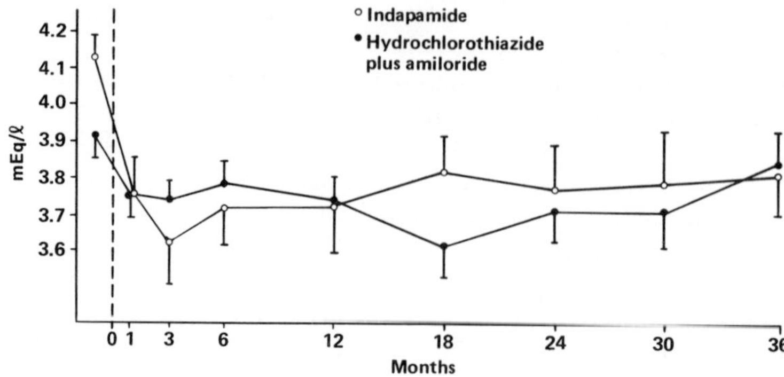

FIGURE 4.   Changes in serum potassium levels in the two groups of patients during 36 months of treatment: mean (±S.E.M.) levels in 24 patients on indapamide (2.5 mg/day) and in 52 patients on hydrochlorothiazide (50 mg/day) plus amiloride (5 mg/day). (From Demanet, J. C., Degante, J. P., and Hubert, C., *Curr. Med. Res. Opin.,* 5(Suppl. 1), 129, 1977. With permission.)

to 48 hr and remained stable thereafter until the dose was discontinued. Plasma concentrations then fell to zero within 48 hr. Both the saluretic effect and the antihypertensive effect is prolonged. Following administration of this material, it is claimed that in addition to its saluretic effect, indapamide has a specific effect on vascular reactivity in experimental hypertension.[23]

Human studies demonstrate that in doses of 2.5 mg, there is a distinct saluretic effect which increases progressively up to doses of 10 mg by mouth, at which dose level there is a very substantial increase in excretion of water, sodium, and chloride.[24]

Clinical studies using this drug have demonstrated conclusively that it is a potent antihypertensive agent, often producing falls of blood pressure which are substantially in excess of those induced by other diuretics. It appears not to induce potassium depletion in long-term studies.[25] In contrast to the benzothiadiazines, it usually induces a fall rather than an increase in pulse rate, and the antihypertensive action of the drug has been reported to persist for up to 10 days following its cessation. The relationship between the magnitude of the diuretic response and the antihypertensive response has not been fully elucidated. Most studies have used doses of 2.5 mg daily, at which dose level, the saluretic effect, although definite, is quite small, yet at this dose level quite marked antihypertensive changes can be demonstrated. It appears possible that this drug may have a dissociation between its diuretic effects and possible effects on vascular responsiveness to sympathetic or other pressor agents. Its current pace in the therapeutics of hypertension is still not fully evaluated, but it appears promising.

c. Bumetanide

Bumetanide was introduced in about 1971, and some clinical studies have been reported.[26] It differs from most other diuretics in not having a chlorine atom ortho to the sulfamoyl group on the aromatic ring. This is of interest, since previously a halogen in this region had been considered necessary for saluretic activity. Bumetanide is a powerful diuretic agent with a predominant action on the ascending limb of the loop of Henle and thus resembles frusemide and ethacrynic acid in its site of action. On a molar basis, it is some 4 times as active as frusemide.[27] It has a rapid onset and a short duration of action. Although it induces some falls of blood pressure, its main clinical usage appears to be for the treatment of edema either of cardiac or of other origin and in pulmonary edema. It is stated that because it is chemically different from existing diuretics, it may be helpful in edema resistant to other drugs like frusemide and

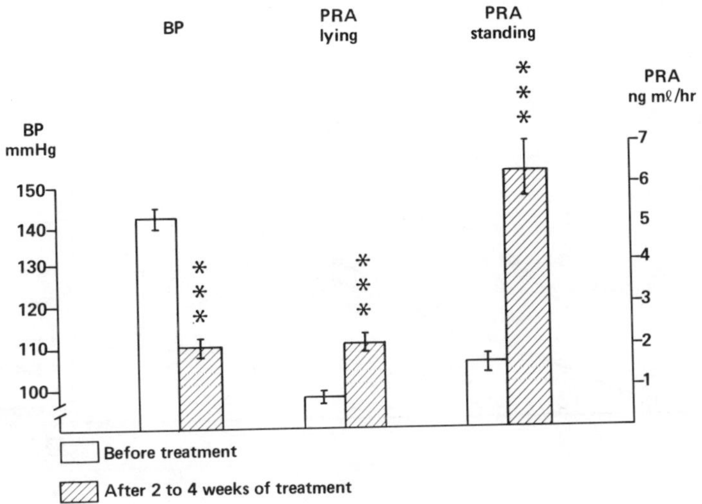

FIGURE 5. Effects of combined antihypertensive therapy including chlorthalidone 100 mg daily on plasma renin activity and blood pressure. (From
Zanchetti, A., Leonetti, G., Morganti, A., Terzoli, L., Schwarz, E., Manfrin, H., and Bernasconi, M., *Systemic Effects of Antihypertensive Agents,*
Sambhi, M., Ed., Stratton Intercontinental, New York, 1976, 251. With permission.)

ethacrynic aid. It induces hyperuricemia and quite marked hypokalemia. It suffers
from the same disadvantages as the other loop diuretics in the treatment of hypertension and is best reserved for patients who are edematous.

III. SELECTION OF PATIENTS FOR DIURETIC THERAPY

In the author's opinion, the use of a diuretic drug is the initial treatment of choice
for all patients with hypertension requiring antihypertensive drug treatment, irrespective of the age of the patient, the severity of the illness, or the presence or absence of
raised or low renin levels in the plasma. As has been previously mentioned, elderly
patients are frequently more sensitive to sodium depletion than younger patients, and
symptoms of postural hypotension may occur due presumably to hypovolemia, so that
smaller doses may need to be used in older patients.

In patients with mild or borderline hypertension, the response to diuretic therapy
alone should be assessed before other drugs are added. In patients with severe hypertension, diuretics and other drugs may be prescribed simultaneously.

The question of the levels of plasma renin in relation to the use of diuretics has been
a matter of some controversy. It was initially claimed that patients with low or suppressed levels of plasma renin responded uniquely well to spironolactone[28] and that
normalization of blood pressure could be achieved in the majority of patients with
aldosterone antagonists alone. There now seems little doubt that a satisfactory response is not confined to spironolactone, but that other diuretic drugs also produce
equally effective falls of blood pressure in patients with low plasma renin levels.[29] In
the author's opinion, there is no very strong evidence to suggest that patients with low
or suppressed plasma renin levels respond better to diuretics than the great majority
of other hypertensive patients, but the evidence for this is not entirely clear one way
or the other.

Given acutely, most diuretics lead to a sharp rise in plasma renin levels (Figure 5),

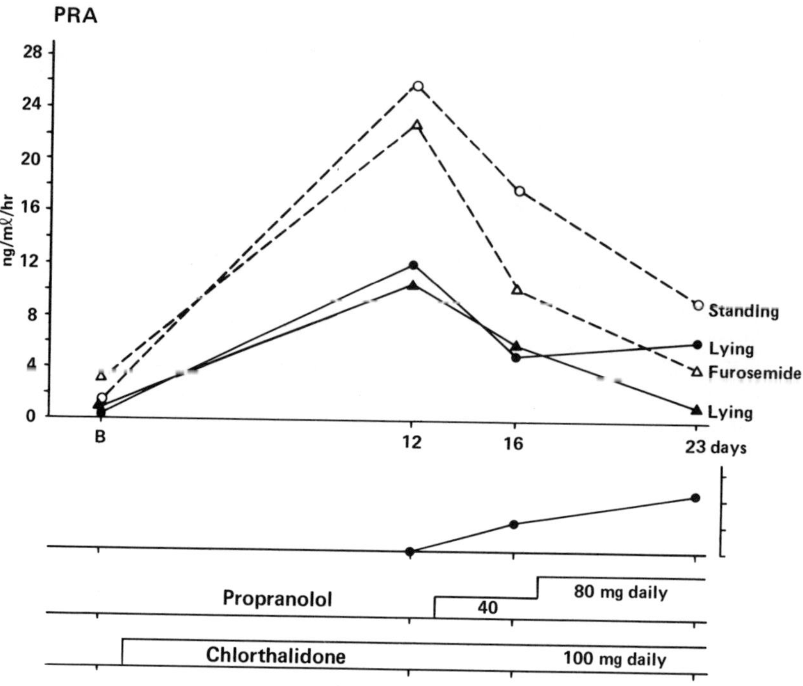

FIGURE 6.   Plasma renin activity in the lying and standing positions and after an i.v. injection of 40 mg furosemide in a hypertensive patient receiving chlorthalidone first and then chlorthalidone plus propranolol. (From Zanchetti, A., Leonetti, G., Morganti, A., Terzoli, L., Schwarz, E., Manfrin, H., and Bernasconi, M., *Systemic Effects of Antihypertensive Agents,* Sambhi, M. Ed., Stratton Intercontinental, New York, 1976, 251. With permission.)

and because it has been suggested that higher levels of plasma renin may be a contributing factor to vascular damage in hypertension,[30,31] the suggestion has been made that diuretic drugs are better avoided in patients with high levels of plasma renin. The balance of evidence also suggests that the renin-stimulating action of diuretic agents continues after several months of treatment, and there is a decrease in plasma renin when the diuretic is stopped[32] (Figure 6).

In spite of the fact that diuretic therapy often raises levels of plasma renin and in spite of the suggestion that high levels may be vasculotoxic, the balance of opinion favors the administration of diuretics, irrespective of whether plasma renin levels are raised or not. This is a pragmatic view since experience has demonstrated that diuretics reduce blood pressure as effectively in patients with high levels of plasma renin as do other drugs and in part reflects the fact that other antihypertensive drugs, whether β-blocking agents or not, tend to lower levels of plasma renin when these have been elevated by diuretics.[32] It is the author's opinion that estimation of plasma renin offers no useful guide as to whether diuretic therapy should be used in the treatment of hypertension.

IV. CHOICE OF DIURETIC

Almost all reports agree that the benzothiadiazine drugs are the most appropriate for the initiation and maintenance of antihypertensive treatment with diuretics. A choice of individual drug is a matter of personal preference, and perhaps the most important consideration is that relating to duration of action. Drugs with a very long duration of action, such as chlorthalidone, seem more likely to induce significant hypokalemia than drugs with a shorter period of action, such as hydrochlorothiazide.[13] On the other hand, drugs with a long duration of action have the advantage that once-daily dosage in always effective, and providing the dose can be reduced to levels which do not induce hypokalemia, longer acting diuretics such as cyclopenthiazide or chlorthalidone may have a marginal advantage over the shorter acting ones.

The combination of potassium-sparing diuretics and benzothiadiazines has proved very effective in practice. The combination of amiloride and hydrochlorothiazide produces a slightly larger diuretic effect than does hydrochlorothiazide alone, and significant hypokalemia during treatment is extremely uncommon. In the author's opinion, this combination diuretic therapy is the best available at present for the initiation of treatment.

The major causes for anxiety in the use of diuretics are the occurrence of rashes and hypersensitivity reactions, which are uncommon. When these occur with an individual benzothiadiazine, they tend to occur also with other members of this group and also with frusemide, and under these circumstances, ethacrynic acid may have to be substituted for the benzothiadiazines. This is as a rule less well tolerated and less effective than the first line diuretics. Hyperuricemia is the second major problem, and there seems to be no particular advantage between one diuretic drug and another in that all when given in effective doses seem to induce hyperuricemia. In patients with hypertensive heart failure or edema from other causes, the benzothiadiazine diuretics may be combined with a shorter acting loop diuretic such as frusemide or bumetamide.

V. β-ADRENOCEPTOR-BLOCKING DRUGS

The report by Prichard and Gillam[33] that propranolol induced useful falls of blood pressure in many hypertensive patients has now been amply confirmed by numerous reports that propranolol and other β-adrenoceptor-blocking agents are effective antihypertensive drugs.[34] Studies have now indicated that in addition to propranolol, pindolol, oxprenolol, metroprolol, atenolol, alprenolol, timolol, sotalol, and numerous other drugs have potent antihypertensive actions. As has been discussed in a previous section, the mode of action of the β-adrenoceptor-blocking drugs in producing an antih-ypertensive effect is not elucidated fully, although the balance of evidence suggests that the most likely cause is a fall in cardiac output, probably combined with an effect on central or peripheral adrenergic control mechanisms. Cardioselectivity, intrinsic sympathomimetic activity, and the presence or absence of membrane-stabilizing effect seem to make little difference in clinical practice to the use of these agents (Figure 7).

Not all hypertensive patients respond to β-adrenoreceptor-blocking drugs. In 30 to 40% of hypertensive patients, control of blood pressure may be dramatically achieved with β-adrenoceptor-blocking drugs alone, with normalization of blood pressure levels, an absence of postural hypotension, and a minimum of side effects. In an additional 30% of patients, β-adrenoceptor-blocking agents, often in large doses, induce useful falls in blood pressure, but other drugs are needed in combination to achieve normalization of blood pressure. A smaller group of patients, probably between 20 to 30%, experience little fall in blood pressure, even when given large doses of these drugs. In the author's opinion, there is no practical method at present available for determining in advance which patients will respond and which will not. Levels of plasma renin, severity of hypertension, age of the patient, and other clinical features, such as a hyperdynamic circulatory state, do not help to distinguish between patients who will respond and those who will not.[35] For this reason, the question as to whether to use this class of drug or not in the treatment of hypertension is one which needs to be based

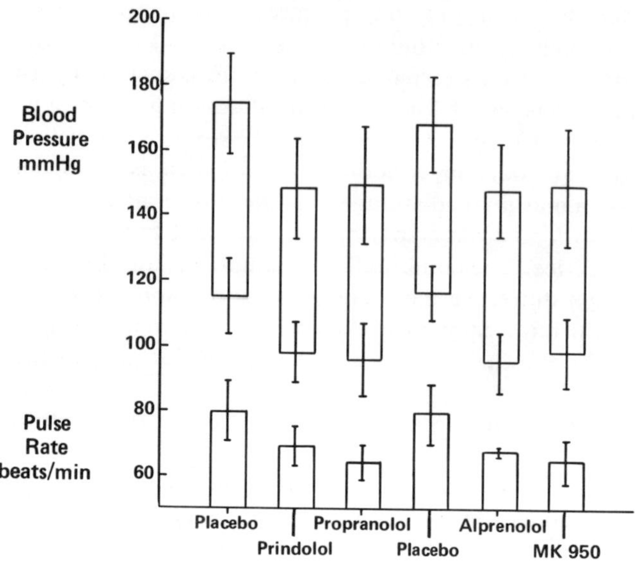

FIGURE 7.   Pulse rate and systolic and diastolic blood pressure (±S.E.M.) in patients during various treatment phases of the double-blind cross-over study which compared the antihypertensive action of MK-950, alprenolol, and pindolol. (From Louis, W. I., Morgan, T. O., Anavekar, S. N., and Doyle, A. E., *Beta-Adrenergic Blocking Agents in the Management of Hypertension and Angina Pectoris,* Magnani, B., Ed., Raven Press, New York, 1974, 25. With permission.)

on practical grounds rather than theoretical considerations. The major advantages of β-adrenoceptor-blocking drugs in clinical practice are, first, that they induce few side effects as a rule and so are well tolerated. Second, they induce falls in blood pressure which are as large in the supine position as in the erect position, and third, that once effective, they appear to remain so, and tolerance is uncommon. The major disadvantages are, first, that they are not effective in all patients and second, that in all patients they induce falls of cardiac output, diminution in myocardial contractility, and pulse rate. These factors determine the indications for this type of drug, and the decision to use them or not needs to be made on the basis of the severity of the hypertension, presence or absence of cardiac involvement, sex of the patient, and age of the patient.

It has already been indicated that the initial treatment of choice for all types of hypertensive patient is a benzothiadiazine diuretic. When these fail to normalize blood pressure, a situation which will obtain in at least 50 to 60% of patients, a β-adrenoceptor-blocking drug is the drug of choice to be added to the regime in the following patients:

1.   Mild or borderline hypertensive patients
2.   Young, sexually active men
3.   Patients with moderate to severe hypertension without evidence of cardiac enlargement or symptoms suggesting incipient heart failure, such as dyspnea on exertion or episodes of paroxysmal nocturnal dyspnea
4.   Patients whose blood pressure remains uncontrolled despite previous attempts to control it with other drugs.
5.   Hypertensive patients with severe angina pectoris

These indications are based on the fact that while manifestations of cardiac decompensation are not common in hypertensive patients following the administratton of these drugs, they occur mostly in patients who have preexisting evidence of cardiac enlargement who fail to respond to the drugs by a fall in blood pressure. They also take account of the lack of other side effects usually induced.

The use of a β-adrenoceptor-blocking drug is best avoided in the following types of patients:

(1) patients with cardiac enlargement or heart failure

(2) patients with a past history of bronchial asthma or with evidence of severe chronic obstructive airway disease

For patients in these categories, drugs not likely to induce a reduction in myocardial contractility or constriction of bronchial smooth muscle should be used in the first instance, in combination with diuretic therapy.

A. Choice of β-Blocking Drug

As has been mentioned in a preceding section, neither cardioselectivity, intrinsic sympathomimetic activity, or membrane-stabilizing effect appear significantly to affect the antihypertensive action of this class of drug. Furthermore, as has been shown in controlled studies, patients who respond to one drug appear to respond equally well to others.[36]

There are marginal differences between drugs in terms of the incidence of side effects and major differences between drugs in terms of pharmacokinetics.

In regard to the incidence of side effects, no clear pattern emerges which conveys any particular advantage to any individual drug.[36] Occasionally, individual patients complain about a side effect such as dreaming or Raynaud's phenomenon with one drug and subsequently state that a change to another drug has improved the symptom, but this is too irregular and not systematic enough to be helpful in choosing between drugs. It is possible that drugs with either intrinsic sympathomimetic activity or cardioselectivity may be somewhat less likely to induce bronchial asthma in susceptible individuals. However, the advantage is marginal and β-adrenoceptor-blocking drugs of all types are best avoided in asthmatic or emphysematous patients. However, in such patients, if control of blood pressure cannot be achieved with other drugs, a cautious trial of either atenolol or metoprolol, or pindolol, may be instituted. A major problem of the use of any of these agents in asthmatic patients is not merely the precipitation of acute asthma, but its failure to respond to β-agonists such as salbutamol if an attack occurs. It is claimed that this is less of a problem with cardioselective agents

Pharmacokinetic considerations are highly relevant to the choice of drug. Drugs such as propranolol and alprenolol, which undergo extensive biotransformation in the liver, induce less predictable responses than drugs such as pindolol or timolol, which are not degraded by the liver. In practice, this means that the time taken to achieve adequate blood levels is both longer and more variable using propranolol or similar drugs than using pindolol or timolol. The effective dose of propranolol in hypertensive patients may be as low as 120 mg daily or as high as 2 to 3 g/day. Since the initial dose levels need to be low, and since stable plasma levels may require 3 to 7 days to achieve, adjustment of the dose of propranolol may take several weeks. By contrast pindolol induces an antihypertensive response within a few hours[37] (Figure 8), and since the effective dose ranges from 15 to 45 mg daily, the extent of the antihypertensive response is usually clear within a few days of initial treatment. Not all patients

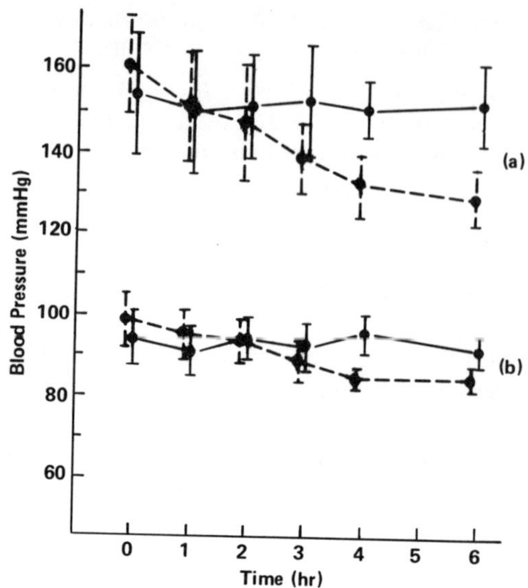

FIGURE 8.   Effects of oral administration of 20
mg of pindolol (broken lines) and placebo (continuous lines) on (a) systolic and (b) diastolic blood pressure in six patients in a double-blind cross-over
study. The points are means with the standard errors
indicated by the vertical lines. (From Anavekar, S.
N., Louis, W. J., Morgan, T. O., Doyle, A. E., and
Johnston, C. I., *Clin. Exp. Pharmacol. Physiol.*, 2,
203, 1975. With permission.)

respond to β-adrenoceptor-blocking drugs, but those who do appear to respond equally
well to all. There are considerable advantages in being able to reach a rapid decision
as to whether an individual patient will respond or not. For this reason, rapidly acting
drugs like pindolol, timolol, or atenolol are considerably easier to use than propranolol
or alprenolol, particularly in the more severely hypertensive patient.

B. Summary of Effects of β-Blocking Drugs in Hypertension

The clinical use of β-adrenoceptor-blocking drugs in hypertension has proved remarkably successful in view of the fact that from the knowledge of their pharmacological properties, it was not expected that they would have antihypertensive properties.
In spite of the fact that some drugs exhibit less bioavailability than others, differences
between β-blocking agents are comparatively marginal. In approximately 30 to 40%
of patients with hypertension, these drugs work extremely effectively and are capable
of normalizing blood pressure levels with no postural component. Drugs whose bioavailability is low, such as propranolol and alprenolol, may need to be used in very
large doses in some patients, but are effective in quite small doses in others. From a
theoretical point of view, any of these drugs might be expected to produce cardiac
decompensation. Clinical experience in general has shown that they do not often do
so, particularly when there is effective control of blood pressure. Unwanted effects of
the drugs relate mainly to their β-adrenoceptor-blocking properties. Apart from cardiac decompensatton, they induce marked peripheral vasoconstriction in some patients, leading to Raynaud's phenomenon, and they may precipitate asthma, presumably by interfering with the action of the autonomic nervous system on bronchial
smooth muscle. Metabolic effects of β-adrenoceptor blockade are usually inconspi-

cuous from a clinical point of view, although they may prevent mobilization of blood glucose and so may prolong hypoglycemia in patients being treated with insulin. Central nervous system side effects are moderately conspicuous. These vary in frequency from drug to drug and presumably relate to the facility with which the drug enters the nervous system. Propranolol and pindolol produce a high incidence of bizarre dreams and there have been reports of depression and suicide[34,36,38] in patients taking propranolol. Whether this latter effect is directly attributable to the drug is by no means certain. The drugs have some conspicuous advantages over other types of antihypertensive drugs in that they do not produce postural hypotension, do not usually interfere with male sexual function, do not as a rule promote fluid retention, and do not induce tolerance.

As has been previously discussed, the precise modes of action of these drugs in producing their antihypertensive action is not resolved. Actions on cardiac output, the peripheral autonomic nervous system, central autonomic nervous system, and renin-angiotensin system may all play a part in different patients in different proportions.

A major but as yet unresolved question is whether for equally effective control of blood pressure, β-adrenoceptor antagonists exert an additional preventive component in the incidence of either sudden death or myocardial infarction. A number of major studies are in progress to evaluate the earlier claims that this is the case. Clearly, if this proves to be so, these drugs, either alone or in combination with benzothiadiazine diuretics, will become firmly established as the treatment of choice, particularly as the treatment of most hypertensive patients is given in the hope of delaying or reducing the incidence of hypertensive vascular disease. Even apart from this possible property, β-adrenoceptor-blocking drugs have substantial advantages over most other classes of antihypertensive drugs in control of recumbent blood pressure and comparative freedom from side effects. At this time, they appear to the author to be the best agents for use, in combination with diuretic therapy.

VI. α-METHYLDOPA

Since its introduction in 1960, α-methyldopa has become probably the most widely used of all antihypertensive drugs. The antihypertensive effect of methyldopa develops rapidly, and a fall in blood pressure can usually be demonstrated after an initial dose within 2 to 4 hr. The sensitivity of individual patients to α-methyldopa varies very considerably. In some patients, as little as 125 mg twice daily in combination with a thiazide diuretic maintains the blood pressure at normal levels, whereas in others, doses up to 6 g daily may be needed. The reasons for these differences in sensitivity are not apparent, but do not seem to relate to pharmacokinetic differences. The drug induces falls of blood pressure both in the recumbent and the erect posture, there usually being some additional fall of blood pressure when the patient stands up.

Most patients who have not experienced normalization of blood pressure levels on diuretics respond by a further fall in blood pressure if methyldopa is added. The initial dose is 250 to 500 mg twice daily, and this may be increased progressively to a total of 4 to 6 g daily. Between 50 to 60% of patients obtain satisfactory control of blood pressure levels with a combination of diuretic and methyldopa in doses of less than 2 g daily. Increasing the dose increases the yield of patients who can be satisfactorily controlled by a further 10 to 15%. There are no particular indices which suggest whether a patient is likely to respond well to methyldopa or not. In general, it is true that most milder patients are more easily treated and respond more readily, but many patients with severe or malignant hypertension also respond readily to small doses of methyldopa, while a few patients with borderline hypertension respond very poorly.

If given without diuretic drugs, methyldopa usually leads to fluid retention which leads to a diminution in the antihypertensive effect. For this reason, the drug is always best combined with a thiazide diuretic. Methyldopa is usually well tolerated. Many patients complain of mild drowsiness, but this is not usually severe. Rarely, a hypersensitivity reaction occurs to methyldopa with a development of a high fever usually within a day or two of commencing the drug treatment.[39] In these patients, later readministration of the drug again induces fever rapidly. Rarely also, methyldopa may induce jaundice,[40] often accompanied by high fever. The precise nature of the liver toxicity is uncertain. Hepatic biopsy usually shows no gross abnormality, and the jaundice usually subsides with the withdrawal of methyldopa, but the syndrome is likely to occur again if the patient is rechallenged with the drug. A positive reaction for antinuclear factor has been reported in a substantial proportion of patients taking methyldopa.[41]

In 1966 to 1967, several reports appeared on the association of positive reactions to the direct Coomb's test in patients being treated with methyldopa, with a small incidence of hemolytic anemia.[41-44] Carstairs et al.[42] reported a positive Coomb's test in 40% of patients taking more than 2 g daily, while Louis et al.[43] found an incidence of 25% in patients taking more than 750 mg daily. Carstairs et al. suggested that a positive Coomb's test usually appeared in the first year of drug treatment.

Few patients who develop a positive Coomb's test develop hemolytic anemia.[44] Carstairs et al.[42] estimated the incidence at only 0.5% of those with a positive Coomb's test.

The mechanism of this complication appears to be a so-called auto-immune process.[44] Antibodies develop which are directed towards antigens on the surface of red cells. It is possible that the antinuclear reaction, hepatotoxicity, and febrile reactions may be other facets of the same process.

Although the frequency of the positive Coomb's reaction is disturbing, hemolytic anemia is sufficiently uncommon, and methyldopa so useful as an antihypertensive agent as to make the small risk acceptable. Hemoglobin levels should be monitored occasionally in patients who develop a positive Coomb's reaction.

Probably the major clinical problem encountered with the use of methyldopa is disturbance of sexual function in the male. Failure of ejaculation and on occasions impotence occur frequently and are common causes of failure of compliance in young sexually active men.

In the author's opinion, until the introduction of β-adrenoceptor-blocking drugs, the drug methyldopa was undoubtedly the drug of choice in combination with a thiazide diuretic. Since β-blocking drugs have been developed, the major choice to be made is between a β-adrenoceptor-blocking drug and α-methyldopa. For patients with severe hypertension, methyldopa probably remains the drug of choice because of its rapid onset of antihypertensive action, ease of use, and lack of effect on myocardial contractility. It is also more predictable in its action than β-adrenoceptor-blocking drugs. In patients with severe hypertension who fail to respond to methyldopa or in patients in whom side effects are severe, β-adrenoceptor-blocking drugs provide a very satisfactory alternative.

VII. CLONIDINE

Clonidine was introduced as an antihypertensive drug in 1966. As has been discussed earlier, there is good evidence that the main antihypertensive effect of clonidine is due to its stimulation of α-adrenoceptors in the medullary inhibitory centers in the brain. Clonidine is active in extremely small doses. After oral administration, the blood pressure begins to fall within 1 to 1½ hr, and the fall of blood pressure is equally large in both the recumbent and the erect positions. The drugs may be administered twice or three times daily, but most patients can maintain a satisfactory control of blood pressure with twice daily administration.

Clonidine is an extremely effective antihypertensive agent in the majority of patients, and probably between 60 to 70% of patients can achieve satisfactory control of blood pressure with clonidine and a diuretic. Tolerance to the drug does not usually occur, at least when it is given with a diuretic, but the main limitation to its clinical use is the high incidence of side effects which are induced. Its major disadvantage is that it induces marked sedation with dryness of the mouth and constipation in most patients. These side effects are dose dependent. Doses of 150 μg twice daily are usually well tolerated without significant side effects, but these doses are effective in normalizing the blood pressure in only a small minority of patients. Increases of dose above 600 μg daily almost always lead to sedation, dry mouth, and constipation. The sedation may be profound and cause patients taking the drug to fall asleep at inappropriate times, such as when driving motor vehicles. Dryness of the mouth appears to be due to a central inhibition of salivary flow and is often very severe. Because of the high incidence of side effects, clonidine is a less satisfactory drug of first choice after the diuretics than either the β-adrenoceptor-blocking drugs or methyldopa in the majority of patients. Its major use is probably as an additive drug in small doses to patients in whom normalization of blood pressure has not been achieved with the previously mentioned drugs. It may then be added in doses of 150 μg twice a day, often with a satisfactory response. Alternatively, advantage may be taken of its sedative properties by prescribing a moderately large dose (300 to 600 μg) at night. This usually leads to some continuation of the antihypertensive effect during the following day, which may add to the actions of drugs such as methyldopa or adrenoceptor-blocking drugs which are given in the morning. A major disadvantage of clonidine is the rebound of blood pressure which has been reported when the drug is discontinued.[45] This phenomenon consists of an exaggerated rise of blood pressure together with tachycardia, palpitations, sweating, and anxiety, associated with an elevation of plasma and urinary catecholamines, which develop usually within 4 to 24 hr of the cessation of the drug. Although this syndrome does not occur frequently, it is nevertheless alarming, both to patient and physician, and is particularly relevant in patients who are suspected of being irregular in their self-administration of drugs.

VIII. LABETALOL

Although labetalol is a β-adrenoceptor-blocking drug, it also possesses α-adrenoceptor-blocking properties. This combination of properties in a single compound appears to be unique, and the therapeutic effects of labetalol are sufficiently different from those of the β-adrenoceptor-blocking drugs to justify it being considered separately.

The therapeutic effects of labetalol differ in several respects from those of the β-adrenoceptor-blocking drugs. It induces less slowing of heart rate than other β-blocking agents and usually induces a rather larger fall of blood pressure in the erect rather than in the supine position. It appears to be effective in a considerable number of patients who respond inadequately to conventional β-adrenoceptor antagonists, and the proportion of patients responding has been considered to be as high as 80%.[46] It appears to be approximately as effective as the combined use of a conventional β-adrenoceptor antagonist and prazosin. It is not at present clear whether the α-receptor-blocking action is on presynaptic receptors as well as the postsynaptic ones, but it has been claimed that the presynaptic receptors are not blocked.[47]

Labetalol is usually well tolerated. Occasionally, patients complain of nausea, but these seem to be a minority, with only 3 of 30 patients complaining of persisting nausea.[48] On the other hand, the incidence of Raynaud's phenomenon is substantially

TABLE 4

The Effects of Labetalol Treatment on Blood Pressure in Previously Treated
Patients

		Previous treatment	Labetalol + diuretic
Lying BP[a]	Systolic	174	159
	Diastolic	109	99
	Pulse	72	74
Standing BP	Systolic	157	140
	Diastolic	105	93
	Pulse	76	81
Exercise BP	Systolic	146	129
	Diastolic	95	82
	Pulse	84	93

[a] Blood pressure.

reduced with labetalol as compared with conventional β-adrenoceptor antagonists, as
is the incidence of sleep disturbances and dreams. A few patients suffer from postural
faintness, but with a few exceptions, this symptom is a minor one. However, examples
of sudden collapse following the first dose have been reported in a small number of
patients.

Louis et al.[48] have reported on the long-term use of this drug in a group of 30 patients with severe hypertension whose diastolic pressures had been originally 115
mmHg or higher. It was found that 23 of these 30 patients had been previously indifferently controlled with other drugs. Of these, 20 were taking either propranolol or
pindolol, 14 were taking methyldopa in a mean dose of 1350 μg daily, 14 were taking
clonidine in a mean dose of 400 μg daily, 12 were taking hydrallazine, and 6 were
taking adrenergic neuron-blocking drugs. The mean consumption of tablets before
beginning labetalol was 12 tablets per patient per day. Ten patients took three different
drugs and fourteen patients four or more. Labetalol was given in combination with a
thiazide diuretic, and adequate control was achieved in 19 of the 21 patients who had
completed 4 weeks treatment without the use of other drugs. The mean dose of labe-
latol used was 1150 μg daily in divided doses. Control of blood pressure was greatly
improved (Table 4).

It seems clear that labetalol appears to have considerable advantages over most other
drugs in the management of the difficult hypertensive patient and in combination with
diuretics, offers a reasonably easy method of control for many patients.

IX. ADRENERGIC BLOCKING DRUGS

This group of drugs include guanethidine, bethanidine, and debrisoquine. These
drugs act by inhibition of the function of postganglionic sympathetic neurons. They
are actively transported into the norepinephrine-containing granules, displacing some
norepinephrine, and acting to produce marked impairment of sympathetic function.
Because these drugs do not readily enter the brain, their action is predominantly peripheral, and by their action on the postganglionic sympathetic neurons they produce
substantial hypotension, with greatly exaggerated falls of blood pressure in the standing position. They usually induce a fall in cardiac output and heart rate, and a further
fall in blood pressure may occur during exercise.

Guanethidine has a very much longer duration of action than bethanidine or debrisoquine. The antihypertensive effects of guanethidine may last for some days after the

drug has been administered for some time, whereas the effects of bethanidine and debrisoquine decline much more rapidly.

They are now used much less frequently than previously, and are usually reserved for patients in whom control of blood pressure has not been achieved with a combination of thiazide diuretic and a β-adrenoceptor-blocking drug, methyldopa, labetalol, or clonidine, or prazosin either alone or in combination. In such patients, adrenergic blocking agents may be added to produce further falls in blood pressure. When used in this way, large doses are not usually needed, so that side effects are correspondingly reduced. The antihypertensive effect of these drugs usually appears within 4 to 6 hr, postural falls of blood pressure are common, and symptoms of postural faintness may occur. Most of the side effects of these drugs relate to their action in blocking sympathetic neuron function. Diarrhea is a common symptom, particularly with guanethidine. Interference with male sexual function is often severe and is manifested particularly as failure of ejaculation, although impotence may also occur. These drugs interact with the tricyclic antidepressants which block the uptake of guanethidine and can prevent or reverse the action of the drug. The adrenergic blocking drugs also potentiate the action of circulating norepinephrine and should not be used in patients with pheochromocytoma. Most patients require an initial dose of 5 mg of guanethidine twice daily, and adjustments to the size of the dose can be made in progressive increments at 2- or 3-day intervals. Few patients require more than 50 mg daily when used in combination with other drugs.

X. GANGLION-BLOCKING DRUGS

Ganglion-blocking drugs were the first type of drug found to be effective in the treatment of hypertension. Because they induce blockade of both sympathetic and parasympathetic ganglia, they induce marked postural hypertension as well as numerous side effects related to parasympathetic ganglion blockade such as constipation, failure of visual accommodation, retention of urine, and impotence. Because of these side effects, ganglion-blocking drugs are seldom used now. In occasional patients who appear to be resistant to most other forms of antihypertensive therapy, these drugs may still be occasionally useful. The ganglion-blocking drug of choice is mecamylamine, which is better absorbed from the GI tract than the quaternary ammonium salts such as hexamethonium. Mecamylamine is best used in combination with other drugs. The initial dose recommended is 2.5 mg twice daily, and the dose can be increased gradually until control of blood pressure is achieved or until the development of side effects limit the use of the drug further.

XI. PRAZOSIN

Prazosin, initially synthesized as a phosphodiesterase inhibitor,[49] with the idea that it might be a vasodilator drug, has more recently been shown to have a selective action in blocking postjunctional α-receptors, with no blockade of the prejunctional receptor.[50] It is a potent antihypertensive agent which has been used as a sole antihypertensive agent in some patients with hypertension. Although it has been claimed that it produces little orthostatic hypertension, there have been numerous reports of collapse following the administration of prazosin, usually with the preliminary doses, and for this reason, initial dose levels need to be low. The usual recommended dose is 0.5 mg three times daily, and the average daily dose is between 6 to 12 mg per day in divided doses, but these doses are usually used in combination with a β-adrenoceptor blocking drug and a thiazide diuretic.

In an open study in 104 patients, Hua et al.[51] reported that prazosin was an effective hypotensive agent which permitted control of the blood pressure in most patients. These authors report that although prazosin was very effective when used on its own even in the control of severe hypertension, its major role in the control of severe hypertension was in combination with a β-adrenoceptor-blocking drug and a thiazide diuretic. These authors further felt that one of the major benefits achieved by combination of a β-adrenoceptor-blocking drug and prazosin was the absence of postural effects and that both agents tended to counteract the side effects of one another. The same authors, however, noted that postural or orthostatic hypotension has been observed in some cases and had noticed other side effects such as drowsiness, tiredness, weakness, nausea, diarrhea, fluid retention, palpitations, and nervousness. Hayes and colleagues[52] attained satisfactory control of blood pressure in 38 out of 50 patients, most of whom had severe hypertension and in most of whom prazosin was given as combined therapy with β-adrenoceptor-blocking agents and diuretics. These authors noted that plasma renin activity fell in the nine patents receiving prazosin alone. These authors also noted that hypertensive cardiac disease and renal impairment did not prevent a satisfactory response. These authors also noted symptoms suggestive of orthostatic hypotension, but concluded that prazosin was a safe and effective antihypertensive agent in the treatment of patients with severe hypertension.

As has been previously mentioned, reports of sudden collapse, presumably due to orthostatic hypotension, have been reported in as many as 1% of patients taking the drug for the first time.[53,54] The balance of evidence suggests that prazosin is best reserved as an additive therapy in patients in whom adequate control of blood pressure has not been achieved with a combination of a diuretic and a β-adrenoceptor-blocking drug.[55] Initial dosage should be small, but it is suggested that the dose may be increased in some patients up to a total of 20 mg a day or more, usually given in divided doses.[55] It appears to be the most effective peripherally acting drug currently available, with the possible exception of minoxidil, but it appears to be somewhat safer than the latter drug. The balance of evidence would sugget that if peripherally acting drug therapy is required, prazosin is preferable either to hydralazine or to minoxidil as additive therapy. It is also likely to displace the adrenergic neuron-blocking agents as the drug of choice after the β-adrenoceptor-blocking drugs, methyldopa and clonidine.

XII. VASODILATOR DRUGS

These drugs act directly on vascular smooth muscle to produce relaxation and dilatation of the small arteries and arterioles. Some also have an action on venous smooth muscle, but some appear not to have this action. Almost all vasodilators produce a fall in blood pressure, which is opposed by the intact baroreceptor mechanisms. In response to the fall in arterial pressure induced by vasodilatation, there is usually an increase in heart rate and cardiac output, which tends to oppose the reduction of blood pressure. There also is usually marked sodium retention with activation of the renin-angiotensin system. Headache presumably due to vasodilatation of the intercranial vessels is also common. Because of these secondary baroreceptor responses, the vasodilator drugs have had a limited place in the treatment of hypertension until the introduction of the β-adrenoceptor-blocking drugs. These latter drugs, however, prevent the occurrence of secondary compensatory mechanisms such as an increase in cardiac output, tachycardia, and sodium retention, so that vasodilator drugs, used in combination with β-adrenoceptor-blocking drugs, have recently regained popularity. Individual drugs are described separately.

A. Hydralazine

Hydralazine is usually used in doses of between 25 mg a day up to a maximum of

200 mg a day in divided doses. It is rapidly absorbed orally, and its antihypertensive effect is usually observed within 1 to 2 hr. It has a half-life in plasma of between 3 and 4 hr. Hydralazine is biotransformed by conjugation with glucuronic acid in the liver and by N-acetylation. Those patients who acetylate drugs slowly have higher serum concentrations of hydralazine than those with more rapid acetylation, and this accounts for variability of doses between patients.[56] The addition of hydralazine to a regime containing a β-receptor-blocking drug usually avoids the high incidence of breathlessness and tachycardia which are observed when β-blocking drugs are not used. Nausea and vomiting are experienced by many patients, and headache is a common symptom.

A major disadvantage of prolonged administration with large doses is the development of a syndrome with joint pain, fever, a positive antinuclear factor, and on occasions, the development of lupus erythamatosus cells.[57] Although this syndrome is uncommon, it may persist for some months after the withdrawal of hydralazine. It is more common in patients who are also slow acetylators. Peripheral neuropathy has been described, and is said to respond to the administration of pyridoxine.[58]

It is the author's opinion that the use of hydralazine can now be very seldom justified in the treatment of hypertension. The drug is not often very effective and has a high incidence of side effects.

B. Minoxidil

This drug is not available in Australia, and the authors have no personal experience of its use. However, minoxidil appears to be a very powerful vasodilator, which appears to have no action on veins, but a powerful action on arterial smooth muscle. It appears to have no action on the sympathetic nervous system, and consequently the unopposed vasodilatation leads to tachycardia, postural hypotension and marked fluid retention. Minoxidil has been reported to concentrate in the arterial wall, and it is claimed that its slow release from these sites explains its prolonged duration of effect. Unlike prazosin, but like hydralazine, it produces a sharp increase in plasma renin activity. The effects on the cardiovascular system and plasma renin are counteracted by the simultaneous use with β-blocking agents.

The dose ranges from 2 to 30 mg and has the advantage that it can be given once daily. A comparison between the effects of minoxidil and hydralazine was reported by Gottlieb et al.[59] The combination of propranolol and minoxidil produced a significantly greater fall in blood pressure than did the combination of propranolol and hydralazine. Sodium retention and tachycardia were controlled with both drugs by the concomitant use of diuretics and β-blockade. There was a larger rise in plasma renin levels with minoxidil. Pettinger and Mitchell[60] have reported the use of minoxidil as an alternative to nephrectomy for refractoy hypertension in patients with malignant hypertension refractory to conventional drugs. In seven patients with advanced renal disease, the blood pressure was reduced to near normal levels in combination with propranolol with remarkably few side effects. There seems little doubt from this and other reports that minoxidil in combination with diuretics to control the fluid retention and β-adrenoceptor-blocking drugs to control the sympathetic reflex responses in the cardiovascular system is an extremely effective antihypertensive agent. In some patients, it induces angina, but this is usually preventable by the simultaneous use of β-blocking drugs. It has two major disadvantages: the first is that it induces marked facial hair growth, which is similar to that seen with the use of diazoxide.[61] Its other major disadvantage is the occurrence of pulmonary hypertension, which has been attributed to the increase in cardiac output.

It is difficult to establish with any certainty the precise place of minoxidil in the currently available spectrum of antihypertensive drugs. Its use has been largely confined to the U.S. and even there it has only been used for patients refractory to other forms of therapy. There seems no doubt that it is superior to hydralazine as an antihypertensive drug, but the side effects may make it less acceptable than prazosin if a peripherally acting drug is needed.

C. Diazoxide

Diazoxide is a nondiuretic benzothiadiazine which acts directly to relax arterial smooth muscle without any significant effect on the venous side of the circulation. Because it is rapidly inactivated by protein binding, the drug is usually administered by i.v. injection as a bolus. Peak plasma and antihypertensive actions occur within a few minutes of administration, and the blood pressure gradually returns to pretreatment levels over the following 4 to 12 hr. The effect is much less marked when it is given by mouth or by continuous i.v. infusion. Like minoxidil and hydralazine, diazoxide induces reflex tachycardia and an increase in cardiac output and also increases plasma renin activity and induces sodium retention.

Because of its rapid action and the need to give it intravenously, diazoxide is usually reserved for the management of hypertensive emergencies. It certainly has a rapid onset of action, but may induce excessive hypotension. It often induces palpitations, sweating, nausea, and vomiting. It is a difficult drug to use because of its potency and prolonged action and is inferior to sodium nitroprusside or i.v. clonidine for use in hypertensive emergencies.

D. Sodium Nitroprusside

Sodium nitroprusside has been known to be an effective antihypertensive agent since 1929. It is a potent smooth muscle relaxant which produces marked vasodilatation in both venous and arterial vascular beds. Probably for this reason, it has a much less marked effect on cardiac output and tachycardia and does not appear to induce so much sodium retention as diazoxide.

Sodium nitroprusside is usually given by i.v. infusion and lowers blood pressure rapidly. The antihypertensive effect disappears within a few minutes of discontinuation of the infusion. It induces nausea, vomiting, and sweating in a few patients, but is generally better tolerated than diazoxide and is much easier to use in an emergency situation in which it is probably the drug of choice.

XIII. THE MANAGEMENT OF SPECIFIC SYNDROMES IN HYPERTENSION

The preceding sections have given a general account of the clinical aspects of hypertension, defined the indications for drug treatment, and contain a description of the drugs available. The present section is intended to be a practical guide to the management of patients presenting with various different hypertensive syndromes. It has to be emphasized that the views expressed are those of the author and are based on experience in treating patients in Australia, New Zealand, and England. Because there are undoubtedly some geographic and racial differences in the manifestations of illness and because there are undoubtedly differences in attitudes and preferences among experienced physicians and in availability of drugs, these views should be interpreted as guidelines which may be useful in managing individual patients.

A. Malignant Hypertension

Malignant hypertension is rare and seems to be becoming rarer. The syndrome consists of very severe hypertension, usually with a diastolic pressure above 130 mmHg, associated with fibrinoid necrosis of small arteries and arterioles. The latter process leads to a variety of focal ischemic manifestations which include retinal cotton wool spots, cerebral infarction or edema, and progressive renal failure due to ischemic necrosis of glomeruli. Although it is far from clear why some patients develop these arterial lesions, while others with apparently equally severe hypertension do not, it has become evident that reduction of blood pressure leads to an abrupt cessation of the development of new arterial lesions. It seems to make no difference by what means the blood pressure is reduced, since the process can be halted by the rice diet, sympathectomy, the use of any effective combination of antihypertensive drugs, or by surgical relief of renal ischemia.

The outlook for the patient with malignant hypertension depends on the extent of ischemic damage which has been sustained by the time treatment begins. The vascular lesions often develop very rapidly, and for this reason, the diagnosis of malignant hypertension demands immediate treatment to prevent further injury developing.

A patient found to have malignant hypertension should be admitted to the hospital at once and should be given antihypertensive drug therapy as soon as possible. Patients are often unwilling to enter the hospital and usually wish to put off admission while they attend to business or social responsibilities, but it is important to regard malignant hypertension as requiring emergency treatment, and every attempt needs to be made to persuade the patient to enter the hospital.

On admission to the hospital, drug therapy should be started immediately. All patients should be given a benzothiadiazine diuretic, and additional antihypertensive drug therapy should be started at the same time. Because it is necessary to reduce the blood pressure as soon as possible, the best course of action is to use a drug with a high probability of achieving an effective response. The drugs of choice are α-methyldopa, an adrenergic neuron-blocking drug, or clonidine. In the author's opinion, methyldopa is the drug of choice, and on admission 1 g of methyldopa should be given orally.

In the author's experience, this initial therapeutic regime is extremely useful because it immediately divides patients into a majority who respond to the methyldopa with a satisfactory fall of blood pressure and a minority who do not. Not uncommonly, this initial dose of methyldopa induces a dramatic fall of blood pressure and occasionally may induce mild hypotensive symptoms, which, however, are never severe if the patient is kept recumbent. Blood pressure needs to be measured at hourly intervals. If a satisfactory response has occurred, the dose of methyldopa can be adjusted subsequently so as to provide satisfactory control of blood pressure with the patient ambulant, but still in hospital and under close observation.

An initial blood sample drawn on admission is necessary to establish whether any degree of renal impairment is present, since this affects immediate management and gives an idea of prognosis. Providing the serum creatinine level is below 2.5 mg% (0.22 mmol/ℓ), the subsequent management of the patient will be e different from that of the average hypertensive patient. Creatinine levels above 3.0 mg% usually imply that drug excretion will be impaired and that drugs will need to be given less frequently than in most patients. If the serum creatinine is considerably elevated (above 10 mg%), the patient has probably already sustained gross renal damage and under these circumstances, renal function may deteriorate further when blood pressure is reduced. If this occurs, consideration will have to be given to admitting the patient to a dialysis or renal transplantation program. The management of patients with renal failure is discussed in more depth later.

Patients with malignant hypertension often have high plasma renin activity, and there is often a low serum potassium, due to hyperaldosteronism secondary to elevation of plasma renin levels. Hyponatremia is also not uncommon, but these changes, in the absence of renal failure, usually revert to normal as control of the blood pressure is achieved.

Once control of the blood pressure has been attained, two considerations become important. First, it is desirable to consider whether an underlying remediable cause is present. In the author's experience, this is not commonly found in the patient whose blood pressure is easily controlled, and this problem will be discussed in more depth in considering the patient who is resistant to treatment. The second consideration, which only becomes relevant once the blood pressure has been reduced, is whether improvements can be made to the therapeutic regime which will minimize side effects and promote compliance. Patients in hospital usually have a different attitude to side effects than outpatient or office patients, and problems of compliance do not usually arise in hospital. For these reasons, unless obvious side effects occur in hospital, it is usually wiser, once control of blood pressure has been achieved and investigations completed, to let the patient go home and arrange to see him within 3 days of leaving the hospital. Further control of blood pressure and adjustments to the therapeutic regime to suit the convenience of the patient are best done on an outpatient basis. Providing control seems adequate, the interval between subsequent visits can be gradually extended, but patients who have had malignant hypertension are usually best seen at intervals of no longer than 4 weeks.

It is not uncommon to find that patients who have been satisfactorily controlled in hopsital may be less satisfactorily controlled at subsequent attendances. Occasionally, the doses needed in hospital prove too large, and hypotensive symptoms develop when the patient is ambulant and active. This usually presents no therapeutic problem, as the dose can be reduced until the excessive falls of blood pressure are overcome. A more common and difficult problem is that of the patient whose blood pressure was well controlled in hospital who develops a recurrence of elevation of blood pressure after discharge. When this occurs, it is never easy to decide whether the patient has discontinued or reduced his dose of tablets, or whether escape of control has developed in spite of adequate compliance. Patients are not always candid about compliance, but if they claim to be following instructions, it is usually wise to assume that this is so and to alter the regime. In this situation, it is usually necessary to give an additional drug, usually a β-adrenoceptor-blocking drug and preferably one with high bioavailability. In this situation, where control of blood pressure needs to be regained quickly, pindolol or timolol are the drugs of choice. For each drug, the dose should be 10 mg thrice daily. Both drugs have the advantage that it becomes evident within 2 to 3 days whether a satisfactory response has occurred. If a satisfactory fall in blood pressure has occurred, the combination of a diuretic, methyldopa, and pindolol or timolol can either be continued, or if side effects from methyldopa are a problem, this can be slowly discontinued with close observation of blood pressure at intervals of a few days. In communities in which propranolol is the only β-adrenoceptor-blocking agent available, rapid control is less easy to achieve. In malignant hypertension escaping from control, propranolol should be given in an initial dose of 40 mg four times daily, and in the absence of a satisfactory response, the dose doubled every third day until a dose of 320 mg is being taken four times daily. If the patient responds to propranolol, further management can be as described above for pindolol and timolol.

As mentioned in an earlier section, about one third of patients with hypertension do not have useful falls of blood pressure in response to β-blocking drugs, and in malignant hypertension, the proportion who fail to respond may be somewhat higher. If after a brief trial no response is obtained, the β-adrenoceptor-blocking drugs should be discontinued and an adrenergic neuron-blocking drug used, as they are effective in reducing the blood pressure in all but a very small number of patients, although at the expense of a fairly high incidence of side effects. It needs to be emphasized that in treating malignant hypertension, control of blood pressure has to be achieved, and while side effects obviously have to be kept at as low a level as possible, both patient and physician need to realize that the illness is so rapidly fatal if inadequately treated that some disadvantages of therapy may have to be accepted as the lesser of two evils.

A significant, although small, minority of patients with malignant hypertension are extremely resistant to most forms of antihypertensive therapy. These patients usually have moderate to marked renal failure, often have high plasma renin activity, and often have some evidence of fluid overload or congestive heart failure. In some patients, large doses of methyldopa, adrenergic blocking drugs, or β-receptor-blocking drugs fail to reduce blood pressure, and even ganglion-blocking drugs are only marginally effective in doses which induce severe side effects. In this unusual situation, minoxidil, in combination with propranolol and a diuretic drug, has been claimed to provide effective control of blood pressure, but the author has had no personal experience of this. An alternative form of treatment for patients with renal failure is hemodialysis with removal of salt and water combined with propranolol. In a few patients, bilateral nephrectomy has been performed, and it is claimed that control of blood pressure can then be readily achieved by sodium restriction.

The possibility of a surgically remediable cause must be considered in patients with malignant hypertension either resistant to treatment or who respond indifferently to antihypertensive drugs.

Renal artery stenosis and pheochromocytoma in particular should be excluded. These are discussed in a later section.

B. Hypertensive Heart Failure

Although hypertensive heart failure used to be a common cause of death, it has now almost disappeared except in patients with advanced renal failure and resistant hypertension or with concomitant myocardial disease. Few patients now present with hypertensive heart failure and those who do usually have either undetected hypertension or have been mismanaged.

The most common presentation is an episode of paroxysmal nocturnal dyspnea. The diastolic pressure usually exceeds 120 mmHg, and there is almost invariably clinical and electrocardiographic evidence of left ventricular hypertrophy. Pulsus alternans is often present as is a presystolic (atrial) triple rhythm.

The most satisfactory initial treatment is the i.v. administration of furosemide, which should be immediately followed by an oral thiazide diuretic. In the author's opinion, methyldopa is the antihypertensive drug of choice in the first instance, although adrenergic blocking drugs are also often effective. The initial dose of methyldopa is 250 mg thrice daily, and the dose may be increased until the blood pressure is controlled. β-Adrenoceptor antagonists should not be used in this situation in the first instance, at least, since if they fail to reduce blood pressure, their negative inotropic action may aggravate the cardiac failure.

Patients who have had hypertensive heart failure are usually very assiduous about taking drugs, as they not uncommonly have a recurrent episode of paroxysmal nocturnal dyspnea if they discontinue them. Cardiac glycosides may be used until the blood pressure has been controlled, but are usually seldom needed subsequently, and their concomitant use with long-term diuretic therapy is better avoided because of the risks of potentiation of arrhythmias by hypokalemia.

Congestive heart failure in the hypertensive patient may be due in part in some patients to myocardial factors, due either to associated coronary disease as following myocardial infarction, or in some patients to a cardiomyopathy. Under these circumstances, the blood pressure may not be extremely high, but reduction of the left ventricular pressure load by reducing blood pressure may still induce substantial resolution of the congestive failure. When myocardial factors appear to be present, cardiac glycosides, in addition to antihypertensive drugs, are usually useful.

In a small number of patients, either aortic incompetence or functional mitral incompetence may develop as a result of left ventricular dilatation, which may further aggravate the severity of the cardiac failure. In most instances, effective control of blood pressure reduces the degree of left ventricular dilatation, and the murmurs may disappear as the heart failure improves.

Once blood pressure has been controlled, the use of β-adrenoceptor-blocking drugs is worth considering. In patients whose blood pressures can be well controlled with these drugs, a recurrence of heart failure is extremely uncommon.

Recently, antihypertensive drugs have been used for the treatment of intractable heart failure in the absence of hypertension, particularly in patients who develop heart failure following soon after a myocardial infarction and particularly in patients with cardiogenic shock. Sodium nitroprusside, infused i.v., has been claimed to improve the short-term prognosis of patients with cardiogenic shock, particularly when combined with counter pulsation. Sodium nitroprusside reduces both the "pre-load" and "after-load" of the left ventricle by relaxing both venous and arterial smooth muscle, and the extent of the response can be controlled accurately by variation in the rate of infusion, since the action of sodium nitroprusside is evanescent.

The use of prazosin orally has also been advocated in similar situations. For the acute situation, prazosin is less desirable than sodium nitroprusside, since it has apparently no actions on veins, the appropriate dose is more difficult to determine, and its duration of action is considerably longer. Prazosin may prove to be useful in the longer term management of patients with severe nonhypertensive congestive heart failure, but its use has not yet been fully evaluated.

C. Cerebral Vascular Accident
1. Cerebral Hemorrhage

There are sound theoretical reasons for attempting to reduce blood pressure in the patient who has suffered an intracerebral hemorrhage, although in practice, the usefulness of this form of treatment is usually limited, partly by the need to use parenteral therapy and partly because the patient may already have sustained severe brain damage. In such patients, it has been the author's practice to use the ganglion-blocking drug, pentolinium, by intramuscular injection to achieve a modest reduction of blood pressure. The initial dose of 5 mg given may induce a fall of blood pressure. Subsequent doses can be given to attempt to keep the systolic blood pressure below 180 mmHg and should be given whenever this level of systolic blood pressure is exceeded.

A similar routine can be adopted in the management of the patient with subarachnoid hemorrhage, particularly in those in whom there is no evidence of neurological damage.

In patients with hypertension who have suffered a subarachnoid hemorrhage, antihypertensive drugs can usually be given by mouth after a few days, once the acute episode appears to be resolving. In such patients, it is necessary to establish by cerebral angiography whether a surgically remediable lesion is present.

There is no firm evidence that antihypertensive drug therapy is useful in patients either with intracerebral or subarachnoid hemorrhage. However, reduction of blood pressure appears to do no harm in such patients, and since it is possible that reduction of blood pressure may limit the rate of bleeding, its use is probably justified. It is important not to reduce the blood pressure too much.

2. Cerebral Infarction

The management of the hypertensive patient with an established hemiplegia of recent onset is best done by the adoption of a conservative attitude. Antihypertensive drug therapy has the disadvantage that reduction of the blood pressure may reduce cerebral blood flow and so lead to extension of the infarction. The evidence that this occurs often is not strong, since the natural history of stroke is so variable. Antihypertensive drug treatment should, in the author's opinion, be reserved for hypertensive patients in whom there are other clear-cut indications for treatment such as heart failure or malignant hypertension, at least until the neurological state appears to have stabilized. In the early stages, an attempt should be made to define the extent of the infarction by computerized tomography.

If antihypertensive therapy is used, it is of great importance that excessive falls of blood pressure are avoided, since not only may this lead to an extension of the infarction, but may also impede mobilization and rehabilitation. The question as to whether long-term antihypertensive thepy is indicated depends on the extent of the residual neurological deficit, the degree of intellectual impairment, and the age of the patient. Young patients with minimal residual deficit should be offered long-term treatment. In old patients, particularly those in whom the residual neurological deficit is extensive, the benefits to be derived from long-term treatment are speculative.

D. The Elderly Patient

The care of the elderly patient with hypertension differs both in detail and in the objectives of treatment than in younger patients. In this context, elderliness is not simply a matter of elapsed age since birth, but has to take account of the presence or absence of other physical or intellectual infirmities.

With increasing age, a number of physical changes occur in the cardiovascular system. The aorta and great vessels commonly become less elastic as elastic tissue is replaced by collagen, with the result that they become less compliant, which leads to a greater systolic pressure for any given left ventricular stroke volume. Similar changes occur within the baroreceptors, which become less sensitive to changes in intravascular pressure. Additionally, the extent of atheroma usually increases with age, leading to an increased liability to intravascular thrombosis. Renal function also deteriorates with age, due to loss of functioning nephrons. These changes usually become clinically significant sometime after the age of 55 years, on the average.

1. Systolic Hypertension

Although a rise in systolic blood pressure is common in patients aged 60 or above, data from the Chicago Stroke Study[62] indicated that in people aged 65 to 74, systolic blood pressures below 180 mmHg with no diastolic hypertension was not significantly associated with any significant increase in death from coronary heart disease or stroke, but systolic blood pressures above 180 mmHg carried about twice the risk of both complications. Whether this fact reflects the high frequency of vascular disease as an underlying cause of systolic hypertension is not certain. There is no clear evidence that antihypertensive therapy alters the incidence.

2. Diastolic Hypertension

Elevation of diastolic blood increases in prevalence with advancing age[63] (Figure 9, Table 5). There is clear evidence that at all ages diastolic hypertension carries an increased risk of vascular complications, and this is true for older patients as well as for younger.

3. Treatment

The overriding consideration in the treatment of hypertension in elderly people is the necessity to avoid doing harm to the patient. Excessive falls of blood pressure may induce cerebral or myocardial ischemia or induce postural faintness or collapse. Older patients appear to be much more sensitive to most antihypertensive drugs than younger

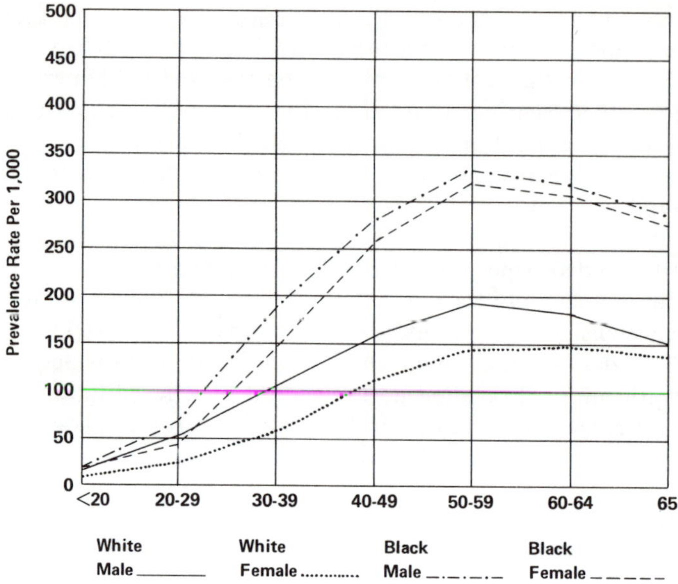

FIGURE 9.   Prevalence of elevated blood pressure at screening (diastolic blood pressure is 95 mmHg). (From Dyer, A. R., Stamler, J., Shekelle, R. B., Schoenberger, J. A., and Farinaro, E., *Med. Clin. N. Am.,* 61, 513, 1977. With permission.)

ones. Even small doses of benzothiadiazine diuretics may sometimes induce significant hypovolemia and postural faintness. β-Adrenoceptor-blocking drugs are usually well tolerated, but induce sleep disturbances and depression more commonly in older patients than in young ones. Methyldopa is usually effective in small doses, but may also induce depression in older patients. Adrenergic blocking drugs (prazosin and labetalol) are usually better avoided unless the hypertension is severe and unresponsive to diuretics, β-adrenoceptor-blocking drugs, or methyldopa. Most elderly patients require small doses of drugs, and resistant hypertension is uncommon except in renovascular hypertension, which may develop in older people as a result of occlusive atherosclerotic disease of the aorta or renal arteries. It may also follow dissection of the abdominal aorta.

It is the author's opinion that treatment of hypertension in persons over the age of 65 is best reserved for those with a diastolic blood pressure exceeding 110 mHg or those who can expect relief from such symptoms as headache, congestive heart failure, or paroxysmal nocturnal dyspnoea. Long-term preventive therapy in old people with marginally elevated blood pressure is better avoided.

E. Transient Cerebral Ischemic Attacks

Recurrent episodes of transient neurological deficit occur not uncommonly in hypertensive patients. When these can be shown to be associated with occlusive disease of the extracranial arteries, surgical relief of the obstruction should be undertaken. In a few patients, such recurrent episodes appear to be related to severe hypertension, and reduction of blood pressure may prevent recurrences. In such patients, however, excessive falls of blood pressure may induce similar episodes. Treatment should be aimed at reducing the blood pressure by a modest amount. Drugs which induce marked postural falls of blood pressure, such as guanethidine, may be dangerous.

TABLE 5

Prevalence of Diastolic Blood Pressure Greater than or Equal to 95 mmHg and Greater than or Equal to 110 mmHg by Age, Sex, and Race. Community Hypertension Evaluation Clinic Program, 1973—1975.

| | % Diastolic ≥ 95 | | | | % Diastolic ≥ 110 | | | |
| | Men | | Women | | Men | | Women | |
Age	White	Black	White	Black	White	Black	White	Black
20—29	5.2	7.0	2.3	4.6	0.7	1.6	0.4	1.1
30—39	10.3	18.2	5.7	14.7	1.8	5.5	1.2	4.5
40—49	15.7	27.7	11.1	25.4	3.4	9.8	2.5	9.1
50—59	19.3	33.4	14.6	31.8	4.5	12.2	3.2	10.9
60—64	18.2	31.8	14.9	31.0	4.2	11.8	3.2	11.2
≥65	15.1	28.6	14.0	27.6	3.3	10.3	3.0	9.2

From Dyer, A. R., Stamler, J., Shekelle, R. B., Schoenberger, J. A., and Farinaro, E., *Med. Clin. N. Am.*, 61, 513, 1977.

F. The Patient Resistant to Drug Therapy

In the author's experience, 70 to 80% of patients with moderate to severe hypertension can be treated easily, with few side effects and with persisting good control of blood pressure. The remaining 20 to 30% present a much more difficult therapeutic problem.

In most hypertensives, satisfactory control of blood pressure can usually be achieved with a benzothiadiazine diuretic, an adrenoceptor-blocking drug, and methyldopa, according to the plan showed in Figure 10. When these three drugs fail to control blood pressure adequately, the sequence shown in Figure 11 is used. Labetalol appears to be the drug currently most likely to be successful in gaining control of blood pressure in patients resistant to the standard drugs. The dose may be increased to 1200 to 1800 mgm daily, if necessary. An alternative to the use of labetalol is a combination of β-adrenoceptor-blocking drug and the selective α-postjunctional receptor-blocking drug, prazosin.

If control is still poor with this combination of drugs, admission to hospital may help to elucidate the situation. In particular, it may allow blood levels of drugs to be assessed to determine whether the problem is one of patient compliance or a pharmacokinetic difficulty, or whether the patient's disease is resistant to treatment because of the presence of underlying renal disease, renovascular hypertension, or pheochromocytoma. In a small number of patients, blood pressure continues to be difficult to control in hospital, but most seem to respond better to antihypertensive drugs in hospital than when ambulant and at home. In patients who fail to respond to the above drugs in hospital, the use of adrenergic blocking drugs or ganglion-blocking drugs may have to be considered.

G. The Hypertensive Emergency

Very few situations in hypertension demand that the blood pressure should be lowered within a few minutes. Parenteral therapy is best avoided in malignant hypertension, and i.v. furosemide is usually very effective in the management of congestive heart failure. Two conditions, namely, dissecting aortic aneurysm and hypertensive encephalopathy are of sufficient severity and urgency to justify immediate reduction of blood pressure. The drug of choice for such situations appears to be sodium nitroprusside, which has the advantage of a rapid onset and offset of action, allowing a

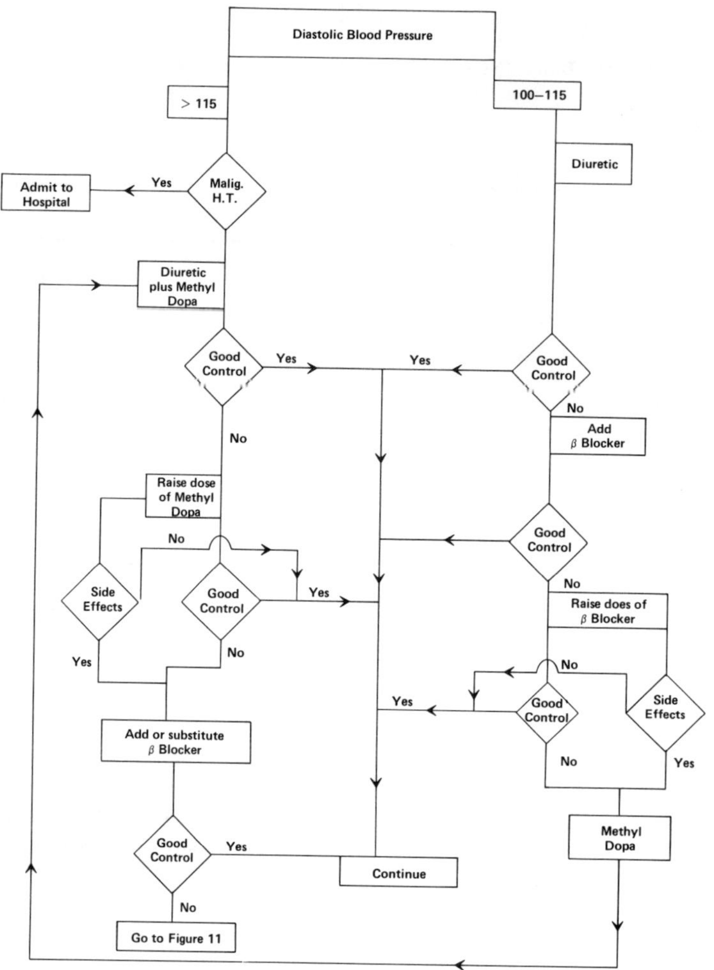

FIGURE 10.   Flow chart showing scheme for treatment of diastolic hypertension.

very precise control of blood pressure to be achieved. Alternatively, a rapid i.v. bolus of diazoxide commonly reduces blood pressure rapidly, but severe hypotension may result, which is sometimes difficult to treat. Clonidine, given slowly i.v. over a period of 5 min in a dose of 0.15 to 0.3 mg is usually an effective antihypertensive agent. The slow administration seems to prevent the rise in blood pressure due to the α-agonist action. Blood pressure usually falls over a period of 5 to 10 min and remains low for several hours, during which time oral antihypertensive therapy can be commenced.

H. Renal Failure

Hypertension is a common manifestation in patients with chronic renal failure due to a variety of underlying kidney diseases. It also is an etiological factor in inducing renal failure, and uncontrolled hypertension may lead to rapid deterioration in renal function in patients with underlying kidney disease.

Three factors complicate the treatment of hypertension associated with chronic renal failure. These are (1) differences in pharmacokinetics due to reduced renal drug excretion, (2) disturbances in extracellular sodium and water, and (3) the renin-angiotensin system.

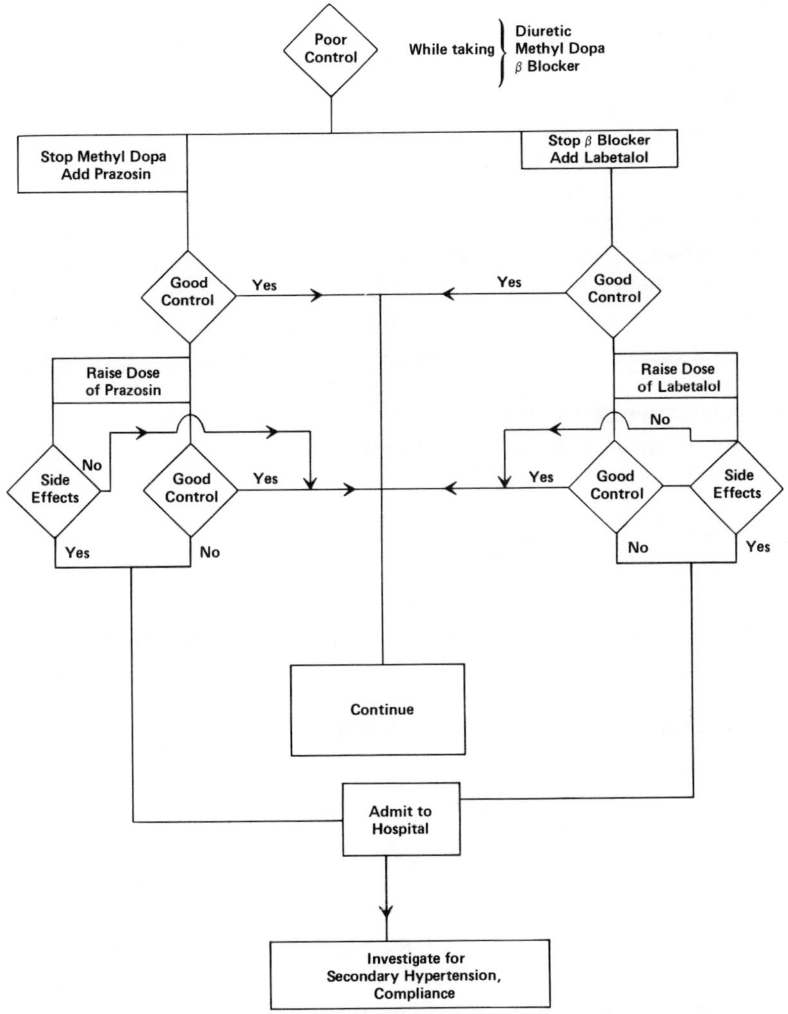

FIGURE 11.   Flow chart showing scheme for treatment of resistant hypertension.

1. Therapeutic Implications of Disturbed Pharmacokinetics in Renal Failure

Many antihypertensive drugs are predominantly excreted in the urine, and such drugs accumulate in patients with chronic renal failure. The drugs involved are the diuretics, methyldopa, clonidine, adrenergic blocking drugs, and the ganglion-blocking drugs. The β-adrenoceptor-blocking drugs predominantly undergo biotransformation in the liver, but propranolol blood levels tend to be higher and of longer duration in patients with renal failure.

The delayed excretion of antihypertensive drugs leads to both enhancement and prolongation of their effects. In patients with severe renal failure, a single dose of a drug may persist for 2 to 3 days. In beginning treatment with antihypertensive drugs in patients with renal failure, once-daily doses are usually prescribed. The effects of an initial once-daily dose level need to be assessed for 3 to 4 days before it becomes evident whether the dose needs to be increased. Increases of dose are best made at intervals of 3 to 4 days. If too large a dose is given, hypotension may persist for 24 to 48 hr after the drug has been stopped. This becomes important during intercurrent infections with fever, in hot weather, or after blood loss, in all of which situations the response to antihypertensive drugs may be considerably enhanced.

2. Variations in Body Fluid Balance

There is an important relationship between extracellular and plasma volume and the effectiveness of these drugs — fluid accumulation leads to loss of response and dehydration to an exaggerated effect. Patients with chronic renal failure have a limited capacity to conserve or excrete salt, and water and variations in body fluid may either enhance or oppose the fall in blood pressure. This is particularly important in patients undergoing long-term dialysis, but is also of relevance in the patient not yet at that stage. Fluid retention due to an increased salt intake may allow the blood pressure to escape from control. If the dose is then raised, a subsequent fall in sodium or water intake is followed by severe hypotension. The practical implication is that the drug treatment of hypertension becomes very difficult if the patient's sodium intake fluctuates much, and an attempt must be made to control diet in these patients.

3. The Renin-Angiotensin System

As will be discussed in more detail in the section on angiotensin-blocking drugs and inhibitors of angiotensin-converting enzyme, the renin-angiotensin system contributes to the maintenance of hypertension in some patients with malignant hypertension, some patients with renal failure, and some patients with renovascular hypertension. In such patients, sodium depletion leads to high circulating angiotensin levels, which reduce the responses to conventional antihypertensive drugs, so that in these patients, the usual enhancement of the effects of these drugs due to sodium loss does not occur. These patients may respond very inadequately to all varieties of conventional antihypertensive drug therapy, often including propranolol.

Additional References relevant to this Chapter are to be found in Volume I, Chapters 1 and 2; and Volume II, Chapters 1, 2, and 3.

REFERENCES

1. **Sackett, D. L., Haynes, R. B., Gibson, E. S., Hackett, B., Taylor, D. W., Roberts, R. S., and Johnson, A. L.,** Randomized clinical trial of strategies for improving medication compliance in primary hypertension, *Lancet,* 1, 1205, 1975.
2. **Finnerty, F. A. Jr., Shaw, L. W., and Himmelsbach, C. K.,** Hypertension in the inner city. II. Detection and follow up, *Circulation,* 47, 76, 1973.
3. **Dollery, C. T.,** Individual differences in response to drugs, in *Advanced Medicine, Topics in Therapeutics,* Breckenridge, A. M., Ed., Pitman Medical, London, 1975.
4. **Kempner, W.,** Treatment of kidney disease and hypertensive vascular disease with rice diet, *N.C. Med. J.,* 5, 125, 1944.
5. **Editorial,** Salt and hypertension, *Lancet,* 1, 1325, 1976.
6. **Hunt, J. C.,** Management and treatment of essential hypertension, in *Hypertension,* Genest, J., Koiw, E., and Kuchel, O., Eds., McGraw-Hill, New York, 1977, 1068.
7. **Morgan, T. O., Adam, W., Gillies, A., Wilson, M., Morgan, G., and Carney, S.,** Hypertension treated by salt restriction, *Lancet,* 1, 227, 1978.
8. **Kirkendall, W. M. and Overturf, M. L.,** Thiazide diuretics and salt consumption in the treatment of hypertension, in *Systemic Effects of Antihypertensive Agents,* Sambhi, M., Ed., Stratton Intercontinental, New York, 1976, 119.
9. **Wilson, I. M. and Freis, E. D.,** Relationship between plasma and extracellular fluid volume depletion and the antihypertensive effect of chlorothiazide, *Circulation,* 20, 1025, 1959.
10. **McQueen, E. G. and Morrison, R. B. I.,** The hypotensive action of diuretic agents, *Lancet,* 1, 1209, 1960.
11. **Leth, A.,** Chances in plasma and extracellular fluid volumes in patients with essential hypertension during long-term treatment with hydrochlorothiazide, *Circulation,* 42, 479, 1970.
12. **Winer, B. M.,** The antihypertensive action of benzothiadiazines, *Circulation,* 23, 211, 1961.

13. **Louis, W. J., Doyle, A. E., Dawborn, J. K., and Johnston, C. I.**, A comparison of chlorothiazide, chlorthalidone and cyclopenthiazide in the treatment of hypertension, *Med. J. Aust.*, 2, 23, 1973.

14. **Dustan, H. P., Tarazi, R. C., and Bravo, E. L.**, Diuretic and diet treatment of hypertension, *Arch. Intern. Med.*, 133, 1007, 1974.

15. **Prichard, B. N. C. and Tuckman, J.**, Management and mechanisms of drug treatment of hypertension, in *Hypertension*, Genest, J., Koiw,E., and Kuchel, O., Eds., McGraw-Hill, New York, 1977, 1085.

16. **Roberts, H. J.**, Potassium chloride and intestinal ulceration, *Lancet*, 2, 1127, 1965.

17. **Baker, D. R., Schrader, W. H., and Hitchcock, C. R.**, Small bowel ulceration apparently associated with thiazide and potassium therapy, *JAMA*, 190, 586, 1964.

18. **Down, P. F., Polak, A., Rao, R., and Mead, J. A.**, Fate of potassium supplements in six out-patients receiving long term diuretics for oedematous disease, *Lancet*, 2, 721, 1972.

19. **Kohner, E. M., Dollery, C. T., Lowy, C., and Schumer, B.**, Effect of diuretic therapy on glucose tolerance in hypertensive patients, *Lancet*, 1, 986, 1971.

20. **Watson, L. S., Fanelli, G. M., Russo, H. F., Sweet, C. S., Ludden, C. T., and Scriabine, A.**, New antihypertensive saluretic-uricosuric Indanone, in *New Antihypertensive Drugs*, Scriabine, A. and Sweet, C. S., Eds., Spectrum Publications, New York, 1976, 307.

21. **Beregi, L. G.**, Antihypertensive and saluretic properties of the indoline and iso-indoline series, *Curr. Med. Res. Opin.*, 5 (Suppl. 1), 3, 1977.

22. **Campbell, D. B. and Phillips, E. M.**, Short term effects and urinary excretion of a new diuretic, indapamide in normal subjects, *Eur. J. Clin. Pharmacol.*, 7, 407, 1974.

23. **Moore, R. A., Seki, T., Oshumi, S., Oheim, K., Kyncl, J., and Desnoyes, P.**, Antihypertensive action of indapamide and review of pharmacology and toxicology, *Curr. Med. Res. Opin.*, 5, (Suppl. 1), 25, 1977.

24. **Onesti, G., Pitone, J., Lowenthal, D. L., Kim, K. E., Affrime, M., Bronstein, B. J., Slurk, J., Valvo, E., Martinez, E., Fernandez, M., and Swartz, C.**, Studies on the natriuretic effect and site of action of indapamide, *Curr. Med. Res. Opin.*, 5 (Suppl. 1), 83, 1977.

25. **Demanet, J. C., Degante, J. P., and Hubert, C.**, Safety and long term efficacy in a long term study of indapamide in essential hypertension, *Curr. Med. Res. Opin.*, 5 (Supp 1), 129, 1977.

26. **Olesen, K. H., Sigurd, B., Steiness, E., and Leth, A.**, Bumetamide, a new potent diuretic. A clinical evaluation in congestive heart failure, *Acta Med. Scand.*, 193, 119, 1973.

27. **Brogden, R. N., Speight, T. M., and Avery, G. S.**, Bumetamide: a preliminary report of its pharmacological properties and therapeutic efficacy in oedema, *Drugs*, 9, 4, 1975.

28. **Spark, R. F. and Melby, J. C.**, Hypertension and low plasma renin activity. Presumptive evidence for mineralocorticoid excess, *Ann. Intern. Med.*, 75, 831, 1971.

29. **Hunyor, S. M., Zweifler, A. J., and Hansson, L.**, Effect of spironolactone and chlorthalidone in essential hypertension: relation to plasma renin activity and plasma volume, *Circulation*, 48 (Suppl. 4), 83, 1973.

30. **Brunner, H. R., Laragh, J. H., Baer, L., Jr., Newton, M. A., Goodwin, F. T., Krakoff, L. R., Bard, R. H., and Bühler, F. R.**, Essential hypertension. Renin and aldosterone, heart attack and stroke, *N. Engl. J. Med.*, 286, 441, 1972.

31. **Brunner, H. R., Sealey, J. E., and Laragh, J.H.**, Renin as a risk factor in hypertension. More evidence, *Am. J. Med.*, 55, 295, 1973.

32. **Zanchetti, A., Leonetti, G., Morganti, A., Terzoli, L., Schwarz, E., Manfrin, H., and Bernasconi, M.**, Longitudinal study of plasma renin activity in hypertensive patients under antihypertensive treatment, including diuretics, in *Systemic Effects of Antihypertensive Agents*, Sambhi, M., Ed., Stratton Intercontinental, New York, 1976, 251.

33. **Prichard, B. N. C. and Gillam, P. M. S.**, Use of propranolol in the treatment of hypertension, *Br. Med. J.*, 2, 725, 1964.

34. **Simpson, F. O.**, Beta-adrenergic blocking drugs in hypertension, *Drugs*, 7, 85, 1974.

35. **Morgan, T. O., Roberts, R., Carney, S. L., Louis, W. J., and Doyle, A. E.**, Beta adrenergic receptor blocking drugs, hypertension and plasma renin, *Br. J. Clin. Pharmacol.*, 2, 159, 1975.

36. **Morgan, T. O., Sabto J., Anavekar, S. N., Louis, W. J., and Doyle, A. E.**, A comparison of beta-adrenergic blocking drugs in the treatment of hypertension, *Postgrad. Med. J.*, 50, 253, 1974.

37. **Anavekar, S. N., Louis, W. J., Morgan, T. O., Doyle, A. E., and Johnston, C. I.**, The Relationship of plasma levels of pindolol in hypertensive patients to effects on blood pressure, plasma renin and plasma noradrenaline levels, *Clin. Exp. Pharmacol. Physiol.*, 2, 203, 1975.

38. **Morgan, T. O., Louis, W. J., Dawborn, J. K., and Doyle, A. E.**, The use of pindolol (Visken) in the treatment of hypertension, *Med. J. Aust.*, 2, 309, 1972.

39. **Gloutz, G. E. and Saslaw, S.**, Methyldopa fever, *Arch. Intern. Med.*, 122, 445, 1968.

40. **Toghill, P. J., Smith, P. G., Benton, P., Brown, R. C., and Matthews, H. L.**, Methyldopa liver damage, *Br. Med. J.*, 3, 545, 1974.

41. Breckenridge, A. M., Dollery, C. T., Worlledge, S. M., Holborn, E. J., and Johnson, G. D., Positive direct Coomb's test and antinuclear factor in patients treated with methyldopa, *Lancet*, 2, 1265, 1967.
42. Carstairs, K. C. A., Breckenridge, A. M., Dollery, C. T., and Worlledge, S. M., Incidence of a positive direct Coomb's test in patients on amethyldopa, *Lancet*, 2, 133, 1966.
43. Louis, W. J., Doyle, A. E., Jerums, G., and Kincaid-Smith, P., Methyldopa and haemolytic anaemia, *Med. J. Aust.*, 2, 104, 1967.
44. Worlledge, S. M., Carstairs, K. C., and Dacie, J. V., Autoimmune haemolytic anaemia associated with amethyldopa therapy, *Lancet*, 2, 135, 1966.
45. Hunyor, S. N., Hansson, L., Harrison, T. S., and Hoobler, S. W., Effects of clonidine withdrawal: possible mechanisms and suggestions for management, *Br. Med. J.*, 2, 209, 1973.
46. Frick, M. H. and Porsti, P., Combined alpha- and beta-adrenoreceptor blockade with labetalol in hypertension, *Br. Med. J.*, 1, 1046, 1976.
47. Blakeley, A. G. H. and Summers, R. J., The effect of AH 5158 on the overflow of transmitter and the uptake of (H)-l-noradrenaline in the cat spleen, *Br. J. Pharmacol.*, 56, 264P, 1976.
48. Louis, W. J., Christophidis, N., Brignell, M., Vijayeskeran, V., McNeil, J., and Vajda, F. J. E., Labetalol: bioavailability, drug plasma levels, plasma renin and catecholamines in acute and chronic treatment of resistant hypertension, *Aust. N.Z. J. Med.*, in press.
49. Hess, H. J., Biochemistry and structure-activity studies with prazosin, in *Prazosin — Evaluation of a New Antihypertensive Agent*, Cotton, D. W. K., Ed., Excerpta Medica, Geneva, 1974, 3.
50. Cambridge, D., Davey, M. J., and Massingham, R., The pharmacology of antihypertensive drugs with special reference to vasodilators and adrenergic blocking agents and prazosin, *Med. J. Aust.*, 2 (Suppl. 2), 3, 1977.
51. Hua, A., MacDonald, S. P., Myers, J. B., and Kincaid-Smith, P., Studies with prazosin — a new effective hypotensive agent. I. Open clinical study of prazosin in combination with other hypotensive agents, *Med. J. Aust.*, 1, 559, 1976.
52. Hayes, J. M., Graham, R. M., O'Connell, B. P., Muir, M. R., Speers, E., and Humphrey, T. J., Experience with prazosin in the treatment of patients with severe hypertension, *Med. J. Aust.*, 1, 562, 1976.
53. Graham, R. M., Thornell, I. R., Gain, J. M., Bagnoli, C., Oates, H. F., and Stokes, G. S., Prazosin: the first dose phenomenon, *Br. Med. J.*, 4, 1293, 1976.
54. Rosendorff, C., Prazosin: severe side effects are dose dependent, *Br. Med. J.*, 3, 508, 1976.
55. Stokes, G. S. and Oates, H. F., Prazosin: new alpha-adrenergic blocking agent in treatment of hypertension, *Cardiovasc. Med.*, 3, 41, 1978.
56. Zacest, R. and Koch-Weser, J., Relation of hydralazine plasma concentration to dosage and hypotensive action, *Clin. Pharmacol. Ther.*, 13, 420, 1972.
57. Perry, H. M., Late toxicity to hydralazine resembling systemic lupus erythematosus or rheumatoid arthritis, *Am. J. Med.*, 54, 58, 1973.
58. Raskin, N. H. and Fishman, R. A., Pyridoxine deficiency neuropathy due to hydralazine, *N. Engl. J. Med.*, 273, 1182, 1965.
59. Gottlieb, T. B., Katz, F. H., and Chidsey, C. A., Combined therapy with vasodilator drugs and beta adrenergic blockade in hypertension. A comparative study of minoxidil and hydralazine, *Circulation*, 45, 571, 1972.
60. Pettinger, W. A. and Mitchell, H. C., Minoxidil: an alternative to nephrectomy for refractory hypertension, *N. Engl. J. Med.*, 289, 167, 1973.
61. Chidsey, C. A., Gottlieb, T. B., Pluss, R. G., Orcutt, J. C., and Weil, J. V., The use of vasodilators and Beta-adrenergic blockade in hypertension, in *Hypertension: Mechanisms and Management*, Onesti, G., Kim, K. E., and Moyer, J. H., Eds., Grune & Stratton, New York, 1973, 357.
62. Shekelle, R., Ostfield, A., and Klawans, H., Hypertension and risk of stroke in an elderly population, *Stroke*, 5, 71, 1974.
63. Dyer, A. R., Stamler, J., Shekelle, R. B., Schoenberger, J. A., and Farinaro, E., Hypertension in the elderly, *Med. Clin. N. Am.*, 61, 513, 1977.

Chapter 5

CLINICAL APPLICATIONS OF AGENTS WHICH BLOCK THE RENIN-ANGIOTENSIN SYSTEM

I. DIAGNOSTIC AND INVESTIGATIONAL

Agents which block the renin-angiotensin system have been used to assess the role of angiotensin in various forms of human hypertension. Mainly, two agents have so far been used for this purpose, the angiotensin-receptor blocker, [Sar[1], Ala[8]]-angiotensin II, hereafter called "saralasin" for brevity, and a synthetic, nonapeptide-converting-enzyme inhibitor, hereafter called "SQ 20881". Although claims have been made that β-adrenoceptor blocking agents produce their hypotensive action by inhibition of renin release and can, therefore, be used to assess the participation of renin in hypertension, it is clear that these agents can lower blood pressure by means other than inhibition of renin release. For this reason, β-adrenoceptor blockers will not be discussed further in this section.

In human hypertension, as in experimental models of hypertension, saralasin and SQ 20881 are usually most effective in patients with raised plasma-renin activity.

Brunner at al.[1] used saralasin infusion in patients with either renovascular, advanced, or malignant hypertension or hypertension associated with pyelonephritis. In eight patients with raised plasma-renin activity, the angiotensin-receptor blocker produced immediate, large falls of blood pressure to near normal levels and was not observed to cause hypotension even when given at ten times the maximal effective dose rate (Figure 1). All of the patients with renovascular hypertension had elevated plasma-renin activity, and all responded to saralasin infusion. Maximum blood pressure reduction was obtained using infusions of the inhibitor at 10 μg/kg/min, and increasing the dose to as much as 100 μg/kg/min did increase the hypotensive effect. Two of the three patients with malignant hypertension had elevated plasma-renin activity, and both responded to saralasin. In all patients, plasma-renin activity rose dramatically after saralasin infusion, indicating the tonic renin-inhibitory effect of angiotensin II in man.

Donker and Leenen[2] reported the use of saralasin infusion in two patients with renovascular hypertension. While on a sodium intake of 100 mmol/day, the analogue produced a decrease in blood pressure of 10 to 20 mmHg, but a much more marked and rapid fall in one of the patients when given after sodium depletion (Figure 2). The use of step-wise infusions between 10 to 100 μg/kg/min in one patient produced acute transient rises in blood pressure and pulse rate. In both patients, the hypertension was subsequently cured by nephrectomy or surgical reconstruction. Interestingly, the authors noted that although plasma-renin activity fell to low values within one day, blood pressure fell slowly over 2 to 3 weeks. This observation suggests that factors other than circulating plasma-renin activity are involved in the maintenance of renal hypertension as discussed in Chapter 1, Volume 2.

The hypotensive effect of saralasin infused at doses up to 100 μg/kg/min in 60 hypertensive patients was assessed after 2 to 3 days of taking a diet containing 10 mmol sodium or 2 hr after 40 mg of i.v. frusemide.[3] Of the patients, 16 had a fall in systolic and diastolic pressures exceeding 10 and 7 mmHg, respectively, during saralasin infusion (Figure 3). Peripheral plasma renin was elevated in 13 of these "responsive" patients. Nine of the ten "saralasin responsive" patients studied by renal arteriography had renal-artery stenosis, and five out of six of the remainder were said to have reduced

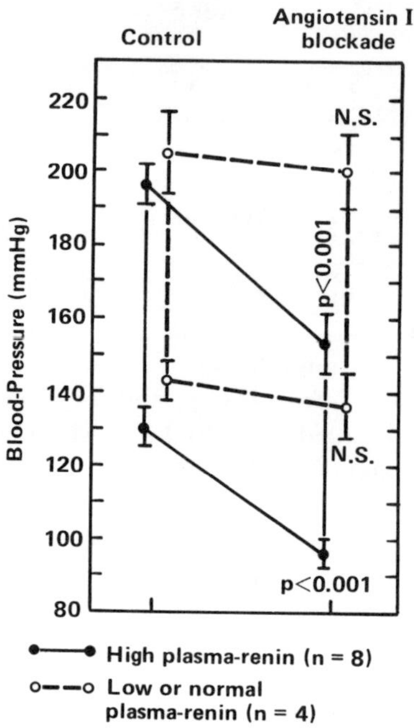

FIGURE 1.   Renin-related blood pressure effect of angiotensin-II blockade by saralasin. In eight hypertensive patients with high renin levels, inhibition of angiotensin II induced marked and highly significant blood pressure reductions. In contrast, no change in blood pressure occurred in the four patients with low or normal renin values. Means and standard errors of systolic and diastolic blood pressure are depicted. P values are derived from a paired *t*-test analysis. N.S. indicates lack of statistical significance. (From Brunner, H. R., Gavras, H., Laragh, J. H., and Keenan, R., *Lancet*, 2, 1045, 1973. With permission.)

renal blood flow to one or both kidneys by isotope renography. Most of these patients had significantly higher levels of renin in the venous blood from the affected side. Four of these "saralasin responsive" patients had relief or reduction of hypertension after unilateral nephrectomy, and eight out of eight responded to propranolol. The authors suggested that saralasin responsiveness was a useful test for curable renal-artery stenosis. However, because of the small number of patients and the difficulty in controlling the predictive factors in these highly selected patients, it is premature to conclude from these data that the saralasin test has predictive value for results of either renal surgery or propranolol treatment. Renal arteriography is still, probably, the only means of excluding renal-artery stenosis and is still needed in patients with high peripheral or renal venous renin levels to define the anatomical lesions. Since most of the "saralasin responsive" patients in the study of Streeten et al.[3] had elevated peripheral plasma renin activity (13 of 16), and all had either elevated peripheral plasma renin activity or renal venous plasma renin activity, it is clear that this test does not add any further information than the renin measurements. However, claims that the test is more convenient or rapid than renin measurements are discussed below.

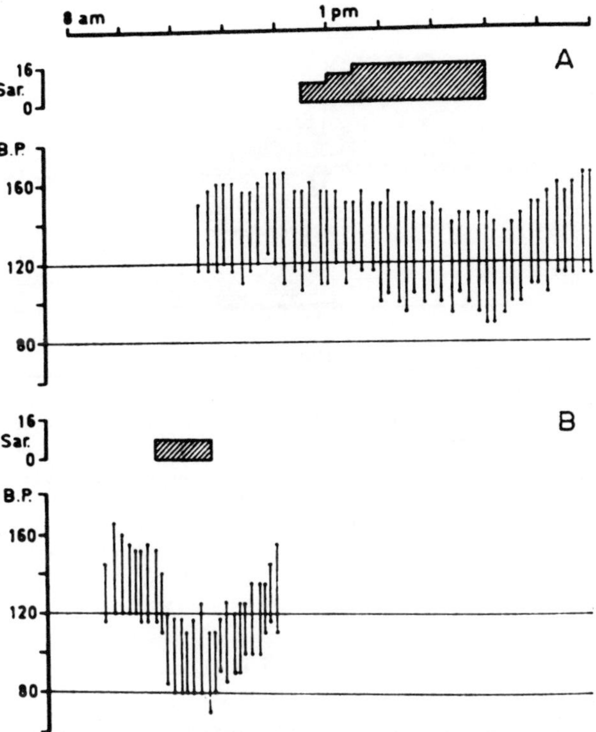

FIGURE 2. Mild hypotensive effect of saralasin infusion (μg/ min) in a patient with renal-artery stenosis. (A) Before sodium depletion and marked effect, (B) after sodium depletion. (From Donker, A. J. M. and Leenen, F. H. H., *Lancet*, 2, 1535, 1974. With permission.)

In a later report, these authors[4] reported the results of saralasin infusion in a larger group of 300 hypertensive patients of whom 31 had depressor responses to the infusion. Again, most of the "saralasin responsive" patients had elevated plasma-renin-activity levels (27 of 31), and 11 of them had unilateral renal artery stenosis. However, only 50% of the whole group of patients with high plasma-renin activity levels had a depressor response to saralasin. It was claimed that only one of the patients with high plasma-renin activity who were unresponsive to saralasin was subsequently found to have renal-artery stenosis. The inference that saralasin-responsiveness might be a better indicator of the presence of "angiotensinogenic hypertension" than measurement of peripheral plasma renin activity is not, however, clearly established by this study.

The use of saralasin given as a rapid i.v. bolus has been reported in 21 hypertensive patients.[5] Frusemide was administered on the evening before the test. Thirteen patients had a marked drop in blood pressure after saralasin, and of these, 11 had renovascular hypertension, and two had "high-renin essential hypertension". Ten of the 13 had elevated peripheral plasma-renin activity (Figure 4). The response to a 10 mg bolus of saralasin correlated well with that to a subsequent infusion of saralasin at 10 μg/kg/ min. In patients who responded to saralasin, blood pressure remained depressed for 30 min after the bolus of inhibitor. The authors argued that this test was a rapid, simple, safe, and inexpensive way to determine the role of angiotensin in sustaining hypertension. There may be potential hazards and difficulties in the bolus saralasin test since occasional, striking, pressor responses have been reported in hypertensives

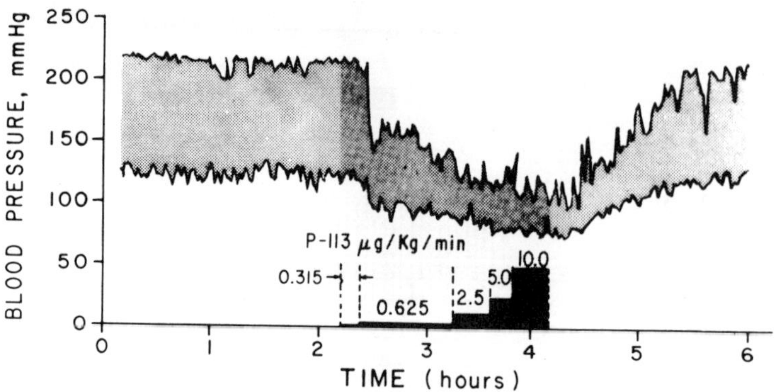

FIGURE 3.   Automatic blood pressure recording during saralasin infusion in a patient with renal-artery stenosis and high plasma-renin activity. Blood pressure fell little, if at all, during saralasin (P-113) infusion at 0.315 µg/kg/min, but fell progressively to normal levels as P-113 infusion was increased to 0.625, 2.5, 5.0 and 10.0 µg/kg/min. During the first hr to 1½ hr after the P-113 infusion was stopped, blood pressure returned gradually to control hypertensive levels. (From Streeten, D. H. P., Anderson, G. H., Freiberg, J. M., and Dalakos, T. G., *N. Engl. J. Med.*, 292, 657, 1975. With permission.)

with low plasma renin.[4] In addition, many patients showed borderline responses which were difficult to interpret with this test.[4]

Saralasin infused at 10 µg/kg/min into 52 hypertensives produced initial transient pressor responses with a slower, more gradual response over 20 min.[6] Most patients with high plasma-renin activity had sustained depressor responses irrespective of sodium intake. In contrast on a normal sodium intake, patients with normal renin had small or no pressor effect, and low-renin patients had more marked pressor responses. After sodium depletion, the usual response to saralasin was depressor, irrespective of pretreatment renin levels.

Later, the same group[7] reported the results of both saralasin infusion and SQ 20881 injection in 39 hypertensive patients. Although both agents produced falls in blood pressure which, overall, correlated well with each other and with the pretreatment plasma renin levels, there were significant differences in the effects of the two agents. Patients with high plasma-renin-activity levels showed large falls in blood pressure with either saralasin or SQ 20881, whereas those with normal plasma-renin activity only showed a fall in blood pressure with SQ 20881. The patients with low plasma-renin activity, including six anephric patients, had pressor responses to saralasin and had no change in blood pressure with SQ 20881 (Figure 5). These results confirm that saralasin is a partial agonist in man and may, therefore, underestimate the involvement of angiotensin in maintenance of blood pressure. Four patients with renal-artery stenosis had elevated peripheral-plasma-renin activity, significant localization of renal venous plasma-renin activity, and marked hypotensive responses to both saralasin and SQ 20881.[7] Dietary sodium intake did not affect the depressor responsiveness of these patients to the two agents.

Saralasin infusion has been used to define two tyes of hypertension in patients with chronic renal failure on maintenance haemodialysis.[8,9] In the group in whom saralasin did not lower blood pressure, removal of fluid by dialysis restored blood pressure to normal. Those patients in whom saralasin did lower blood presure were unresponsive to dialysis-induced weight loss, but responded to a β-adrenoceptor blocker and a vasodilator[8] or to bilateral nephrectomy.[9]

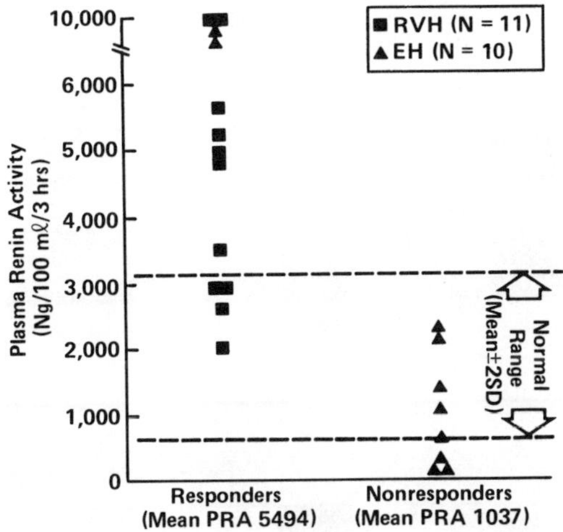

FIGURE 4.   Plasma-renin activity in hypertensive patients who were responsive or unresponsive to a bolus injection of saralasin. (From Marks, L. S., Maxwell, M. H., and Kaufman, J. J., *Lancet*, 2, 784, 1975. With permission.)

Baer et al.[10] infused saralasin in 20 hypertensive patients who were taking a normal sodium diet. Twelve of the patients had falls of diastolic blood pressure ranging from 10 to 40 mmHg. Of these, 11 had radiological evidence of renal-artery stenosis, lateralized renal-vein renin levels, suppression of renin release from the contralateral kidney, and elevated peripheral plasma-renin activity. In this study of highly selected patients therefore, the depressor response to saralasin infusion correlated well with the presence of high plasma-renin levels and was most often found in patients with significant unilateral renal-artery stenosis.

However, the saralasin test is not uniformly successful in identifying patients with significant renal-artery stenosis. The results seem to be influenced by sodium status and the levels of peripheral plasma-renin activity before the test. Thomas et al.[11] reported two patients with renovascular hypertension, in both cases due to fibromuscular hyperplasia of the right renal artery. Both patients were apparently taking normal diets and had low or normal levels of peripheral-plasma-renin activity. Saralasin infusion failed to lower the blood pressure in either patient although both had a sustained reduction of blood pressure after autotransplantation of their affected kidneys.

The effect of sodium status on the response to saralasin infusion was investigated in 14 patients with essential hypertension.[12] After mild sodium depletion, approximately equal numbers of patients had a fall, no change, or a rise in blood pressure during the infusion. These groups corresponded to those with high, normal, or low plasma-renin-activity levels before the infusion. The degree of sodium loss achieved was related to the elevation of plasma-renin activity. When the low plasma-renin-activity group was subjected to protracted sodium depletion, plasma-renin activity rose, and saralasin infusion then induced falls in blood pressure. These results agree with the animal experiments and other human investigations previously discussed. It is clear that responsiveness of normal and hypertensive animals and man to angiotensin-receptor blockage is critically dependent on sodium intake. It is, therefore, meaningless to categorize patients as having angiotensin-dependent hypertension without reference to sodium status (Figure 6). Angiotensin dependence of blood pressure can apparently occur in either normal subjects or in diseased patients whenever they become volume or sodium depleted.

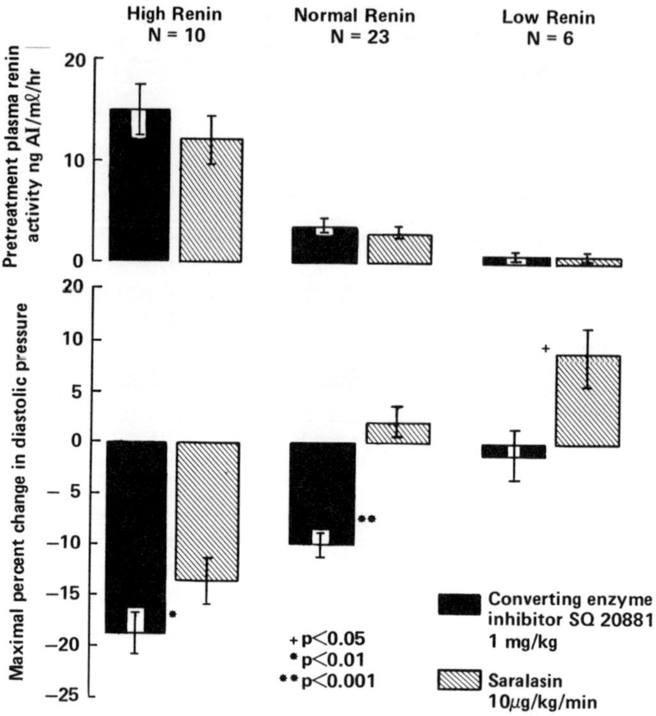

FIGURE 5.   Levels of plasma-renin activity for each renin subgroup prior to angiotensin blockade (upper panel), and the maximal induced per cent change in diastolic pressure for each treatment group directly below (lower panel). Mean values ± standard error are shown for renin and blood pressure measurements. (From Case, D. B., Wallace, J. M., Keim, H. J., Weber, M. A., Drayer, J. I. M., White, R. P., Sealey, J. E., Laragh, J. H., *Am. J. Med.*, 61, 790, 1976. With permission.)

The responses of a group of patients with apparently significant renovascular hypertension to saralasin infusion (10 μg/kg/min) has been compared while sodium replete and deplete.[13] In the sodium replete state, blood pressure was unchanged by infusion of saralasin for 1 hr. However, after sodium depletion, the drug induced large falls in blood pressure, frequently to normal levels. This drop of blood pressure was due to a fall in total peripheral resistance. Although there were small early increases in heart rate and cardiac output, these were not sustained and returned to below control values during the hypotensive period. This interesting lack of reflex tachycardia during saralasin-induced hypotension has been noted by other investigators[14] and could represent blockade of some of the autonomic effects of angiotensin.

The results of infusing saralasin into 418 untreated hypertensive subjects 4 hr after they were given 40 mg of i.v. frusemide revealed that the change in the blood pressure during the infusion correlated inversely with the plasma-renin activity before the procedure (Figure 7). A pressor response occurred in 23% of the subjects and was associated with low initial plasma-renin-activity values. In normal subjects taking low sodium, unrestricted, or high sodium diets, saralasin caused, respectively, a fall, no change, or a rise in blood pressure. The hypertensive patients who showed rises in blood pressure with saralasin also had greater sensitivity to the pressor effect of angiotensin II.

There are several possible mechanisms for the pressor effect of saralasin. Evidence that the analogue is a partial agonist on vascular smooth muscle, particularly of the

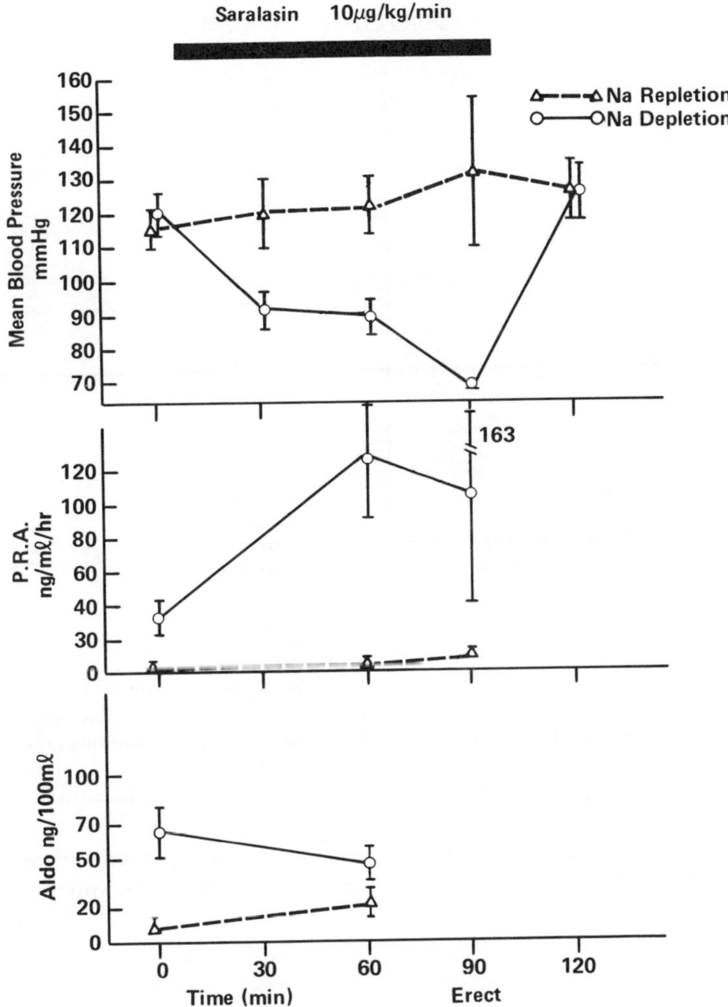

FIGURE 6.   Changes in blood pressure (BP), plasma-renin activity (PRA), and plasma aldosterone (Aldo) during infusion of the angiotensin antagonist in the sodium-depleted and sodium-repleted state in five hypertensive patients. Means and standard errors are shown. (From Gavras, H., Ribeiro, A. B., Gavras, I., and Brunner, H. R., *N. Engl. J. Med.*, 295, 1278, 1976. With permission.)

kidney, was discussed in Volume II, Chapter 1. In addition, various position-8-substituted analogues of angiotensin can release adrenal catecholamines in vitro,[16,17] and saralasin has been reported to induce a hypertensive crisis in a patient with phaeochromocytoma. During the acute pressor response to saralasin in man, plasma norepinephrine concentration rises.[19,20] This suggests that the analogue may either enhance norepinephrine release or inhibit its uptake by sympathetic nerve terminals, either of which could contribute to its acute pressor effect.

Diuretic treatment was used before saralasin testing in some studies.[4,5,15] The interpretation of the results of this combined diuretic-saralasin test is complicated. It is probable that the magnitude of the diuresis achieved, responsiveness of renin release to volume contraction, and hence, the elevation of plasma angiotensin II achieved all can affect the final response to saralasin in these studies. Thus, the degree of sodium deprivation has been shown to affect the results of saralasin testing in hypertensives[12]

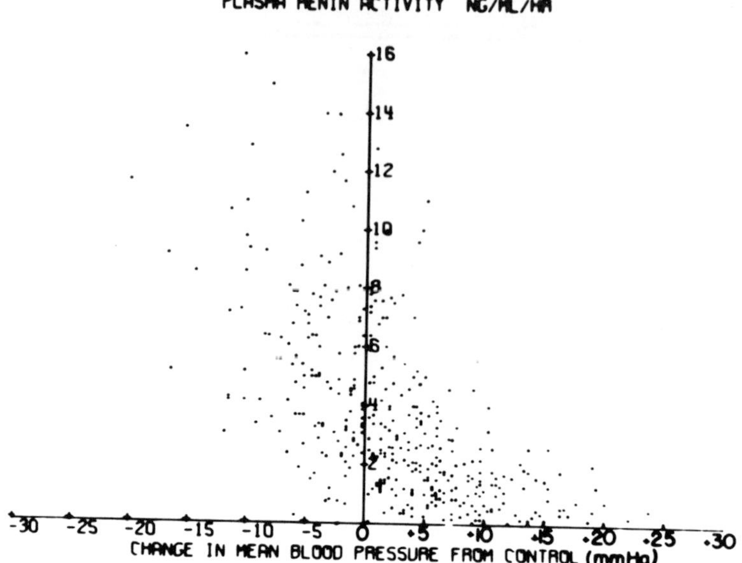

FIGURE 7.   Correlation of changes in mean blood pressure induced by saralasin, 5 μg/kg/min (horizontal axis) with stimulated plasma-renin activity vertical axis) in 418 hypertensive subjects. The mean blood pressures of all readings during and for 6 min after saralasin infusion at 5.0 μg/kg/min were averaged. If a transient rise in blood pressure occurred during the first 6 min of this saralasin infusion, it was not included in the average. (From Anderson, G. H., Streeton, D. H. P., and Dalakos, T. G., *Circ. Res.*, 40, 243, 1977. With permission.)

or normals.[15] A remarkably close relationship has been reported between the basal (presaralasin) plasma angiotensin II concentration and the subsequent fall in blood pressure (Figure 8).[21]

Currently, there is no convincing evidence that testing the acute depressor response to angiotensin-receptor blockers or converting-enzyme inhibitors does anything more than identify patients with high plasma renin and angiotensin II levels at the time of the test. The case for their use as diagnostic tests in hypertension depends on arguments for their rapidity and convenience. Measurements of plasma levels of renin and angiotensin II under standardized conditions probably provide the same information as the use of saralasin or SQ 20881. Although the risks of using these agents appear quite low, they cannot be ignored. There is considerable confusion and controversy as to the use of diuretics before administration of these agents in diagnostic tests. Diuretics complicate the interpretation of the pathophysiological mechanisms involved in responsiveness to blocking agents. Those who use diuretics argue that the combined test has diagnostic value.

An interesting diagnostic use of saralasin as an adjunct to the diagnosis of renal hypertension was suggested by Pettinger and Mitchell.[22] They proposed on theoretical grounds that saralasin should augment any difference in renal venous-renin secretion in patients with renal-artery stenosis, and that the inhibitor might be more effective in aiding lateralization than other hypotensive agents.

At present, it appears that the use of blocking agents is an important research tool in understanding the mechanisms of hypertension. Further evaluation is needed to define the place of these tests in routine clinical use.

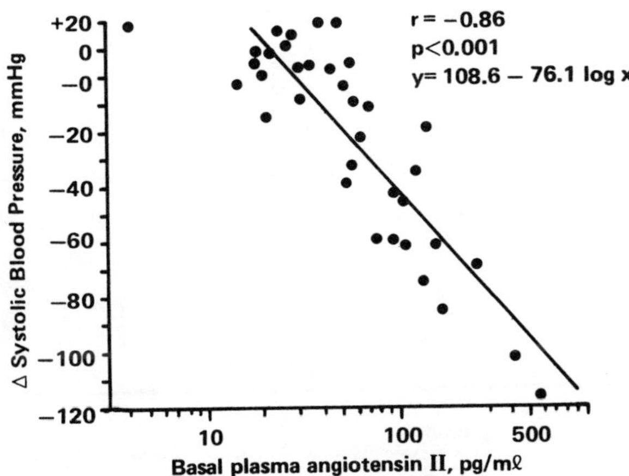

FIGURE 8.   Change in systolic arterial pressure on saralasin administration in relation to the basal (presaralasin) plasma-angiotensin-II level in a group of patients with hypertension of diverse causes. (From Brown, J. J., Brown, W. C. B., Fraser, R., Lever, A. F., Morton, J. J., Robertson, J. I. S., Rosei, E. A., and Trust, P. M., *Prog. Biochem. Pharmacol.*, 12, 230, 1976. With permission.)

II. TREATMENT

A. Severe or Malignant Hypertension

Johnson et al.[23] treated 12 patients with severe hypertension (two with grade IV retinopathy, six with grade III retinopathy, three with dialysis-resistant hypertension associated with chronic renal failure, and one with high-renin essential hypertension) with the converting-enzyme inhibitor SQ 20881 for 5 to 7 days. The drug was given initially as an i.v. bolus of 0.125 mg/kg, and the dose was then doubled every 3 hr until blood pressure was controlled or a maximum dose of 4 mg/kg reached. In nine of the 12 patients, the blood pressure fell virtually to normal after starting the inhibitor. In two of the patients who initially responded only partially, addition of frusemide 40 mg/day produced falls of blood pressure to normal. Of the eight patients with elevated plasma renin activity, all responded well to SQ 20881.

Gavras et al.[24] administered SQ 20881 to four patients with malignant hypertension and 19 with moderately severe hypertension of diverse causes. Sixteen of the 23 had falls in blood pressure with the inhibitor. Blood pressure started to fall within minutes of the adminisration of SQ 20881 as an i.v. bolus and continued to fall further for 1 to 2 hr. A maximum effect was obtained with a dose of 1 mg/kg, and further increases up to 4 mg/kg prolonged the duration, but not the magnitude, of the effect. The longest hypotensive effect lasted for 16 hr. The four patients with malignant hypertension had striking falls of blood pressure from 221/151 (± 6/5) to 172/107 (± 7/5) mmHg, and 12 of the remaining patients responded. None of four patients with primary aldosteronism responded to the inhibitor. Six of the patients were studied before and after sodium depletion. Although blood pressure did not change with this maneuver, the hypotensive response to SQ 20881 was potentiated.

In contrast to these results obtained with SQ 20881, the angiotensin receptor blocker [Sar¹, Ile⁸]-angiotensin II only lowered blood pressure in one of five patients with malignant hypertension.[25] The likely reason that less patients respond to [Sar¹, Ile⁸]-angiotensin II than to SQ 20881 is that this angiotensin analogue is a partial pressor agonist.

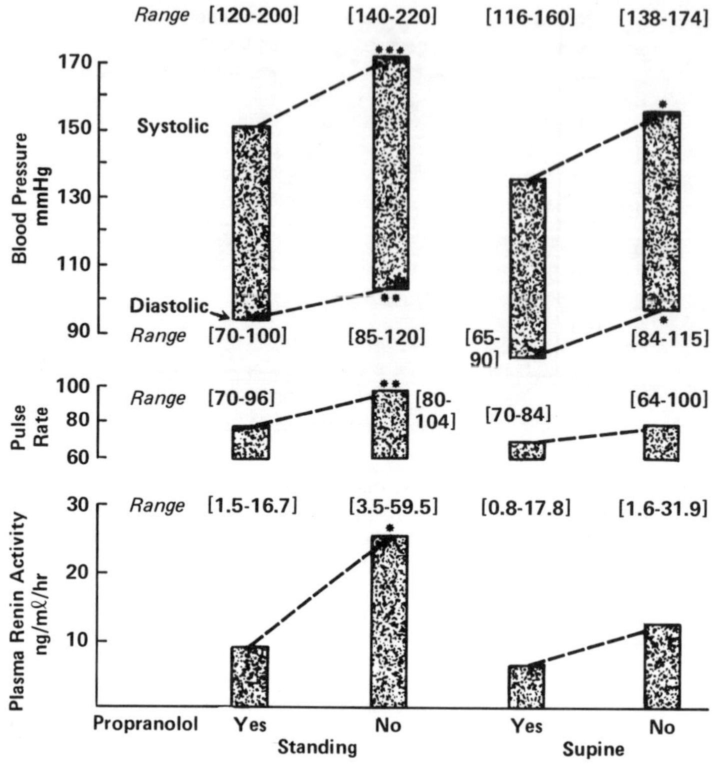

FIGURE 9.   Effect of propranolol withdrawal on blood pressure, pulse
rate, and plasma-renin activity in seven minoxidil-treated patients supine and
standing (*P < 0.05; **P < 0.01; ***P < 0.001). (From Pettinger, W. A.
and Mitchell, H. C., *N. Engl. J. Med.*, 292, 1214, 1975. With permission.)

Although most patients apparently do not have angiotensin-dependent hypertension,
it may become so after treatment with diuretics. In addition, vasodilator drugs may
induce a state where angiotensin plays a role in maintenance of blood pressure. Saralasin infusion has been used to evaluate the role of angiotensin in the interaction of
the vasodilator, minoxidil, and the β-adrenoceptor blocker, propranolol.[14] In seven
patients initially treated with both drugs, propranolol was withdrawn, leading to a rise
in blood pressure and plasma-renin activity (Figure 9). At this stage, five of the seven
patients showed hypotensive responses to saralasin infusion and clearly had an angiotensin-dependent component in their hypertension. After resumption of propranolol,
blood pressure and plasma-renin activity fell, and the hypotensive response to saralasin
was impaired or abolished. These results indicate that in patients treated with a vasodilator angiotensin may contribute to the maintenance of blood pressure. The use of
a β-adrenoceptor blocker concurrently with the vasodilator leads to the suppression of
renin release and loss of the angiotensin-dependence of blood pressure.

At least in this situation, there is some evidence that part of the hypotensive action
of propranolol is mediated by blockade of renin release. This aspect of β-adrenoceptor
blockers is discussed further in Volume I, Chapter 2.

These results indicate that in patients treated with either vasodilators, diuretics, or
both there may be compensatory increases in the activity of the renin-angiotensin system. Although there may have been little or no evidence for participation of angiotensin in blood-pressure maintenance before treatment, these patients may subsequently
have a significant contribution from angiotensin. At this stage, there may be valid

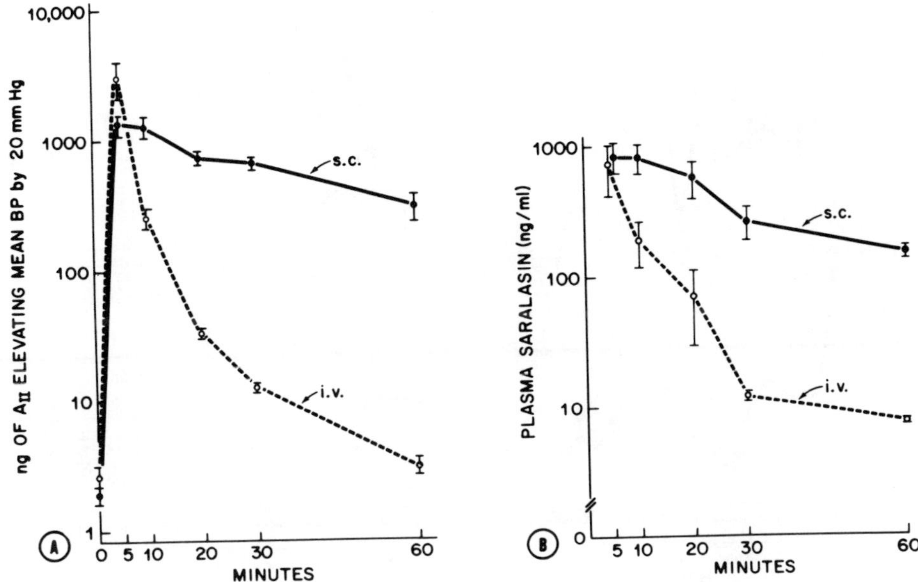

FIGURE 10.   (A) Kinetics of angiotensin by saralasin in the rat. A dose of 10 mg/kg was administered i.v. in saline and s.c. in Pharmagel A. A_{II}, angiotensin II. (B) Kinetics of saralasin in the rat as determined by radioimmunoassay. A dose of 10 mg/kg was administered i.v. in saline or s.c. in Pharmagel A. (From Pettinger, W. A., Keeton, K., and Tanaka, K., *Clin. Pharmacol. Ther.*, 17, 146, 1975. With permission.)

B. Therapeutic Combinations of Angiotensin Blockers with Diuretics or Vasodilators

theoretical and practical reasons to add an agent which blocks the action of the renin-angiotensin system. At present, there are no orally active angiotensin-receptor blocking agents suitable for this purpose. A recently developed orally active converting-enzyme inhibitor discussed in Volume II, Chapter 1 could be the prototype of new drugs whose antihypertensive application, in conjunction with other drugs, could be very broad.

It seems possible that the greatest therapeutic application of agents which block the renin-angiotensin system might be in hypertensive patients being treated with other drug combinations. Less common applications might be in patients with other high-renin forms of hypertension, such as that associated with accelerated or malignant hypertension or renal-artery stenosis.

III. PHARMACOKINETICS

There are very few reports relating the plasma levels of the peptide blockers of the renin-angiotensin system to their biological effects. This is probably due to the technical difficulties of measuring low concentrations of these compounds in biological fluids.

A radioimmunoassay for saralasin has been developed which shows very little cross-reactivity to angiotensin I, angiotensin II, or [des Asp^1]-angiotensin II and is sufficiently sensitive for pharmacokinetic studies.[26] The antibody specificity was directed to the C-terminus of the molecule and cross-reactivity occurred with other 8-alanyl-substituted angiotensin derivatives, was greatly reduced with Ile^8-analogues, but not markedly affected by modifications at the N-terminus. After injection of saralasin, 10 mg/kg into rats, the pharmacological half-life was followed by serial determinations of angiotensin-I dose-response curves and its chemical half-life by plasma-saralasin assays. When the peptide was injected i.v., the pharmacological half-life was 3.9 min. which agreed well with the chemical half-life in plasma of 4.2 min (Figure 10A). After

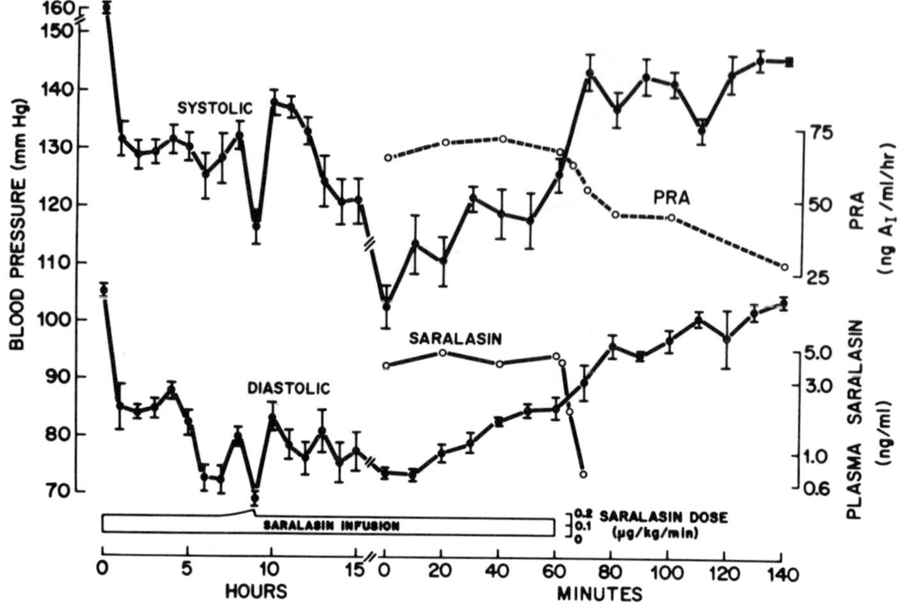

FIGURE 11.   The antihypertensive effect of overnight infusion of saralasin in a 64-year-old male with hypertension poorly controlled by multiple drugs and associated with high PRA levels. (From Pettinger, W. A., Keeton, K., and Tanaka, K., *Clin. Pharmacol. Ther.*, 17, 146, 1975. With permission.)

s.c. injection of saralasin suspended in gelatin, both the half-lives were prolonged to 23 and 20 min, respectively (Figure 10B).

Saralasin was infused at 0.1 to 20μg/kg/min into nine hypertensive patients whose blood pressure was poorly controlled on multiple antihypertensive drugs.[26] In 3 of the patients, blood pressure fell to normal, and this effect could be sustained during a 15 hr infusion in 1 patient (Figure 11). On terminating the infusion in three responsive patients, blood pressure promptly returned to control values with half-lives of systolic and diastolic pressure of 7.8 ± 0.9 and 8.5 ± 1.5 min, respectively. The disappearance of plasma saralasin after stopping the infusion was 5.0 ± 0.4 minutes. Similarly, after bolus injections of the drug varying from 1 to 100 μg/kg, the biochemical half-life of 3.6 ± 0.6 min was comparable to the half-life of return of systolic and diastolic pressure to control levels of 4.1 ± 0.5 and 4.3 ± 0.5 min, respectively.[26]

These results show a good correlation between biological and chemical half-lives of saralasin and suggest that the drug has a rapid, short-lived effect directly related to its plasma concentration. There was no detectable difference in the pharmacokinetics of the drug between the patients responsive or unresponsive to the hypotensive effects of the drug, indicating that differences in metabolism of the peptide are not responsible for differences in response.

IV. A NEW CLASS OF ORALLY ACTIVE CONVERTING-ENZYME INHIBITORS

The design and synthesis of a new class of potent orally active converting-enzyme inhibitors by the Squibb group[27] was a triumph of molecular pharmacology and was described in Volume II, Chapter 1. These compounds have considerable experimental application and may prove to be of therapeutic importance. The most potent member of this group is a substituted amino acid, D-2-methyl-3-mercaptopropanoyl-L-proline

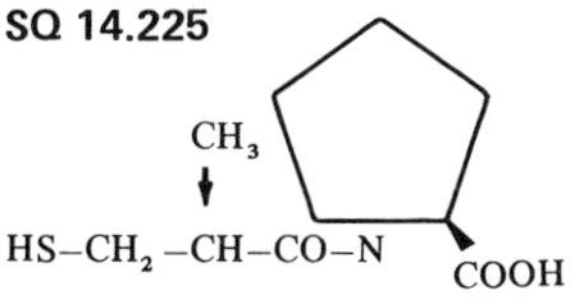

SQ 14.225

CH$_3$

HS–CH$_2$–CH–CO–N   COOH

FIGURE 12.   Structure of SQ
14225   (D-2-methyl-3-mercap-
topropanoyl-L-proline).

(SQ 142252, Figure 12). In 14 male volunteers, SQ 14225 caused a significant blockade of converting enzyme within 15 min of oral administration.[28] The magnitude and duration of the effect was dose-related, and after 20 mg, complete blockade was observed for at least 2 hr and partial inhibition for 4 hr (Figure 13). No adverse effects of the drug were noted. Basal blood pressure and heart rate were not altered. Plasma renin rose after larger doses of the drug (5 to 20 mg). The pressor responsiveness to angiotensin II was not altered.

There have recently been three reports concerning the use of this drug in the treatment of hypertension. Gavras et al.[29] treated six patients with essential hypertension and six patients with renovascular hypertension. Treatment was discontinued in one patient who developed fever, tachycardia, bronchospasm, and a maculopapular rash 7 days after beginning treatment. Seven patients took the drug for 20 to 30 days, and four patients with previously refractory hypertension continued to take the drug. In all patients, the diastolic blood pressure fell to less than 95 mmHg in hospital. In the patients with essential hypertension, the blood pressure fell from a mean of 166/110 mmHg to a mean of 136/91 mmHg, while in the patients with renovascular hypertension, the pressure fell from 189/109 to 135/84 mmHg. There was no correlation between the pretreatment levels of plasma renin and the hypotensive response. Patients categorized as low- , normal- , and high-renin types, responded equally well to the drug (Figure 14). With the one exception noted above, there were no adverse reactions. Plasma-renin activity rose very considerably during treatment, the rise in PRA occurring within three hr of the ingestion of the first dose. There was a correlation between the fall in mean blood pressure and the rise in PRA (Figure 15). There was a tendency for the PRA to fall with continued treatment, although in all cases, the levels remained substantially above the pretreatment levels. There was no significant change in sodium balance, and the serum sodium was unaltered. However, serum potassium increased because potassium excretion fell. Plasma aldosterone levels also fell substantially.

Brunner et al.[30] noted very similar findings in a group of patients who included six patients with renal failure. Fourteen patients were treated chronically for periods up to 6 months with satisfactory control of blood pressure. These workers also found that the concomitant use of diuretics enhanced the depressor responses to SQ 14225.

Bravo et al.[31] found similar changes in 17 patients given SQ 14225. They also found that the falls in blood pressure were due predominantly to falls in total peripheral resistance, with little change in cardiac index. Baroreceptor responses were not altered.

These preliminary results indicate that the use of an angiotensin converting-enzyme inhibitor promises to be a major advance in antihypertensive drug treatment. Many of the effects of this interesting compound clearly relate to inhibition of converting enzyme. However, the exact mechanism by which the fall in blood pressure is induced is not certain, The fact that patients with low plasma-renin levels respond as well as those with high suggests that a fall in circulating levels of angiotensin II is unlikely to be the whole explanation for the antihypertensive effect. Other possible explanations are accumulation of bradykinin, inhibition of angiotensin II formation at some local

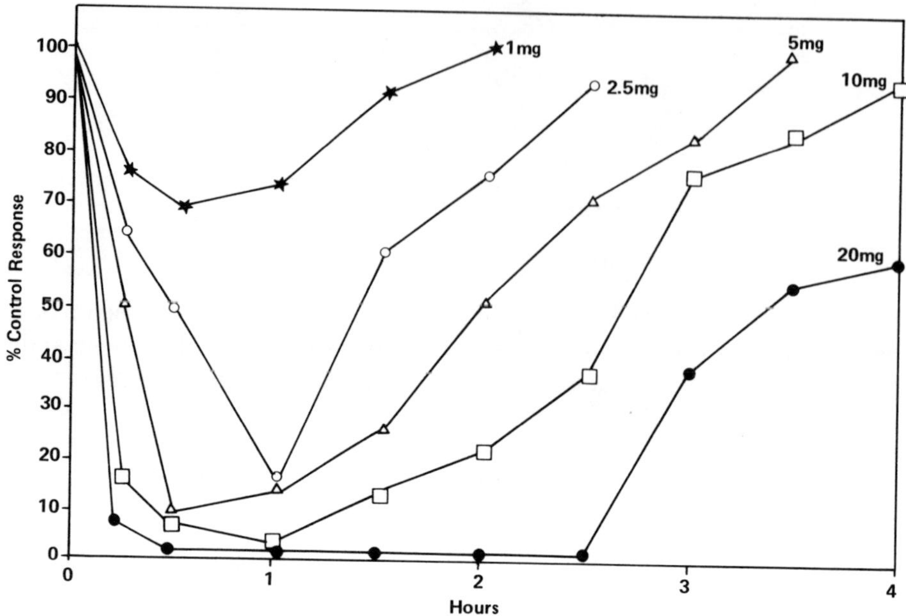

FIGURE 13.   Inhibition of systolic pressor responses to angiotensin I in 14 healthy men after incremental doses of oral SQ 14225. Values on the ordinate represent percentage of control response obtained before administration of the angiotensin-converting-enzyme inhibitor (time 0). Mean responses of three men are shown for each dose except 20 mg where data are derived from 2 volunteers only. (From Ferguson, R. K., Turini, G. A., Brunner, H. R., Gavras, H., and McKinstry, J, *Lancet*, 1, 775, 1977. With permission.)

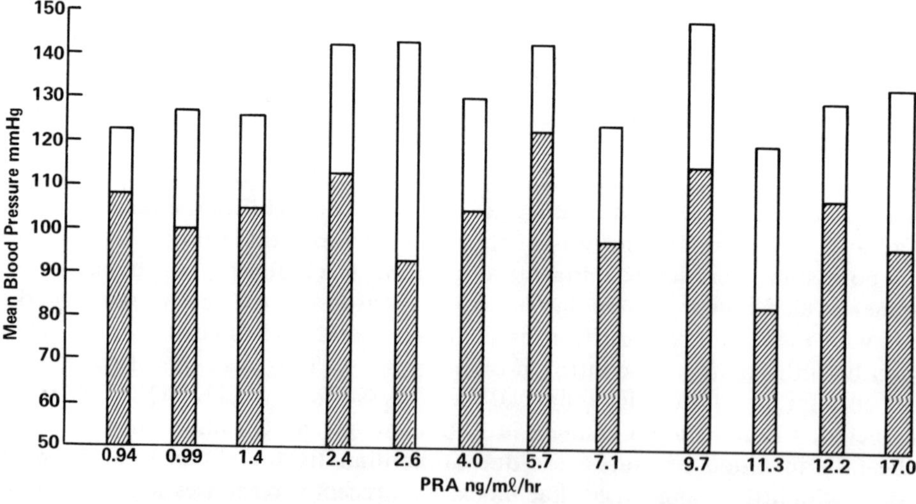

FIGURE 14.   Mean blood pressure (BP) before and during (hatched area) converting-enzyme inhibition with SQ 14225 in relation to pretreatment plasma-renin activity (PRA) in individual patients. (From Gavras, H., Brunner, H. R., Turini, G. A., Kershaw, G. R., Tifft, C. P., Cuttelod, S., Gavras, I., Vukovich, R. A., and McKinstry, D. N., *N. Engl. J. Med.*, 298, 991, 1978. With permission.)

site within the vascular system or brain, or the reduction in aldosterone levels noted by all workers.

The enhancement of the effects of SQ 14225 by the concomitant use of diuretics is

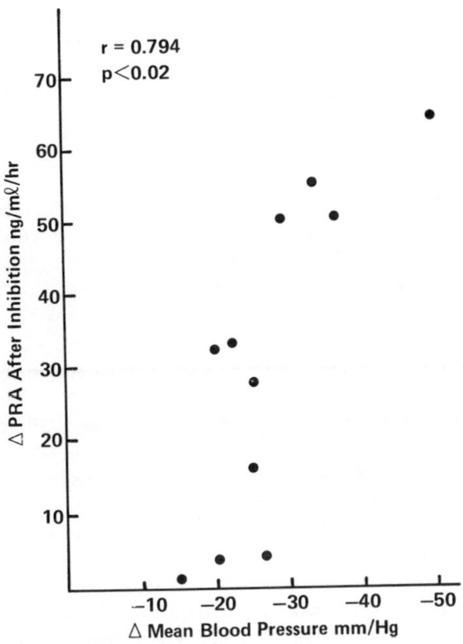

FIGURE 15.   Correlation between fall in mean blood pressure (BP) and rise in plasma-renin activity (PRA) during converting-enzyme inhibition with SQ 14225. (From Gavras, H., Brunner, H. R., Turini, G. A., Kershaw, G. R., Tifft, C. P., Cuttelod, S., Gavras, I., Vukovich, R. A., and McKinstry, D. N., *N. Engl. J. Med.*, 298, 991, 1978. With permission.)

probably related to the renin-angiotensin system. It is consistent with the observations of Leonetti et al.[32] and of Ibsen et al.,[33] both of whom have reported that the use of diuretics leads, in some patients, to elevations of plasma-renin activity and to an enhanced response to the angiotensin-receptor blocking agent saralasin. These observations suggest that the antihypertensive effect of diuretic drugs may be limited in some patients by the development of angiotensin-dependent hypertension, which would no doubt lead to exaggerated depressor responses to inhibition of angiotensin converting enzyme.

Provided that this compound has low toxicity, it seems likely that it will prove useful, not only in patients with refractory angiotensin-dependent hypertension but also possibly in the treatment of essential hypertension. It seems likely, also, that the use of this compound will give further insight into the pathogenesis of hypertension.

REFERENCES

1. Brunner, H. R., Gavras, H., Laragh, J. H., and Keenan, R., Angiotensin-II blockade in man by Sar¹-Ala⁸-angiotensin II for understanding and treatment of high blood pressure, *Lancet*, 2, 1045, 1973.
2. Donker, A. J. M. and Leenen, F. H. H., Infusion of angiotensin-II analogue in two patients with unilateral renovascular hypertension, *Lancet*, 2, 1535, 1974.

3. Streeten, D. H. P., Anderson, G. H., Freiberg, J. M., and Dalakos, T. G., Use of an angiotensin II antagonist (saralasin) in the recognition of "angiotensinogenic" hypertension, *N. Engl. J. Med.,* 292, 657, 1975.

4. Streeten, D. H. P., Anderson, G. H., and Dalakos, T. G., Angiotensin blockade: its clinical significance, *Am. J. Med.,* 60, 817, 1976.

5. Marks, L. S., Maxwell, M. H., and Kaufman, J. J., Saralasin bolus test. Rapid screening procedure for renin-mediated hypertension, *Lancet,* 2, 784, 1975.

6. Case, D. B., Wallace, J. M., Keim, H. J., Sealey, J. E., and Laragh, J. H., Usefulness and limitations of saralasin, a partial competitive agonist of angiotensin II for evaluation of renin and sodium factors in hypertensive patients, *Am. J. Med.,* 60, 825, 1976.

7. Case, D. B., Wallace, J. M., Keim, H. J., Weber, M. A., Drayer, J. I. M., White, R. P., Sealey, J. E., and Laragh, J. H., Estimating renin participation in hypertension: superiority of converting enzyme inhibitor over saralasin, *Am. J. Med.,* 61, 790, 1976.

8. MacGregor, G. A. and Dawes, P. M., Angiotensin II blockade in hypertensive dialysis patients, *Prog. Biochem. Pharmacol.,* 12, 190, 1976.

9. Lifschitz, M. D., Kirschenbaum, M. A., Rosenblatt, S. G., and Gibney, R., Effect of saralasin in hypertensive patients on chronic hemodialysis, *Ann. Intern. Med.,* 88, 23, 1978.

10. Baer, L., Parra-Carrillo, J. Z., Radichevich, I., and Williams, G. S., Detection of renovascular hypertension with angiotensin II blockade, *Ann. Intern. Med.,* 86, 257, 1977.

11. Thomas, D., Ball, S. G., and Lee, M. R., Failure of saralasin to predict a response to surgery in renovascular hypertension, *Lancet,* 1, 724, 1977.

12. Gavras, H., Ribeiro, A. B., Gavras, I., and Brunner, H. R., Reciprocal relation between renin dependency and sodium dependency in essential hypertension, *N. Engl. J. Med.,* 295, 1278, 1976.

13. Fagard, R., Amery, A., Lijnen, P., Reybrouck, T., and Billiet, L., Haemodynamic effects of Sar¹-Ala⁸-angiotensin II in patients with renovascular hypertension, *Prog. Biochem. Pharmacol.,* 12, 242, 1976.

14. Pettinger, W. A. and Mitchell, H. C., Renin release, saralasin and the vasodilator-beta-blocker drug interaction in man, *N. Engl. J. Med.,* 292, 1214, 1975.

15. Anderson, G. H., Streeton, D. H. P., and Dalakos, T. G., Pressor response to 1-Sar-8-Ala-angiotensin II (saralasin) in hypertensive patients, *Circ. Res.,* 40, 243, 1977.

16. Peach, M. J. and Ober, M. J., Inhibition of angiotensin-induced adrenal catecholamine release by 8-substituted analogs of angiotensin II, *J. Pharmacol. Exp. Ther.,* 190, 49, 1974.

17. Peach, M. J. and Ackerly, J. A., Angiotensin antagonists and the adrenal cortex and medulla, *Fed. Proc. Fed. Am. Soc. Exp. Biol.,* 35, 2502, 1976.

18. Dunn, F. G., de Carvalho, J. G. R., Kem, D. C., Higgins, J. R., and Frohlich, E. D., Phaeochromocytoma crisis induced by saralasin, *N. Engl. J. Med.,* 295, 605, 1976.

19. Vlachakis, N. D., Ribeiro, A. B., and Krakoff, L. R., Effect of saralasin upon plasma catecholamines in hypertensive patients, *Am. Heart J.,* 95, 78, 1978.

20. McGrath, B. P., Ledingham, J. G. G., and Benedict, C. R., Plasma catecholamines and the pressor response to Sar¹-Ala⁸-angiotensin II in man, *Clin. Sci. Mol. Med.,* 53, 341, 1977.

21. Brown, J. J., Brown, W. C. B., Fraser, R., Lever, A. F., Morton, J. J., Robertson, J. I. S., Rosei, E. A., and Trust, P. M., The effects of the angiotensin II antagonist saralasin on blood pressure and plasma aldosterone in man in relation to the prevailing plasma angiotensin II concentration, *Prog. Biochem. Pharmacol.,* 12, 230, 1976.

22. Pettinger, W. A. and Mitchell, H. C., Angiotensin antagonists as diagnostic and pharmacologic tools, *Prog. Biochem. Pharmacol.,* 12, 203, 1976.

23. Johnson, J. G., Black, W. D., Vukovich, R. A., Hatch, F. E., Friedman, B. I., Blackwell, C. F., Shenouda, A. N., Share, L., Shade, R. E. Acchiardo, S. R., and Muirhead, F. E., Treatment of patients with severe hypertension by inhibition of angiotensin converting enzyme, *Clin, Sci. Mol. Med.,* 48, 53s, 1975.

24. Gavras, H., Brunner, H. R., Laragh, J. H., Gavras, I., and Vukovich, R. A., The use of angiotensin-converting enzyme inhibitor in the diagnosis and treatment of hypertension, *Clin. Sci. Mol. Med.,* 48, 57s, 1975.

25. Yamamoto, T., Doi, K., Ogihara, T., Ichihara, K., Hata, T., and Kumahara, Y., Changes of blood pressure, plasma renin activity and plasma aldosterone concentration following the infusion of Sar¹-Ile⁸angiotensin II in hypertensive, fluid and electrolyte disorders, *Prog. Biochem. Pharmacol.,* 12, 174, 1976.

26. Pettinger, W. A., Keeton, K., and Tanaka, K., Radioimmunoassay and pharmacokinetics of saralasin in the rat and hypertensive patients, *Clin. Pharmacol. Ther.,* 17, 146, 1975.

27. Cushman, D. W., Chung, H. S., Sabo, E. F., and Ondetti, M. A., Design of potent competitive inhibitors of angiotensin-converting enzyme. Carboxylalkanoyl and mercaptoalkanoyl amino acids, *Biochemistry,* 16, 5484, 1977.

28. Ferguson, R. K., Turini, G. A., Brunner, H. R., Gavras, H., and McKinstry, D., A specific orally active inhibitor of angiotensin-converting enzyme in man, *Lancet*, 1, 775, 1977.

29. Gavras, H., Brunner, H. R., Turini, G. A., Kershaw, G. R., Tifft, C. P., Cuttelod, S., Gavras, I., Vukovich, R. A., and McKinstry, D. N., Antihypertensive effect of the oral angiotensin converting-enzyme inhibitor, SQ 14225 in man, *N. Engl. J. Med.*, 298, 991, 1978.

30. Brunner, H. R., Turini, G. A., Waeber, B., Chappuis, P., and McKinstry, D. N., Long-term treatment of hypertension in man by an orally active converting enzyme inhibitor, *Clin. Sci. Mol. Med.*, (Suppl.), in press, 1978.

31. Bravo, E. L., Tarazi, R. C., Cody, R. J., and Fouad, F. M., Converting enzyme inhibition with an orally active compound in hypertensive man, *Clin. Sci. Mol. Med.*, (Suppl.), in press, 1978.

32. Leonetti, G., Tergoli, L., Sala, C., Bianchini, C., Sernesi, L., and Zanchetti, A., Relationship between the hypotensive and renin-stmulating actions of diuretic therapy in hypertensive patients, *Clin. Sci. Mol. Med.*, (Suppl.), in press, 1978.

33. Ibsen, H., Leth, A., Hollnagel, H., Kappelgaard, A. M., Damjaer Nielsen, M., and Giese, J., Functional significance of angiotensin II in essential hypertension — plasma angiotensin II concentration as a predictor of response to thiazide treatment, *Clin. Sci. Mol. Med.*, (Suppl.), in press, 1978.

Chapter 6

REMEDIABLE SECONDARY HYPERTENSION

I. INTRODUCTION

The mechanisms which lead to high blood pressure are complex, and those which cause essential hypertension in man have not yet been finally unravelled. In human hypertension, however, there are a number of clearly definable pathological processes which may lead to high blood pressure; successful treatment of these conditions often rapidly reverses the hypertension. Examples of such processes are stenosis of the major renal arteries or their branches, renin secreting tumors, primary aldosteronism, phaeochromocytoma, and coarctation of the aorta. In most of these examples, surgical correction is often possible, and often such treatment is followed by a cure. These patients form an important minority in the hypertensive population. Although together they probably account for <10% of human hypertension, they are important for two reasons. First, they confirm that, in some instances, hypertension may be the result of a single process, which leads to the hope that other patients now classified as having essential hypertension may ultimately prove to have an isolated and treatable cause. Second, they are important because they confirm that in hypertension, as in other diseases, cure of the underlying pathological process is preferable to symptomatic relief, however effective this may be in most patients. The present chapter reviews the diagnosis and management of these disorders.

II. RENAL ARTERY STENOSIS (RENOVASCULAR HYPERTENSION)

Partial obstruction of the renal arterial supply to the kidney often causes hypertension in experimental animals, and there is clear evidence that, in man, this pathological process may likewise cause hypertension. A distinction needs to be made between those cases in which the arterial obstruction causes the hypertension and those in whom renal artery stenosis, although demonstrable, is not apparently responsible for the rise in blood pressure.

Estimates of the frequency of renovascular hypertension vary with the type of referral pattern and the extent of the investigation carried out. However, in the Cooperative Study of Renovascular Hypertension,[1] renal arterial lesions were found in 36% of 2442 hypertensive patients; of these, 63% were due to atherosclerotic lesions, and 32% were due to arterial dysplasias. Atherosclerotic lesions were much more common in the patients aged above 50, while arterial dysplasias occurred much more frequently below the age of 40 and were particularly common in women. This incidence of renal arterial lesions probably does not reflect the frequency of true renovascular hypertension, for Holley et al.,[2] in an autopsy study of normotensive patients at the Mayo Clinic, reported moderate-to-severe renal arterial stenosis in 49% of 256 patients. Eyler et al.[3] found radiological evidence of renal arterial abnormalities in about one third of normotensive patients and in almost two thirds of hypertensive patients. These data make it evident that the finding of renal arterial obstruction of moderate or severe degree does not necessarily indicate a causal relationship for the hypertension. Foster and Oates,[4] on the basis of radiology, with split renal function tests and renal venous renin assays, found an incidence of renovascular hypertension in 16% of their hypertensive population, which was, however, highly selected because of the particular expertise of this group. Estimates of the incidence of renovascular hypertension suggest that about 4 to 5% of the hypertensive population may have true renovascular hypertension.[5]

The diagnosis of renovascular hypertension can occasionally be made clinically, but more often, radiological and functional studies are needed to establish the diagnosis.

A. Clinical Manifestations

There are few, if any, clinical characteristics which are absolutely reliable indications that renovascular hypertension is present. Probably, the most comprehensive studies of large numbers of patients are those of the Cooperative Study,[6] of Maxwell et al.,[7] and of Shapiro et al.[8] The single most valuable sign appears to be the presence of an abdominal bruit; patients with renovascular hypertension had an audible bruit in the upper abdomen six to nine times as often as did patients with essential hypertension,[6] although as the authors point out, since essential hypertension is much more common, a bruit is probably more common in patients without renal artery stenosis than those with the lesion.

A reliable history of the recent onset of hypertension is not always easy to elicit[9] and, even when it is present, does not reliably indicate the presence of renovascular hypertension. Similarly, although fibromuscular hyperplasia occurs more commonly in females below 40 and atherosclerotic lesions in males above 50 years of age, almost 20% of patients with essential hypertension develop hypertension before the age of 20 years or after the age of 50.[6] Renovascular hypertension, while often severe and often accompanied by proteinuria, often lacks these features, while, on the other hand, they may occur in essential hypertension. In the author's experience, it is possible to define a group of patients in whom the probability of finding true renovascular hypertension is high. The combination of severe hypertension, an abdominal bruit, proteinuria, hypokalaemia, elevated plasma renin levels, and resistance to most antihypertensive drugs strongly suggests the possibility that renovascular hypertension may be present. Even, however, with this combination of signs, investigation reveals no evidence of renal artery stenosis in about one half of the patients studied.

B. Radiological Features

Intravenous urography often gives a clue to the presence of underlying renal artery stenosis. When the stenosis is unilateral or much more severe on one side than the other, the renal shadow is often reduced in size on the side of the lesion. Differences in renal length exceeding 2 cm do not commonly occur in essential hypertension. Perhaps of more value is the rate of dye excretion, and, for this reason, films need to be taken at 1, 2, 3, and 5 min after the intravenous injection of contrast material. Opacification of the renal calyceal system is usually evident within 1 to 2 min of the injection, and, in the absence of arterial obstruction, both sides become opacified at about the same time. Severe renal artery stenosis may delay the appearance of contrast material for up to 5 min on the affected side. Difference in the density of opacification between the two sides is often an additional useful indication of the presence of arterial obstruction; the density is higher in the affected than the nonaffected side. The difference in density may not be as obvious if the urogram is performed when the patient has been deprived of water for some hours, but can be quite striking if urography is performed during a diuresis, in which case the density of the calyceal opacification on the unaffected side is usually markedly reduced, whereas the inability of the affected kidney to increase water excretion results in a dense pyelogram.

Intravenous urography is a reliable investigation in patients with severe, functionally significant stenosis of one main renal artery, and it is extremely unusual to find a normal pyelogram in this condition. However, it is less reliable in bilateral renal artery stenosis, in patients with stenosis of renal artery segmental branches, or in the presence of multiple main arteries.

Renal arteriography is an essential investigation in patients in whom renovascular hypertension is considered likely to be present. Even in skilled hands, this investigation has a small morbidity, mainly minor and involving injury to the femoral artery into which the arterial catheter is inserted. Renal arteriography should, therefore, only be performed when remedial surgery is being seriously contemplated. It is indicated in all patients in whom drug treatment is difficult and in any patient below the age of 40 years with severe hypertension in whom no other obvious etiological factor is discernible. The investigation should not be performed in patients over the age of 40 years whose blood pressure can be readily controlled by drug treatment since, in these patients, the yield of positive results is very low, and the indications for remediable surgery are controversial.

Unless there is obvious occlusive arterial disease of the lower aorta and femoral arteries, renal angiography is best performed by retrograde catheterization of the abdominal aorta from a femoral artery. When this approach is made difficult by lower aortic disease, catheterization via the brachial artery is usually feasible and is considerably safer than translumbar arteriography, which carries a substantial morbidity and a small mortality.

Contrast medium is injected initially into the abdominal aorta above the origins of the renal arteries. Subsequently, selective renal angiography can be performed (if the initial study suggests that it is necessary) by introducing the catheter into the main renal arteries. Atherosclerotic stenoses characteristically occur at, or close to, the origins of the main renal arteries. Poststenotic dilatation is common. These stenoses are characteristically localized. Fibromuscular hyperplasia of the renal arteries may be unilateral or bilateral and may involve both the main renal arteries and their major branches. A detailed description of these lesions is beyond the scope of this book. The pathological features of renal arterial lesions have been extensively reviewed by Harrison and McCormack,[10] and the radiological features by Bookstein et al.[11]

C. Functional Studies

As has already been indicated, the demonstration of a stenosing lesion in one or both renal arteries does not imply that the lesion is necessarily causing or contributing to the hypertension and does not imply that its relief will cure or ameliorate the hypertension. Functional studies have been devised to evaluate the probability of a cause-and-effect relationship between renovascular disease and the hypertension, mainly to allow selection of those patients likely to be cured by surgery.

1. Split Renal Function Tests

Reduction in renal blood flow leads to avid reabsorption of both water and sodium in the proximal tubule, as described in Chapter 1, even though the glomerular filtration rate may remain normal or only slightly reduced. White[12] and Mueller et al.[13] reported that, in dogs, a clipped kidney excreted significantly less water and sodium than the normal contralateral kidney. This observation was exploited for clinical purposes by Connor et al.[14] Urine collected by bilateral ureteric catheterizaton shows a decreased volume, a reduced sodium concentration, and an increased concentration of creatinine (plus inulin and *p*-amino hippuric acid) from the affected kidney. There is no doubt that this investigation has a high predictive value in that a positive result almost invariably correlates closely with cure of hypertension following surgery. The main disadvantages of the study are technical. Leakage of urine around the ureteric catheters, bleeding, and very low urine flow rates often make interpretation of the data difficult. The test involves epidural anesthesia and is extremely uncomfortable for the patient. Much of the same information can be obtained in a less invasive way by the water

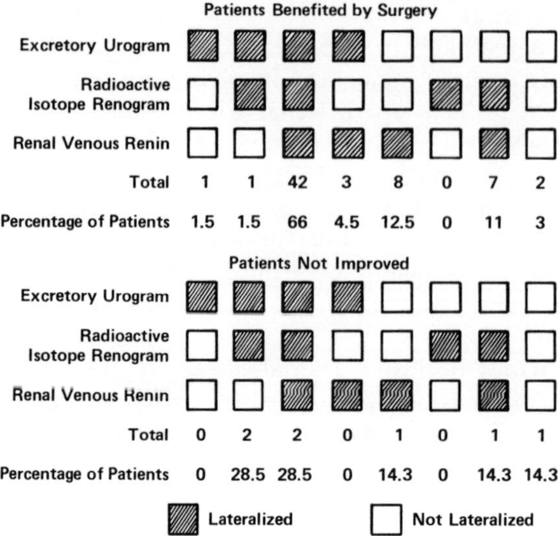

FIGURE 1. Distribution of patients benefited or improved by surgical treatment for renal hypertension according to lateralization of excretory urography, isotope renography, and renal venous renin activity. (From Juncos, L. I., Strong, C. G., and Hunt, J. C., *Arch. Intern. Med.*, 134, 655, 1974. With permission.)

load excretion urogram. Split renal function studies have been abandoned by our group and by many others mainly because of the technical difficulties, and because differential renal venous estimations of plasma renin give comparable predictive results.

2. Plasma Renin Activity

Estimation of plasma renin activity from peripheral venous blood is of little value in the evaluation of renovascular hypertension. Although in many instances they are elevated and can almost always be elevated by sodium depletion, there are many patients with normal values of plasma renin activity in peripheral or inferior vena caval blood who respond well to surgery. Thus, Strong et al.[15] found that peripheral plasma renin levels correlated with the surgical result in only 23% of cases.

Estimations of plasma renin activity in the venous blood from both kidneys seems to be the most reliable method of predicting the results of surgery, particularly if the study is performed after a period of sodium depletion.[15] In patients likely to be cured or improved by surgery, the renin concentration in venous blood from the affected side exceeds that from the unaffected side by a ratio of 1:5:1 or greater. Juncos et al.[16] reported that lateralization by this method successfully predicted the outcome of surgery in 66 of 74 patients; in five of those not successfully lateralized, bilateral lesions were present (Figure 1).

III. INFUSION OF ANGIOTENSIN ANTAGONISTS

The angiotensin analogue, [Sar,[1] Ile[8]]-angiotensin II (saralasin), has been shown to act as a competitive inhibitor of angiotensin II. Experimental data reported by Pals et al.[17] show that saralasin competitively inhibits the effects of angiotensin II on rabbit aortic strips and in the pithed rat infused with angiotensin II. In the acute phase of hypertension following aortic ligation between the two renal arteries in rats, it produced a dose-dependent fall in blood pressure. In the chronic phase, the fall in blood pressure was much smaller. It had no effect in the spontaneously hypertensive rat, normotensive rate, or rats made hypertensive by Deoxycorticosterone acetate (DOCA) implantation.

In man, infusions of saralasin cause falls of blood pressure which relate closely to pre-existing plasma angiotensin II plasma levels.[18]

It has been claimed that saralasin infusion causes a fall in blood pressure in patients whose hypertension is renin dependent, and the use of saralasin infusion has been suggested as a possible screening device to predict the response to surgery in renovascular hypertension (Streeten et al.[19]). The number of patients studied so far is not large, and a complication in interpretation has been the use of sodium depletion prior to saralasin infusion to increase renin dependency. Even under these circumstances, only one half of the patients in Streeten's series with high plasma renin levels showed a fall in blood pressure during saralasin infusion, including one with renal artery stenosis. Thomas et al.[20] report two patients with renal artery stenosis in whom saralasin failed to induce a fall in blood pressure, even after sodium depletion. In both of these patients, subsequent surgery, performed on the basis of renal venous renin levels, proved curative. It is evident that, although saralasin infusions commonly induce falls in blood pressure in patients with renovascular hypertension, some patients fail to respond. Moreover, since many patients with high renin levels, but without renovascular hypertension, also respond, the value of this study remains uncertain.

The effects of angiotensin antagonists have been reviewed more extensively in Volume II, Chapter 5.

IV. RESULTS OF TREATMENT

When hypertension is severe, and the response to drug treatment is poor, surgical relief of renal artery stenosis is obviously the treatment of choice, irrespective of other considerations. Elderly patients with atherosclerotic lesions of the renal arteries are unattractive surgical candidates because of the presence of widespread vascular disease, but even in these patients, surgical treatment carries less risk and is more likely to prolong life than medical management. In patients with less severe hypertension or in those who have had a satisfactory response to antihypertensive drug treatment, a choice has to be made between continuing medical management and surgery. In patients in whom the findings are unequivocal, repair of the obstruction, either by endarterectomy, bypass, or autotransplantation, is indicated. In older patients, continuing treatment with antihypertensive drugs may be considered as an alternative to surgery, but if these are not entirely satisfactory, surgery should be undertaken.

Hunt et al.[21] have reviewed the long-term results of surgical and medical management of renal artery stenosis (Tables 1 and 2). The results indicate clearly that more medically treated patients died than surgically treated, and the incidence of myocardial infarction, stroke, and renal failure were all higher in medically treated than in surgically treated cases (Table 3). This may reflect, in part, the lower blood pressures achieved in the surgically treated patients. Following successful surgery, improvement is rapid in most cases, although, in a few, a progressive fall of blood pressure may continue for some months or years[16] (Table 4).

V. RENIN-SECRETING TUMORS

A small number of benign tumors of the kidney have been described which secrete

TABLE 1

Results of Surgical Treatment for Renal Artery Stenosis with Hypertension (100 Cases)

| | Follow-up interval for type of stenosis, range and mean (year) | | | | | |
| | Atheromatous (37 patients) | | | Fibromuscular (63 patients) | | |
	1—6	5—10	7—12	1—8	5—12	7—14
Status of patients	(3.6)	(7.0)	(8.8)	(3.0)	(7.0)	(8.8)
Surviving	37	29	26	62	60	58
<90 mmHg diastolic blood pressure with medication						
None	14	13	12	41	39	39
Mild	14	14	12	15	16	15
Taking sympatholytic agents	9	2	2	6	5	4

From Hunt, J. C., Sheps, S. G., Harrison, E. G., Strong, C. G., and Bernatz, P. E., *Arch. Intern. Med.*, 133, 988, 1974.

TABLE 2

Results of Medical Treatment for Renal Artery Stenosis with Hypertension (114 cases)

| | Follow-up interval for type of stenosis, range and mean (years) | | | | | |
| | Atheromatous (44 patients) | | | Fibromuscular (70 patients) | | |
	1—8	5—12	7—14	1—8	5—12	7—14
Status of patients	(3.8)	(7.1)	(9.0)	(3.9)	(7.2)	(9.1)
Dead	3	16	27	0	5	12
Subjected to surgery	2	7	7	2	9	9
Surviving with medication	39	21	10	68	56	49
Blood pressure						
Control[a]	33	15	9	59	48	43
Unsatisfactory	6	6	1	9	8	6

[a] Blood pressure <100 mmHg diastolic most of the time.

From Hunt, J. C., Sheps, S. G., Harrison, E. G., Strong, C. G., and Bernatz, P. E., *Arch. Intern. Med.*, 133, 988, 1974.

renin and lead to hypertension.[22-26] These tumors appear to be adenomas of juxtaglomerular cell tissue and contain high concentrations of renin. The clinical characteristics consist of severe hypertension associated with polyuria, hypokalemia, and very high levels of plasma renin. Most of the patients have been young. In all, the renal arterial tree was normal. The tumors have all been small and, in some cases, have escaped detection radiologically, and in all cases removal of the tumor and in most cases the kidney bearing it have been followed by a prompt fall in blood pressure.

TABLE 3

Cause of Death in 55 Cases of Renal Artery Stenosis with Hypertension

Type of lesion and treatment	No. of patients	Myocardial infarction	Stroke	Renal failure	Other causes
Atheromatous					
Surgical	11	5	3	2	1
Medical	27	18	4	4	1
Fibromuscular					
Surgical	5	1	1	1	2
Medical	12	3	4	4	1
Total	55	27	12	11	5

From Hunt, J. C. Sheps, S. G., Harrison, E. G., Strong, C. G., and Bernatz, P. E., *Arch. Intern. Med.,* 133, 988, 1974.

The diagnosis should be suspected in patients with hypokalemia associated with high plasma renin levels who have no evidence of renovascular hypertension. Renal venous renin levels, in all cases, reveal an abnormally high renin content in the blood from one kidney.

VI. PRIMARY ALDOSTERONISM (CONN'S SYNDROME)

Hypersecretion of aldosterone, due either to an adrenal cortical adenoma or to multinodular hyperplasia of the zona glomerulosa, is now well recognized as a cause of hypertension in man. It appears that the sequence of events is that the excess aldosterone secretion leads to increased sodium reabsorption in the distal collecting tubules with a consequent increase in extracellular fluid volume and an increased urinary potassium excretion. The consequences of this are the development of hypertension and suppression of plasma renin levels, both, presumably, as a result of sodium retention and volume expansion. The precise mechanism by which the hypertension develops is not clear, but may be analogous to the experimental DOCA-salt hypertension in the rat, in which there is early evidence of participation of the autonomic nervous system (Chapter 4). Alternatively, it may be due to increased cardiac output in the early stages[27] or due to the effects of the sodium ion in vascular smooth muscle.[28] It appears that both hypertension and suppression of plasma renin activity appear early in the course of the disease, and it is thought that, in some instances, these may precede significant hypokalemia.[29] The possibility that minor degrees of hyperaldosteronism may be a relatively frequent cause of apparently essential hypertension, particularly in low-renin hypertension, has been discussed in Volume I, Chapter 1. This possibility can not be fully excluded, but, at present, for clinical purposes, the classical syndrome of hypertension, suppressed plasma renin, and persistent hypokalemia with evidence of excess production of aldosterone are needed for the diagnosis of primary aldosteronism.

A. Clinical Features

There are some distinctive clinical features of primary aldosteronism, all of which, however, may not be present, and, in many patients, the only clinical features are those of essential hypertension. The elevation of blood pressure may be modest or severe[30] (Figure 2), and the extent of end organ involvement appears to depend mainly on the height of the blood pressure. Cardiomegaly, myocardial infarction, and stroke may

TABLE 4

Overall Results of Surgery in Renal Hypertension at Different Follow-Up Intervals

	Period of follow-up (months after operation)							
Patients' postoperative status	6	12	18	24	30	36	42	48
No. (and %) cured	48(64.0)	44(59.5)	36(55.3)	24(48.9)	18(58.0)	14(53.8)	11(68.7)	8(100)
No. (and %) improved	20(16.6)	23(31.0)	23(35.4)	19(38.6)	10(32.3)	10(38.5)	5(31.3)	0(0)
No. (and %) benefited by surgery	68(90.6)	67(90.5)	59(90.7)	43(87.7)	28(90.3)	24(92.3)	16(100)	8(100)
No. (and %) unimproved	7(9.4)	7(9.5)	6(9.3)	6(12.3)	3(9.7)	2(7.7)	0(0)	0(0)

Note: For those treated in the latter parts of the 3-year period, a relatively shorter period of follow-up was available.

From Juncos, L. I., Strong, C. G., and Hunt, J. C., *Arch. Intern. Med.,* 134, 655, 1974.

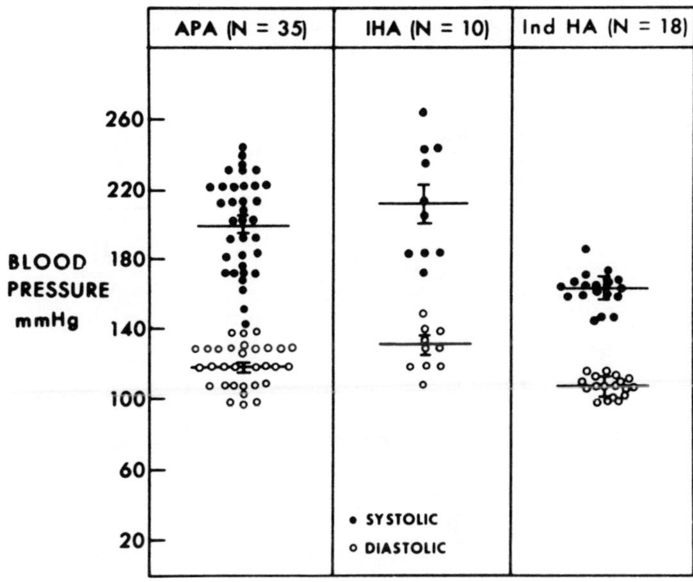

FIGURE 2. Preoperative blood pressure levels in patients with the syndrome of primary aldosteronism (mean ± standard error). (From Biglieri, E. G., Stocklgt, J. R., and Schambelan, M., *Am. J. Med.*, 52, 623, 1972. With permission.)

occur; malignant hypertension with retinal hemorrhages, cotton-wool spots, and papilledema have been reported,[31] but are apparently very rare.

The distinctive clinical features relate to the hypokalemia and to the associated alkalosis. Polyuria, nocturia, and thirst are common symptoms. Muscular weakness, often episodic, is common in advanced cases, and tetany, manifested by carpopedal spasm and by positive Chvostek and Trousseau's signs, may be present.

B. Laboratory Investigations

The classic biochemical features of primary aldosteronism are hypokalemia, elevation of plasma bicarbonate, hypernatremia, suppression of plasma renin activity, and increased excretion or plasma levels of aldosterone. Biglien et al.,[30] whose data are shown in Figures 3, 4 and 5, separated patients with primary aldosteronism into three groups. Those with a cortical adenoma comprised the majority. In these, hypokalemia was invariable, the highest value of serum potassium being 3.5 mmol/l and the mean for the whole group at 2.7 mmol/l. In this group, the serum sodium and bicarbonate levels and aldosterone excretion was higher than in the other two groups, and plasma renin levels were lower. There was, however, some overlap between the aldosterone group and those with idiopathic hyperaldosteronism who had either nodular hyperplasia or microscopic hyperplasia of the zona glomerulosa of the adrenal cortex. These authors stressed that no single biochemical parameter or clinical feature allowed the certain distinction between primary aldosteronism due to adenoma and those with nodular hyperplasia. Similar findings have been reported by Ferris et al.,[32] who also found that, although most of the biochemical abnormalities were more pronounced in patients with adenomata than in those with hyperplasia, there was considerable overlap of the variables. These workers found that a multidimensional computer-assisted quadric analysis enabled complete separation of the tumor and nontumor groups (Figure 6).

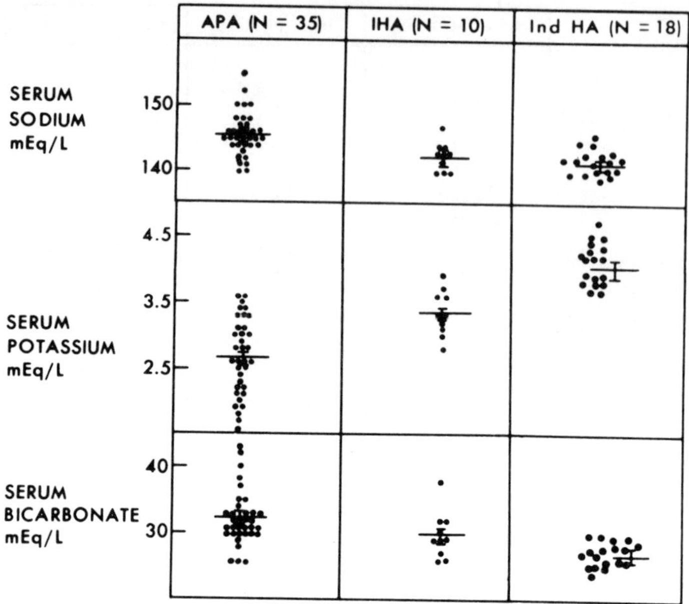

FIGURE 3.   Preoperative serum electrolyte concentrations in patients with the syndrome of primary aldosteronism (mean ± standard error). (From Biglieri, E. G., Stockigt, J. R., and Schambelan, M., *Am. J. Med.*, 52, 623, 1972. With permission.)

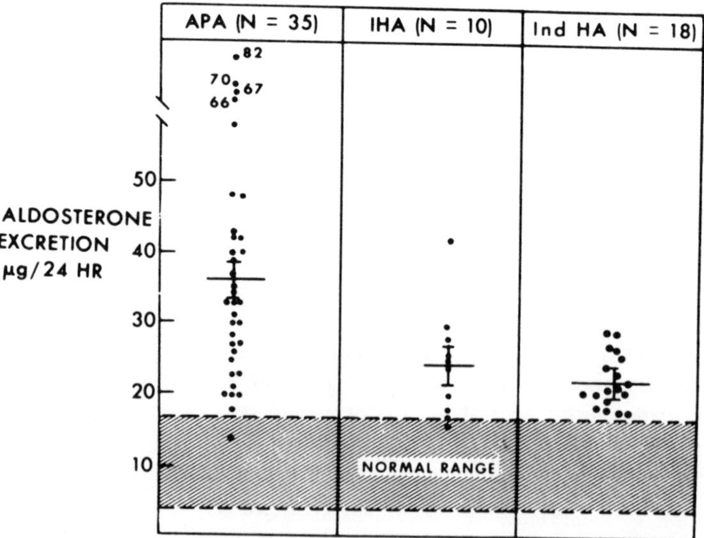

FIGURE 4.   Preoperative aldosterone excretion in patients with the syndrome of primary aldosteronism (mean ± standard error). (From Biglieri, E. G., Stockigt, J. R., and Schambelan, M., *Am. J. Med.*, 52, 623, 1972. With permission.)

The effects of administration of DOCA on aldosterone excretion has been reported by Biglieri et al.[30] in patients with primary aldosteronism. DOCA administration did not suppress aldosterone excretion in patients with adrenocortical adenomata. In patients with nodular hyperplasia, aldosterone excretion was suppressed in only two of

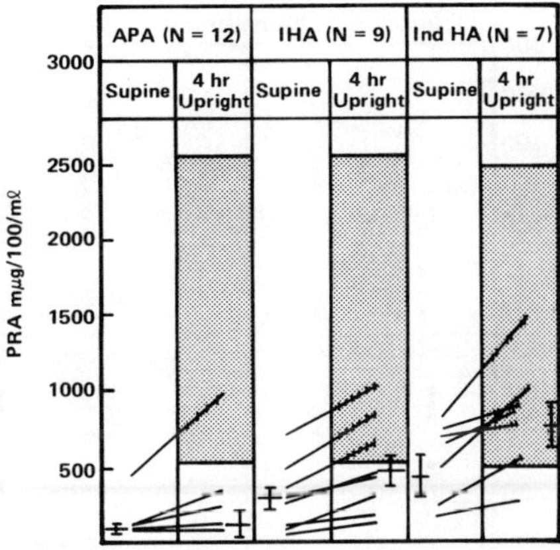

FIGURE 5. Plasma renin activity (PRA) (bioassay) in patients with the syndrome of primary aldosteronism in the supine and standing positions after 3 days of sodium restriction (less than 20 mEq/day) (mean ± standard error). Stippled areas represent the normal range. (From Biglieri, E. G., Stockigt, R., and Schambelan, M., *Am. J. Med.*, 52, 623, 1972. With permission.)

ten patients studied, suggesting that this test is not of value. Biglieri et al.[30] have also described a group, which they designate as indeterminate hyperaldosteronism, who have little evidence of potassium depletion and partly suppressed plasma renin levels with modestly increased aldosterone excretion, which can be fully suppressed by DOCA administration. Since this group of patients has seldom been subjected to adrenal exploration, it is somewhat uncertain whether this group has true primary aldosteronism.

C. Management

The distinction between patients who have primary aldosteromas and those with multinodular hyperplasia is of some importance. Patients with adrenocortical adenoma often respond extremely well to removal of the tumor, with regression of the abnormal biochemical findings and a fall in blood pressure. Conn[33] claims that 70 to 80% of patients with adenomata removed surgically are cured within a period of 3 years from operation and that a further 15 to 20% have a fall in blood pressure, but not to normal, while the remaining group have no response. In the majority of instances, the blood pressure response occurs in the first few weeks postoperatively, but in a few, the fall in blood pressure takes 2 to 3 years to become maximal. Patients with elevated blood urea levels are less likely to have a satisfactory surgical response.[34] Brown et al.[34] have reported that prolonged postoperative treatment with spironolactone in doses of 50 to 400 mg daily (mean 254 mg daily) induced a highly significant reduction in both systolic and diastolic blood pressures in patients with hyperaldosteronism (Figure 7). The drug was equally effective in controlling blood pressure in patients with a cortical adenoma and in patients with multinodular hyperplasia. In both groups of patients, some failed to respond or responded inadequately. Diastolic pressure fell to 95 mm Hg or less in 52 of 67 patients. In 11 patients, the fall in blood pressure was considerably less, and, in 4, no change in blood pressure occurred. There was a close relationship between the antihypertensive effect of spironolactone and that induced by surgery in 32 patients in this series.

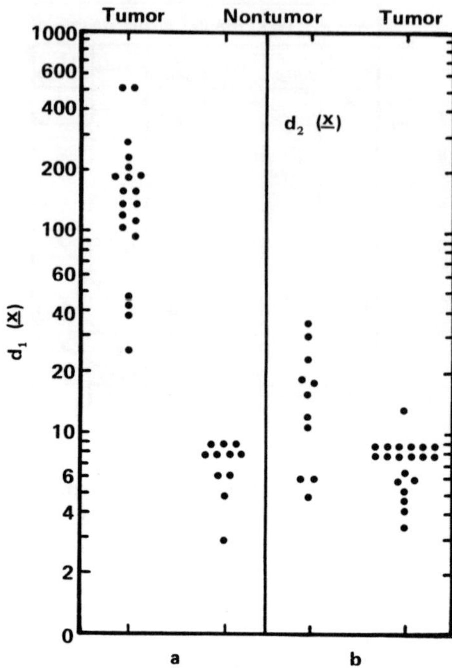

FIGURE 6. Separation by multidimensional computer-assisted quadric analysis of the features of tumor and nontumor patients with primary aldosteronism. (a) Distance of individual patients from center of nontumor quadric, (b) distance of individual patients from center of tumor quadric. (From Ferris, J. B., Brown, J. J., Fraser, R., Kay, A. W., Neville, A. M., O'Muircheartaigh, I. G., Robertson, J. I. S., Symington, T., and Lever, A. F., *Lancet*, 2, 995, 1970. With permission.)

It is evident, therefore, that in patients with a solitary adenoma, the overall responses to removal of the adenoma are satisfactory, particularly in the majority who appear to have a good preoperative antihypertensive response to spironolactone. Because removal of a solitary adenoma is comparatively straightforward and is usually not followed by prolonged insufficiency, surgical removal appears to be the treatment of choice for these patients. Preoperative lateralization of the adenoma can usually be accomplished by adrenal venography,[35] by measurement of aldosterone in adrenal venous blood,[36] or by measurement of the uptake of radioactive cholesterol using scintillation scanning.[37]

The management of patients with multinodular hyperplasia is much less clearcut. Since the lesions are bilateral, unilateral adrenalectomy is seldom effective, and either bilateral adrenalectomy or 80% adrenalectomy is the usual surgical management. Not all patients have satisfactory falls of blood pressure, even following bilateral total adrenalectomy; these are usually those whose blood pressure does not fall preoperatively with spironolactone or amiloride. In view of the satisfactory response to spironolactone in many of these patients, and the fact that those who do not respond to spironolactone are likely to have poor responses to surgery, bilateral adrenalectomy is now seldom performed in most centers.

Long-term treatment with spironolactone induces a reduction in weight, a decrease

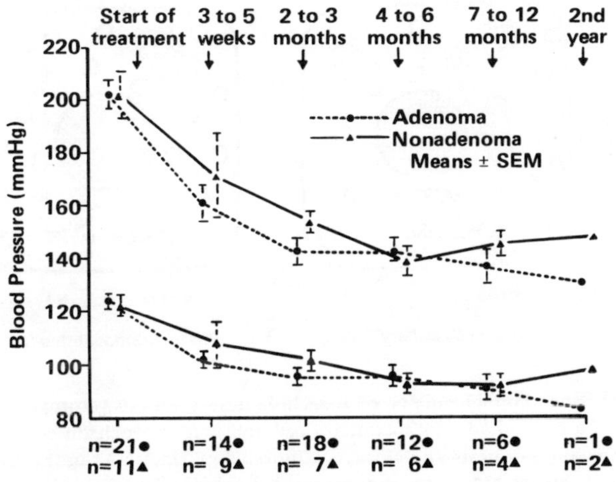

FIGURE 7.   Comparison of preoperative response to spironolactone in 21 patients subsequently shown to have an adrenocortical adenoma with that in 11 patients who did not have
a tumor. The number in each group reviewed at the various
intervals is shown. (From Brown, J. J., Davies, D. L., Freis,
J. B., Fraser, R., Haywood, E., Lever, A. F., and Robertson,
J. I. S., *Br. Med. J.*, 2, 729, 1972. With permission.)

in total body water exchangeable sodium, and an increase in exchangeable potassium.
Plasma renin levels usually rise, sometimes to above the normal range, and aldosterone
excretion either increases or remains unchanged.[34] The changes in plasma electrolytes
in hyperaldosteronism are corrected whether or not the blood pressure falls.

In patients whose blood pressures are not reduced by spironolactone, the drug
should be continued to correct the biochemical abnormalities, and additional antihypertensive drugs should be used to control the hypertension. A few patients do not
respond readily to antihypertensive drug therapy, but the majority can be managed
with no great difficulty.

D. Summary

Although in many patients, there seems to be a clear relationship between hypersecretion of aldosterone and hypertension, a number of unsolved difficulties remain to
be explained. These include the fact that some patients with hyperaldosteronism fail
to respond either to surgery or to spironolactone. While this may be due to the development of secondary changes either in the vascular system or in the kidney, this has
not been proven. The pathogenesis of multinodular hyperplasia of the adrenal cortex
is quite unsolved. The stimulus-inducing hyperplasia does not appear to be either angiotensin or ACTH. Finally, the question as to whether low-renin hypertension is
sometimes due to an excessive production of aldosterone and if so, for what reason
and how frequently, remains controversial, as does the question as to whether true
primary aldosteronism is ever associated with normal levels of serum potassium.

VII. PHAEOCHROMOCYTOMA

Phaeochromocytoma is a rare cause of hypertension. These tumors originate from
chromaffin tissue and synthesize and secrete catecholamines at a high rate. The tumors
are not innervated. The storage of catecholamines within the chromaffin vesicles appears to be normal, but there is a high rate of catecholamine synthesis,[38] which appears

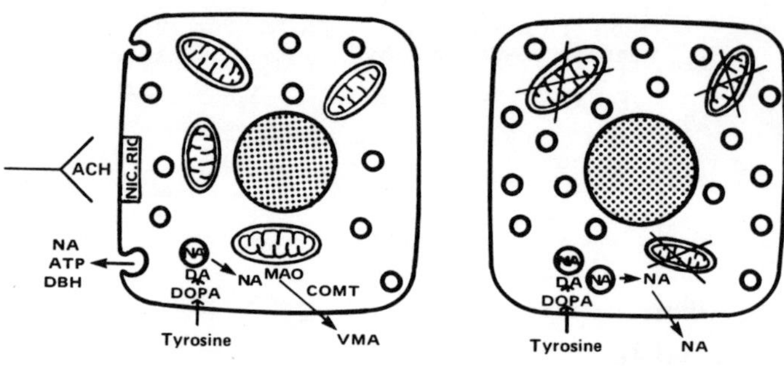

FIGURE 8.   Topochemistry of catecholamine synthesis, storage, and release in a normal adrenal medullary cell and in a phaeochromocytoma cell. After the synthesis and storage of norepinephrine (NA) in the medullary cell, excess NA in the cytoplasm is catabolized by mitochondrial monoamine oxidase (MAO) and possibly cytoplasmic catechol-O-methyltransferase (COMT) to an inactive metabolite that diffuses out of the cell. Release of NA together with ATP and dopamine-β-hydroxylase (DβH) is by nerve-mediated exocytosis from the storage vesicles. After synthesis and storage of NA in the noninnervated phaeochromocytoma cells, excess NA in the cytoplasm formed by excess synthesis is not as extensively catabolized by MAO due to reduced levels of this enzyme, and, therefore, free NA, but not DβH, diffuses out of the cell and into the circulation. (From Louis, W. J., Jarrott, B., and Doyle, A. E., *Pathophysiology and Management of Arterial Hypertension,* Berglund, G., Hansson, K., and Werko, L., Eds., Lundgren and Souer, A. B., Mölndal, Sweden, 1975, 16. With permission.)

to be due to the fact that, in these tumors, the normal inhibitory feedback process by which catecholamine levels inhibit tyrosine hydroxylase activity appears not to operate.

It appears that, in phaeochromocytoma, release of catecholamines is due to diffusion rather than to an exocytotic process, since although plasma catecholamines are elevated, there is no corresponding increase in dopamine-β-hydroxylase.[39] Louis et al.[40] reported that tyrosine hydroxylase, dopa-decarboxylase, and dopamine-β-hydroxylase activities were all 3 to 10 times higher in phaeochromocytoma tissue than in normal adrenal medullary tissue. Activity of monoamine oxidase was only a quarter of that found in normal medullary tissue. The activity of succinate dehydrogenase, a mitochondrial marker, was also reduced, suggesting a reduced number or severe damage to mitochondria in this tumor (Figure 8).

The elevated levels of all the enzymes of the biosynthetic pathway in tumor tissue, together with the reduced activity of monoamine oxidase, would account for the high free level of norepinephrine in the cytoplasm of the tumors and for the fact that newly synthesized norepinephrine is capable of bypassing the saturated stores in the vesicles, thus passing directly into the circulation. It would also explain the fact that provocative agents, such as glucagon and histamine, caused increased catecholamine release by increasing tumor blood flow.

The symptoms and clinical manifestations of phaeochromocytoma are due to the fact that these tumors release large amounts of norepinephrine and often epinephrine into the circulation.

A. Clinical Features

Phaeochromocytoma may occur at any age and with approximately equal frequency in males and females. About 2% of phaeochromocytoma cases are extra-abdominal,

TABLE 5

Mean Plasma Norepinephrine and Blood Pressure Levels in the Various Patient Groups

Patient group	Plasma norepinephrine (ng/ml ± SD)	Systolic blood pressure (mmHg ± SD)	Diastolic blood pressure (mmHg ± SD)
Normotensive (n = 14)	0.20 ± 0.22	128 ± 0.22	77 ± 7.1
Essential hypertension (n = 28)	0.40 ± 0.21[a]	158.1 ± 12.2[a]	104.9 ± 10.1[a]
Labile hypertension (n = 9)	0.22 ± 0.15	104.5 ± 45.9[b]	80 ± 7.6
Depression (n = 5)	0.74 ± 0.09[a]	137 ± 7.2[b]	86 ± 6.3[b]
Phaeochromocytoma (n = 15)	11.1 ± 11.8[a]	183 ± 43.4[a]	116 ± 28.9[a]

[a] Significantly different from normotensive levels; $p < 0.01$.
[b] $p < 0.05$.

mostly within the chest; estimates of the incidence of extra-adrenal tumors vary from 6%[41] to 20%.[42] Multiple tumors are often present.[42] There is a well documented familial incidence often associated with medullary cell carcinomas of the thyroid gland.

The hypertension may be paroxysmal or persistent. In patients with paroxysmal hypertension, the blood pressure is usually nearly normal between attacks. In this group of patients, episodes of headache, sweating, palpitations, which may be rapid or slow, pallor, nausea, trembling, and anxiety occur. The symptoms usually begin abruptly and usually persist for 30 min or less. In a few patients, there may be acute pulmonary edema, hypertensive fits with loss of consciousness, or pain resembling that due to myocardial infarction. The attacks may occur spontaneously, but may be induced by various precipitating factors, such as sneezing, pressure on the abdomen, or coitus.

Less commonly, persistent hypertension may be present, but, in such patients, a careful history usually reveals the presence of paroxysmal symptoms similar to those described above.

Phaeochromocytoma is associated with neurofibromatosis in approximately 10% of tumors.[41] In children, tumors are particularly likely to be multiple. Blood pressure may be normal or slightly raised between attacks and is often very high during paroxysms, often reaching levels such as 280/160 mmHg.

B. Diagnosis

The diagnosis of phaeochromocytoma depends on the demonstration of elevated levels of catecholamines in blood or urine or on the finding of increased metabolic products of catecholamines in the urine. Measurement of urinary norepinephrine and epinephrine is the simplest and, probably, the most reliable assay available. Combined catecholamine excretion is measured in a 24-hr urinary sample by a fluorimetric analysis.[44] It is necessary to ensure that the patient has not taken either l-dopa or α-methyldopa for at least 72 hr before the urine collection. Alternatively, total metanephrine excretion is claimed to be a reliable index of total catecholamine metabolism.[45] Plasma catecholamine and norepinephrine levels are also a reliable diagnostic index (Table 5).[40] Urinary excretion and plasma levels of catecholamines or their metabolites are consistently elevated in patients with phaeochromocytoma, even between episodes of paroxysmal hypertension.

A number of provocative tests for phaeochromocytoma have been described. These include the administration of histamine,[46] tyramine,[47] and glucagon.[48] They have two disadvantages: first, that false-negative and false-positive results occur, although not with great frequency, and second, that the magnitude of the rise in blood pressure may be occasionally extreme. They should be reserved for patients in whom the clinical suspicion that a tumor is present is high, but in whom catecholamine levels are normal. These tests are now seldom used.

Preoperative localization of the tumor is important, since the tumors may be multiple and extra-adrenal. Localization is best performed, if facilities are available, by multiple sampling at various sites from the inferior cava and, if necessary, the superior vena cava.[49] Localization by angiography is best deferred until the presence of a phaechromocytoma has been established biochemically and treatment has been commenced with a combination of an α- and a β-adrenoceptor antagonist, as this minimizes the risk of hypertensive reactions. If the tumor is found to be excreting epinephrine as well as norepinephrine, the probability is overwhelming that it is within the adrenal,[50] although one case of an extra-adrenal tumor which secreted epinephrine has been reported.[51]

The rise in blood pressure during a hypertensive crisis is best managed by the intravenous administration of the α-receptor blocking drug, phentolamine. A dose of 5 mg is usually sufficient to block the hypertensive response, but, if this is not fully effective, the dose can be increased.

The definitive treatment of choice is surgical removal of the tumor. Preoperatively, the blood pressure should be controlled by the combined use of phenoxybenzamine in a dose of 10 to 20 mg twice daily and propranolol in a dose of 10 to 40 mg four times daily. These drugs should be used for about 2 weeks preoperatively and continued until the operation commences. This regime usually prevents the extreme rises of blood pressure which occur during handling of the tumor and may prevent the very large fall of blood pressure which occurs when the tumor is removed. If this fails, phentolamine can be used to control the hypertensive response during handling of the tumor, and the hypotensive response following removal of the tumor can be treated by a slow infusion of angiotensin II in a dose of up to 40 μg/min. It is of interest that successful removal of the tumor leads to an immediate and maintained return of the blood pressure to normal levels, in contrast to the situation in primary aldosteronism.

Phaeochromocytoma is occasionally malignant, and metastases may occur. In such patients, the hypertension can be controlled by the use of tyrosine hydroxylase-blocking drug, α-methyltyrosine,[52] which blocks the biosynthetic pathway by preventing the hydroxylation of tyrosine to deoxy phenyl alanine (DOPA). α-Methyltyrosine acts very rapidly, and both blood pressure and catecholamine excretion fall, usually within 24 to 48 hr.

Recently, the use of labetalol, the combined β- and α-adrenoceptor-blocking drug, has been described in the treatment of patients with phaeochromocytoma.[53] Five patients with phaeochromocytoma were treated with this drug. In four of these patients, the blood pressure could be easily controlled, and, in two of these, the drug provided satisfactory cover during surgical removal of the tumor. The use of labetalol in malignant phaeochromocytoma does not seem to have been described, but it would seem likely that this drug might be preferable to α-methyltyrosine, since the latter induces crystalluria on prolonged administration.

VIII. COARCTATION OF THE AORTA

Coarctation of the aorta consists of a narrowing or, occasionally, an occlusion of the aorta just distal to the origin of the left subclavian artery. It is associated with both systolic and diastolic hypertension in the upper part of the body and, usually, with lower pressures in the trunk and legs. The cause of the hypertension is not clear. It may be renal in origin.

A. Clinical Features

The clasical findings are the presence of hypertension, which may be mild or severe, in the arms and delayed and weak femoral pulses with a reduced blood pressure in the legs; collateral vessels are common and may be best seen in the region of the scapulae. There is commonly an ejection systolic murmur at the base of the heart, which can also be heard above the left scapula.

Patients are often free of symptoms; in severe obstruction, left ventricular enlargement and occasionally heart failure occurs, particularly in infants. Intermittent claudication is sometimes present.

Investigation reveals electrocardiographic and radiological evidence of left ventricular hypertrophy, and the chest film may show rib notching due to the enlarged intercostal arteries. The diagnosis can be confirmed by aortic arch angiography.

Complications include infective endarteritis, dissecting aneurysm, and heart failure. Resection of the coarctation is best undertaken after the pubertal growth has occurred. A fall of blood pressure usually occurs postoperatively, but the blood pressure may remain higher than usual.

REFERENCES

1. **Foster, J. H., Maxwell, M. H., and Franklin, S. S.,** Renovascular occlusive disease. Results of operative treatment, *JAMA,* 231, 1043, 1975.
2. **Holley, K. E., Hunt, J. C., and Brown, A. L., Kincaid, O. W., and Sheps, S. G.,** Renal artery stenosis. A clinical pathological study in normotensive and hypertensive patients, *Am. J. Med.,* 37, 14, 1964.
3. **Eyler, W. R., Clark, M. D., Garman, J. E., Rian, R. C., and Meininger, D. E.,** Angiography of the renal areas including a comparative study of renal arterial stenoses in patients with and without hypertension, *Radiology,* 78, 879, 1962.
4. **Foster, J. H. and Oates, J.,** Recognition and management of renovascular hypertension, in *Hypertension: Mechanisms, Diagnosis and Management,* Davis, J. O., Laragh, J. H., and Selwyn, A., Eds., Hospital Practice, New York, 1977, 245.
5. **Genest, J., Boucher, R., Rojo-Ortega, J. M., Roy, P., Lefebvre, R., Cartier, P., Nowaczynski, W., and Kuchel, O.,** Renovascular hypertension, in *Hypertension,* Genest, J., Koiw, E., and Kuchel, O., Eds., McGraw-Hill, 1977, 815.
6. **Simon, N., Franklin, S. S., Bleifer, K. H., and Maxwell, M. H.,** Clinical characteristics of renovascular hypertension, *JAMA,* 220, 1209, 1972.
7. **Maxwell, M. H., Kaufman, J. J., and Bleifer, K. H.,** Stenosing lesions of the renal arteries. Clinical manifestations, *Postgrad. Med.,* 40, 247, 1966.
8. **Shapiro, A. P., Perez-Stable, E., and Scheib, E. T., Brown, K., Montsos, S. E., Berg, G., and Misage, J. R.,** Renal artery stenosis and hypertension. Observations on current status of therapy from a study of 115 patients, *Am. J. Med.,* 47, 175, 1969.
9. **Perloff, D., Sokolow, H., Wylie, E. J., Smith, D. R., and Palubinskas, A. J.,** Hypertension secondary to renal artery occlusive disease, *Circulation,* 24, 1286, 1961.
10. **Harrison, E. G. and McCormack, L. J.,** Pathologic classification of renal arterial disease in renovascular hypertension, *Mayo Clin. Proc.,* 46, 161, 1971.
11. **Bookstein, J. J., Abrams, H. L., Buenger, R. E., Lecky, J., Franklin, S. S., Reis, M. D., Bleifer, K. H., Klatte, E. C., and Maxwell, M. H.,** Radiologic aspects of renovascular hypertension. I. Aims and methods of the radiology study group, *JAMA,* 220, 1218, 1972.
12. **White, H. L.,** The excretion of sodium in relation to glomerular filtration, in *Renal Function,* Bradley, S. E., Ed., Josiah Macey Foundation, New York, 1950, 127.
13. **Mueller, B. B., Surtshin, A., Carlin, M. R., and White, H. L.,** Glomerular and tubular influences on sodium and water excretion, *Am. J. Physiol.,* 165, 411, 1951.

14. Connor, T. B., Thomas, W. C., Haddock, L., and Howard, J. E., Unilateral renal disease as a cause of hypertension. Its detection by ureteral catheterization studies, *Ann. Intern. Med.*, 52, 544, 1960.

15. Strong, C. G., Hunt, J. C., Sheps, S. G., Tucker, R. M., and Bernatz, P. E., Renal venous renin activity. Enhancement of sensitivity of lateralization by sodium depletion, *Am. J. Cardiol.*, 27, 602, 1971.

16. Juncos, L. I., Strong, C. G., and Hunt, J. C., Prediction of results of surgery for renal and renovascular hypertension, *Arch. Intern. Med.*, 134, 655, 1974.

17. Pals, D. T., Masucci, F. D., Denning, G. S., Sipos, F., and Fessler, D. C., Role of the pressor action of angiotensin II in experimental hypertension, *Circ. Res.*, 29, 673, 1971.

18. Brown, J. J., Brown, W. C. B., Fraser, R., Lever, A. F., Morton, J. J., Robertson, J. I. S., Agabiti-Rosei, E., Free, M., and Trust, P. M., Effects of infusing angiotensin II antagonist saralasin on arterial blood pressure and on plasma concentrations of aldosterone, renin and angiotensin II in normal subjects and selected hypertensive patients, in *Systemic Effects of Antihypertensive Agents*, Sambhi, M. P., Ed., Stratton Intercontinental, New York, 1976, 499.

19. Streeten, D. H. P., Anderson, G. H., Dalakos, T. G., Freiberg, J. N., and Schroeder, E. T., The therapeutic potential of angiotensin antagonists, in *Systemic Effects of Antihypertensive Agents*, Sambhi, M. P., Ed., Stratton Interconinental, New York, 1976, 517.

20. Thomas, R. D., Ball, S. G., and Lee, M. R., Failure of saralasin to predict a response to surgery in renovascular hypertension, *Lancet*, 1, 724, 1977.

21. Hunt, J. C., Sheps, S. G., Harrison, E. G., Strong, C. G., and Bernatz, P. E., Renal and renovascular hypertension. A reasoned approach to diagnosis and management, *Arch. Intern. Med.*, 133, 988, 1974.

22. Robertson, P. W., Klidjian, A., Harding, L. K., Walters, G., Lee, M. R., and Robb-Smith, A. H. T., Hypertension due to a renin-secreting tumour, *Am. J. Med.*, 43, 963, 1967.

23. Kihara, I., Kitamura, S., Hoshino, T., Hitoshi, S., and Watanabe, T., A hitherto unreported vascular tumour of the kidney. A proposal of "juxtaglomerular cell tumour", *Acta. Pathol. Jpn.*, 18, 197, 1968.

24. Schambelan, M., Howes, E. L., Jr., Stockigt, J. R., Naokes, C. A., and Biglieri, E. G., Role of renin and aldosterone in hypertension due to a renin-secreting tumour, *Am. J. Med.*, 55, 86, 1973.

25. Bonnin, J. M., Hodge, R. L., and Lumbers, E. R., A renin secreting renal tumour associated with hypertension, *Aust. N. Z. J. Med.*, 2, 178, 1972.

26. Brown, J. J., Fraser, R., Lever, A. F., Morton, J. J., Robertson, J. I. S., Tree, M., Bell, P. R. F., Davidson, J. K., and Ruthven, I. S., Hypertension and secondary aldosteronism associated with a renin-secreting juxtaglomerular-cell tumour, *Lancet*, 2, 1128, 1973.

27. Guyton, A. C., Coleman, T. G., and Granger, H. J., Circulation: overall regulation, *Annu. Rev. Physiol.*, 34, 13, 1972.

28. Friedman, S. M., An ion exchange approach to the problem of intracellular sodium in the hypertensive process, *Circ. Res.*, 34 and 35 (Suppl. 1), 123, 1974.

29. Conn, J. W., Cohen, E. L., Rovner, D. R., and Nesbit, R. M., Normokaleamic primary aldosteronism. A detectable cause of curable "essential" hypertension, *JAMA*, 193, 200, 1965.

30. Biglieri, E. G., Stockigt, J. R., and Schambelan, M., Adrenal mineralocorticoids causing hypertension, *Am. J. Med.*, 52, 623, 1972.

31. Kaplan, N., Primary aldosteronism with malignant hypertension, *N. Engl. J. Med.*, 269, 1282, 1963.

32. Ferris, J. B., Brown, J. J., Fraser, R., Kay, A. W., Neville, A. M., O'Muircheartaigh, I. G., Robertson, J. I. S., Symington, T., and Lever, A. F., Hypertension with aldosterone excess and low plasma-renin: preoperative distinction between patients with and without adrenocortical tumour, *Lancet*, 2, 995, 1970.

33. Conn, J. W., Primary aldosteronism, in *Hypertension*, Genest, J., Koiw, E., and Kuchel, O., Eds., McGraw-Hill, New York, 1977, 768.

34. Brown, J. J., Davies, D. L., Freis, J. B., Fraser, R., Haywood, E., Lever, A. F., and Robertson, J. I. S., Comparison of surgery and prolonged spironolactone therapy in patients with hypertension, aldosterone excess, and low plasma renin, *Br. Med. J.*, 2, 729, 1972.

35. Conn, J. W., Rovner, D. R., Cohen, E. L., Bookstein, J. J., Cerny, J. C., and Lucas, C. P., The preoperative diagnosis of primary aldosteronism. Including a comparison of operative findings and preoperative tumour localization by adrenal phlebography, *Arch. Intern. Med.*, 123, 113, 1969.

36. Scoggins, B. A., Oddie, C. J., Hare, W. S. C., and Coghlan, J. P., Preoperative lateralization in primary aldosteronism, *Ann. Intern. Med.*, 76, 891, 1972.

37. Conn, J. W., Beierwaltes, W. H., Lieberman, L. M., Ansari, A. N., Cohen, E. L., Bookstein, J. J., and Herwig, K. R., Primary aldosteronism: preoperative tumour visualization by scintillation scanning, *J. Clin. Endocrinol. Metab.*, 33, 713, 1971.

38. Winkler, H. and Smith, A. D., Catecholamines in phaeochromocytoma, *Lancet*, 1, 793, 1968.

39. Geffen, L. B., Rush, R. A., Louis, W. J., and Doyle, A. E., Plasma catecholamine and dopamine β hydroxylase amounts in phaeochromocytoma, *Clin. Sci.*, 49, 421, 1973.
40. Louis, W. J., Jarrott, B., and Doyle, A. E., The role of the autonomic nervous sytem in human hypertension: studies in essential hypertension and in phaeochromocytoma, in *Pathophysiology and Management of Arterial Hypertension,* Berglund, G., Hansson, K., and Wĕrko, L., Eds., Lundgren and Söuer, AB, Mölndal, Sweden, 1975, 16.
41. McNeill, A. D., Groden, B. M., and Neville, A. M., Intrathoracic phaeochromocytoma, *Br. J. Surg.,* 57, 457, 1970.
42. Sullivan, J. M., Phaeochromocytoma, *Arch. Surg. (Chicago),* 104, 130, 1972.
43. Wolf, R. L. and Mendlowitz, M., Clinical experiences with phaeochromocytoma, *Cardiovasc. Clin.,* 1, 158, 1969.
44. Crout, J. R. and Sjoerdsma, A., Catecholamines in the localization of phaeochromocytoma, *Circulation,* 22, 516, 1960.
45. Gitlow, S. E., Pertsemlidis, D., and Pertani, L. M., Management of patients with pheochromocytoma, *Am. Heart J.,* 82, 557, 1971.
46. Chapman, W. P. and Singh, M., Evaluation of tests used in the diagnosis of pheochromocytoma, *Mod. Concepts Cardiovasc. Dis.,* 23, 221, 1954.
47. Engelman, K. and Sjoerdsma, A., A new test for pheochromocytoma. Pressor responsiveness to tyramine, *JAMA,* 189, 81, 1964.
48. Lawrence, A. M., Glucagon provocative test for pheochromocytoma, *Ann. Intern. Med.,* 66, 1091, 1967.
49. Wilson, A. C., Bennett, R. C., Niall, J. F., Clareborough, J. K., Doyle, A. E., and Louis, W. J., An unusual case of intrathoracic phaeochromocytoma, *Aust. N. Z. J. Surg.,* 44, 27, 1974.
50. Wurtman, R. J., Catecholamines, *N. Engl. J. Med.,* 273, 746, 1965.
51. Engelman, K. and Hammond, W. G., Adrenaline production by an intrathoracic phaeochromocytoma, *Lancet,* 1, 609, 1968.
52. Sjoerdsma, A., Engelman, K., Spector, S., and Udenfriend, S., Inhibition of catecholamine synthesis in man with alpha-methyl-tyrosine, an inhibitor of tyrosine hydroxylase, *Lancet,* 2, 1092, 1965.
53. Agabiti-Rosei, E., Brown, J. J., Lever, A. F., and Robertson, J. I. S., Treatment of phaeochromocytoma and of clonidine withdrawal hypertension with Labetalol, *Br. J. Clin. Pharmacol.,* 3 (Suppl. 3), 809, 1976.

INDEX

A

C